Hypertension: New Frontiers

Hypertension: New Frontiers

Editor: Gilbert Wheeler

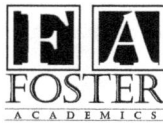

FA

FOSTER
ACADEMICS

www.fosteracademics.com

www.fosteracademics.com

FA FOSTER
ACADEMICS

Cataloging-in-Publication Data

Hypertension : new frontiers / edited by Gilbert Wheeler.
        p. cm.
Includes bibliographical references and index.
ISBN 978-1-63242-897-4
1. Hypertension. 2. Blood circulation disorders. 3. Hypertension--Diagnosis.
4. Hypertension--Treatment. I. Wheeler, Gilbert.
RC685.H8 H97 2020
616.132--dc23

Foster Academics,
118-35 Queens Blvd., Suite 400,
Forest Hills, NY 11375, USA

ISBN 978-1-63242-897-4 (Hardback)

Contents

Preface

In my initial years as a student, I used to run to the library at every possible instance to grab a book and learn something new. Books were my primary source of knowledge and I would not have come such a long way without all that I learnt from them. Thus, when I was approached to edit this book; I became understandably nostalgic. It was an absolute honor to be considered worthy of guiding the current generation as well as those to come. I put all my knowledge and hard work into making this book most beneficial for its readers.

Hypertension or high blood pressure is a medical condition characterized by persistently elevated levels of blood pressure in the arteries. It can contribute to the incidence of heart failure, stroke, coronary artery disease, atrial fibrillation, chronic kidney disease, etc. Some people with hypertension experience headaches, lightheadedness, tinnitus, vertigo, fainting episodes or altered vision. Blood pressure rises with age. Several environmental and genetic factors influence blood pressure. 35 genetic loci have been identified so far with an influence on blood pressure. Lack of exercise, obesity, high salt intake and depression contribute to hypertension. Various clinical conditions may also cause hypertension, such as kidney disease, hypothyroidism and hyperthyroidism, Cushing's syndrome, Conn's syndrome, renal artery stenosis, etc. Lifestyle changes are considered as effective as antihypertensive medication. Adopting physical exercise regimens, use of stress reduction techniques, dietary changes with increased potassium and low sodium, etc. are some of the changes for the management of this condition. In case of extremely elevated blood pressure, it should be reduced rapidly in order to stop organ damage. The various studies that are constantly contributing towards advancing management strategies for hypertension are examined in detail in this book. In this book, using case studies and examples, constant effort has been made to make the understanding of hypertension as easy and informative as possible, for the readers.

I wish to thank my publisher for supporting me at every step. I would also like to thank all the authors who have contributed their researches in this book. I hope this book will be a valuable contribution to the progress of the field.

Editor

Blood Pressure Response to Zofenopril or Irbesartan Each Combined with Hydrochlorothiazide in High-Risk Hypertensives Uncontrolled by Monotherapy

Ettore Malacco,[1] Stefano Omboni,[2] and Gianfranco Parati[3]

[1]L. Sacco Hospital, 20157 Milano, Italy
[2]Italian Institute of Telemedicine, Solbiate Arno, 21048 Varese, Italy
[3]Istituto Auxologico Italiano and University of Milano-Bicocca, 20149 Milano, Italy

Correspondence should be addressed to Ettore Malacco; ettore.malacco@tiscali.it

Academic Editor: Francesco Cappuccio

In this randomized, double-blind, controlled, parallel group study (ZENITH), 434 essential hypertensives with additional cardiovascular risk factors, uncontrolled by a previous monotherapy, were treated for 18 weeks with zofenopril 30 or 60 mg plus hydrochlorothiazide (HCTZ) 12.5 mg or irbesartan 150 or 300 mg plus HCTZ. Rate of office blood pressure (BP) response (zofenopril: 68% versus irbesartan: 70%; $p = 0.778$) and 24-hour BP response (zofenopril: 85% versus irbesartan: 84%; $p = 0.781$) was similar between the two treatment groups. Cardiac and renal damage was equally reduced by both treatments, whereas the rate of carotid plaque regression was significantly larger with zofenopril. In conclusion, uncontrolled monotherapy treated hypertensives effectively respond to a combination of zofenopril or irbesartan plus a thiazide diuretic, in terms of either BP response or target organ damage progression.

1. Introduction

Hypertension is a major modifiable risk factor for cardiovascular morbidity and mortality [1]. Effective control of high blood pressure (BP) by pharmacological treatment substantially reduces the risk of developing major cardiovascular complications, including myocardial infarction, stroke, heart failure, and kidney disease [2]. However, in most hypertensive patients and particularly in those with associated cardiovascular risk factors or at high risk for cardiovascular events, a combination therapy based on at least two drugs is required in order to achieve the recommended BP goals [3]. As a matter of fact, clinical studies and large meta-analyses have demonstrated that combination therapy allows significant improvements of both systolic BP (SBP) and diastolic BP (DBP) control in 70–80% of treated hypertensive patients [4–7], the use of combination treatment being characterized by a greater antihypertensive efficacy than the doubling of

the monotherapy dose [8, 9]. For these reasons guidelines on management of hypertension currently recommend the use of two-drug combinations also as a first line therapy [3].

The association of an Angiotensin Converting Enzyme- (ACE-) inhibitor and a diuretic is amongst the preferred two-drug combinations, because the ACE-inhibitor antagonizes the counterregulatory system activity triggered by the diuretic and this results in an improvement of the efficacy and tolerability of the single drug components [3, 10].

Zofenopril calcium, a prodrug of the active compound zofenoprilat, is an ACE-inhibitor which has been successfully and safely employed in the treatment of essential hypertension [11] and acute myocardial infarction or heart failure [12], also in subgroups of patients with high BP [13, 14]. In subjects with essential hypertension zofenopril has been shown to be as effective as beta-blockers [15], diuretics [16], calcium channel blockers [17], other ACE-inhibitors [18, 19], and Angiotensin Receptor Blockers (ARBs) [20, 21].

Zofenopril has also been proved to be effective when given in combination with a thiazide diuretic [22, 23]. However, so far, only a limited fraction of subjects has been tested with the highest dose of zofenopril (60 mg) plus the diuretic, no direct comparative data on the antihypertensive efficacy and safety of the zofenopril plus hydrochlorothiazide combination versus that of an ARB plus a diuretic exist, and no information on the possible benefit of the two-drug combination on cardiovascular and renal damage is yet available. The present study was planned and conducted in order to bridge this void, by selecting essential hypertensive patients not controlled by a previous monotherapy, and with one or more additional cardiovascular risk factors.

2. Methods

2.1. Study Population. Essential hypertensive subjects of both genders, aged 18 to 75 years, with at least one additional cardiovascular risk factor, and taking one antihypertensive medication among ACE-inhibitors, ARBs, calcium channel blockers, diuretics, and beta-blockers, in the last 3 months, but not adequately controlled (sitting office SBP ≥140 mmHg and/or sitting office DBP ≥90 mmHg), were eligible for study participation. The following cardiovascular risk factors were considered among the inclusion criteria [3]: (a) current smoking; (b) elevated total cholesterol (>190 mg/dL) or specific lipid-lowering drug treatment; (c) elevated Low Density Lipoprotein (LDL) cholesterol (>115 mg/dL) or specific lipid-lowering drug treatment; (d) low High Density Lipoprotein (HDL) cholesterol (<40 mg/dL in males and <46 mg/dL in females) or specific lipid-lowering drug treatment; (e) fasting plasma glucose between 102 and 125 mg/dL or being on specific drug treatment for hyperglycemia; (f) diabetes mellitus (fasting plasma glucose ≥126 mg/dL) controlled by diet or specific antidiabetic therapy; (g) abdominal obesity: waist circumference ≥102 cm in males and ≥88 cm in females, or Body Mass Index (BMI) between 25 and 29.9 kg/m^2; and (h) family history of premature cardiovascular disease (males at age <55 years and females at age <65 years).

Patients were excluded if they had (a) secondary or malignant hypertension; (b) orthostatic hypotension (office SBP drop upon standing ≥20 mmHg); (c) history of heart failure requiring medical treatment; (d) myocardial infarction or cerebrovascular accidents in the previous 6 months; (e) hemodynamically significant cardiac valve disease; (f) severe or clinically significant systemic, renal, hepatic, neurological, or psychiatric disease; (g) obesity (BMI ≥30 kg/m^2); (h) large (circumference >32 cm) or tiny upper arm (circumference <24 cm); (i) known hypersensitivity to ACE-inhibitors, ARBs, or thiazide diuretics.

Pregnant women and breastfeeding mothers were excluded as well. Premenopausal women with childbearing potential had to practice an effective method of birth control and were required to have a negative urine pregnancy test.

The study was conducted according to Good Clinical Practice guidelines and the Declaration of Helsinki, and the protocol was approved by the ethics committees of the centers involved. Written informed consent was obtained from all patients prior to their inclusion into the study.

2.2. Study Design. This was an Italian, multicenter, randomized, double-blind, parallel group study, conducted at 34 Italian hospitals. The first patient was enrolled in May 2009 and the last patient was enrolled in January 2012. Patients were randomized 1:1, using a centralized, computer-generated randomization list in blocks of 4. The study consisted of a 2-week run-in period during which current monotherapy was continued unchanged, followed by 18 weeks of double-blind treatment with zofenopril or irbesartan at the initial doses of 30 and 150 mg combined with hydrochlorothiazide 12.5 mg. Study drugs were given orally and once daily (between 9 and 11 a.m.) with a glass of water. The two study treatments were supplied as identical oral tablets (overencapsulation technique). After the first 6 and 12 weeks of active treatment the dose of zofenopril and irbesartan had to be doubled, respectively, to 60 and 300 mg, if office SBP was ≥140 mmHg or office DBP was ≥90 mmHg in nondiabetic patients and if office SBP was ≥130 mmHg or office DBP was ≥80 mmHg in diabetic patients or in patients with at least 3 cardiovascular risk factors.

At the screening visit informed consent was obtained, medical history was collected, and a physical examination, BP and heart rate measurements, and laboratory tests (blood count, glucose, total, LDL, and HDL cholesterol, triglycerides, uric acid, creatinine, sodium and potassium, transaminases and γ-GT, total bilirubin, urinalysis, and urine pregnancy test) were assessed. At randomization visit, 2 weeks after inclusion, a 12-lead ECG, an echocardiogram, and a carotid ultrasonography were carried out. Physical examination and BP and heart rate measurements were repeated at each visit (6, 12, and 18 weeks after randomization), while an ECG, an echocardiogram, and a carotid ultrasonography were assessed again and laboratory tests (including urine pregnancy test) were rechecked at the end of the 18 weeks of double-blind treatment. Adverse events, use of concomitant medications, and compliance with treatment were assessed at each visit. At the end of the 2-week run-in period and of the 18 weeks of double-blind treatment BP was also measured by 24-hour ambulatory monitoring.

The study also included a 30-week double-blind follow-up period for patients uptitrated to the high drug dose of zofenopril or irbesartan during the first 18 weeks. During this period patients were seen initially after 6 weeks and then every 8 weeks: office BP was measured at each visit, whereas a 24-hour ambulatory BP monitoring was performed at the end of the 30 weeks.

2.3. Office BP and Heart Rate Measurement. BP and heart rate were measured in the office by a validated, automatic, electronic, upper-arm sphygmomanometer (A&D UA-767PC, A&D Company Limited, Tokyo, Japan) [24], approximately 24 hours after the last placebo or drug intake. The arm cuff was kept at the heart level during every BP measurement. Three measurements, taken at 2 min intervals, after 5 min of rest in the sitting position were averaged and used as the office BP reference value. BP and heart rate values were taken also after 1 and 4 minutes of standing.

2.4. Ambulatory BP Measurements. Ambulatory BP monitoring was performed at randomization and the final visit, noninvasively over the 24 hours by an oscillometric, validated, automatic, electronic device (A&D TM-2430, A&D Company Limited, Tokyo, Japan) [25]. The monitoring cuff was wrapped around the nondominant arm and the patient was asked to keep her/his arm still during the automatic BP measurements. The device was programmed to provide automatic readings every 15 min throughout the whole monitoring period. Each recording started in the morning, immediately after office BP assessment and administration of placebo or active treatment. Patients were then sent home and asked to come back 24 hours later. They were instructed to attend their usual activities during the monitoring period, avoiding strenuous exercise, and to keep the arm extended and immobile during the automatic cuff inflations. Results of the recording were read by connecting the BP measuring device to a wireless interface which sent data to a centralized data management center through the mobile telephone network and the web [26]. Traces had to be analyzed in real time and in case of a bad quality recording (see below) the investigator was contacted in order to repeat the recording in the next two days, whenever possible.

2.5. Echocardiography. In order to obtain reliable and accurate tests, echocardiograms were performed by operators trained and certified during a course held at the coordinating center before study initiation. Echocardiograms were obtained with the subject in left lateral decubitus, after 30 minutes of rest. Only one certified physician in each center was responsible for recording the echocardiograms. Left ventricular internal diameters, left ventricular posterior wall thickness, and interventricular septum thickness were measured monodimensionally from the longitudinal parasternal view previously identified bidimensionally, according to the indications of the American Society of Echocardiography [27]. Left ventricular mass was calculated according to the Penn Method [28] and indexed to body surface area by using the formula of D. Du Bois and E. F. Du Bois [29]. Left ventricular hypertrophy was considered to be present if the left ventricular mass index (LVMI) exceeded 125 g/m^2 in males or 110 g/m^2 in females [3]. Since LVMIs were calculated locally only by few centers and using different algorithms, they were recalculated centrally and blindly from the original measures, before the database lock.

2.6. Carotid Ultrasonography. Also in case of carotid ultrasonography, in order to obtain reliable and accurate reports, the test was performed by operators trained and certified during a course held at the coordinating center prior to study initiation. Patients were examined in the supine positions by B-mode carotid scans. The carotid arteries were interrogated using an ultrasound system with a linear-array transducer operating at a fundamental frequency of at least 7 MHz. Examinations of carotid artery and measurement of intima-media thickness (IMT) were obtained manually at different carotid sites (common, bifurcation, external, and internal carotid artery), from at least 3 different angles of incidence in each segment, as recommended by current guidelines

[30]. The three measurements taken at each segment were averaged and the average was used as the reference for each segment. Ultrasound scans were performed by only one certified sonographer at each referral center and were read locally. Data were expressed as the maximum IMT at each carotid segment explored. Atherosclerotic plaque was defined as an IMT >1.3 mm in any of the segments examined [30, 31]. The choice of 1.3 mm was done because at the time the protocol was devised and implemented on field this was the threshold recommended by guidelines and this was used as a reference for patients' management by the investigators at each study site [31].

2.7. Data Analysis. The primary efficacy study end-point was the intertreatment comparison in the rate of office sitting BP response (<140/90 mmHg in nondiabetics and <130/80 mmHg in diabetics or high-risk patients, or SBP reduction ≥20 mmHg or DBP reduction ≥10 mmHg) at the end of the 18 weeks of double-blind treatment.

This was a noninferiority trial and thus the hypothesis was that zofenopril plus hydrochlorothiazide and irbesartan plus hydrochlorothiazide had to be defined as equivalent in case of a difference <10% in the rate of responders after 18 weeks of treatment. This choice was based on previous evidence on response rate in zofenopril- and irbesartan-based studies [20, 21, 32, 33], and its appropriateness has been documented in a twin study, recently published [34]. Using a one-sided two-group large-sample normal approximation test of proportions at the 2.5% level, with a power of 80%, the estimated minimum number of patients to be randomized was 446 (including a 10% drop-out rate), 223 for each treatment group.

Analysis was performed on patients valid for intention-to-treat analysis, defined as all randomized patients receiving at least one dose of active treatment drug and having at least one office BP measurement after randomization. The last observation carried forward method was used for patients prematurely leaving the study. The per-protocol population included all randomized patients completing the 18-week double-blind study period without major protocol violations and was used for confirmatory analysis.

Secondary study end-points included intertreatment comparison of (a) changes in sitting office SBP and DBP after 18 weeks of treatment; (b) percentage of patients with an average 24-hour BP <130/80 mmHg or a SBP reduction ≥10 mmHg or a DBP reduction ≥5 mmHg at study end; (c) changes in LVMI with treatment and percentage of patients with cardiac damage at study end (LVMI ≥125 g/m^2 in males or ≥110 g/m^2 in females) [3]; (d) changes in albumin-creatinine ratio and microalbuminuria with treatment and percentage of patients with renal damage at study end (albumin-creatinine ratio ≥22 mg/g for males and ≥31 mg/g for females or microalbuminuria, evaluated quantitatively or semiquantitatively by dipstick, between 30 and 300 mg/24 h) [3]; (e) changes in maximum IMT with treatment and percentage of patients with vascular damage at study end (maximum IMT >1.3 mm in any district) [30, 31]. Rate of office BP responders, office and 24-hour SBP and DBP changes from baseline, and changes in cardiac, renal, and vascular damage from baseline at week 48 were the study end-points for the double-blind extension phase.

The analysis of 24-hour BP recordings was preceded by removal of artifacts according to previously described editing criteria [35]. Recordings were considered valid when no more than 1 hour was missing over the 24 hours and when at least 70% of expected measurements were available.

For the primary study end-point and for the changes in sitting office SBP and DBP a subgroup analysis was also done, considering subjects taking the low dose of both drugs (zofenopril 30 mg and irbesartan 150 mg). For the primary end-point, this subgroup analysis was applied to all subjects and also to those with mild (office SBP 140–159 mmHg and DBP 90–99 mmHg) and moderate-severe hypertension (office SBP ≥160 mmHg and DBP ≥100 mmHg).

Safety analysis was applied to all randomized patients, by calculating the incidence of adverse events and changes in laboratory data or ECG during the study.

Intertreatment differences for the primary study end-point were tested using a chi-square test, correcting by the center effect: the 95% confidence interval of the difference in proportion was calculated and the lower bound was compared with the 10% noninferiority limit. The same analysis was applied to secondary end-points with a discrete distribution, while differences between the two randomization groups for continuous variables were tested by analysis of variance, or, in the case of target organ damage measures, by analysis of covariance (continuous variables) or logistic regression analysis (discrete variables), by adjusting for the baseline value and other potentially confounding variables (age, gender, abdominal obesity, HDL cholesterol, family history for premature cardiovascular disease, baseline BP, and BP changes with treatment). The rates of patients experiencing an adverse event were compared between the two treatment groups by a logistic regression analysis, taking into account treatment and confounding variables. The level of statistical significance was kept at 0.05 throughout the whole study. Data are shown as mean ±SD, as mean and 95% confidence interval, and as absolute (n) or relative (%) frequency.

3. Results

3.1. Baseline Demographic and Clinical Data. A total of 560 patients were screened, but 98 were lost during the run-in period. Thus the number of patients randomized to one of the two treatment arms was 462: 389 of these patients completed the 18-week double-blind randomized phase, while 73 discontinued the study because of consent withdrawal ($n = 29$), adverse events ($n = 16$), loss to follow-up ($n = 10$), lack of compliance with study procedures ($n = 8$), decision of the investigator ($n = 5$), or protocol violation ($n = 5$). A flow diagram of the patients throughout the study is presented in Figure 1.

Overall 434 patients were valid for the intention-to-treat analysis (213 in the zofenopril plus hydrochlorothiazide and 221 in the irbesartan plus hydrochlorothiazide treatment group) and 302 for the per-protocol analysis (146 in the zofenopril plus hydrochlorothiazide and 156 in the irbesartan

plus hydrochlorothiazide treatment group). 229 out of 438 patients undergoing ambulatory BP monitoring at baseline had valid recordings and were included in this subgroup analysis (113 randomized to zofenopril plus hydrochlorothiazide and 116 to irbesartan plus hydrochlorothiazide).

A total of 244 patients, uptitrated to the high drug dose of zofenopril ($n = 130$) or irbesartan ($n = 114$), entered the double-blind extension phase and were followed for 30 weeks; 223 of them were included in the intention-to-treat analysis for this period (119 in the zofenopril plus hydrochlorothiazide and 104 in the irbesartan plus hydrochlorothiazide treatment group). The number of patients with valid ambulatory BP recordings at the end of the extension phase was 50 in the zofenopril and 44 in the irbesartan group.

As shown in Table 1, patients randomized to zofenopril plus hydrochlorothiazide were homogeneous for baseline demographic and clinical characteristics. This was the case also for the subgroup of patients included in the ambulatory BP monitoring analysis (data not shown). Most of the enrolled subjects had at least 3 major cardiovascular risk factors and were thus classified as being at high or very high cardiovascular risk.

3.2. Drug Dosing. The full dose of zofenopril (60 mg) in combination with hydrochlorothiazide was taken at the end of the study by 55.9% of patients randomized to this drug, while the full dose of irbesartan (300 mg) was taken by 47.1% of patients ($p = 0.066$).

3.3. Sitting Office BP Responders. As shown in Figure 2, the primary study end-point (proportion of patients with office BP <140/90 mmHg in case of nondiabetics and <130/80 mmHg in case of diabetics or high-risk patients, or SBP reduction ≥20 mmHg or DBP reduction ≥10 mmHg) was achieved by the end of the 18 weeks of double-blind treatment by a similar proportion of patients treated with zofenopril plus hydrochlorothiazide (68.2%) and irbesartan plus hydrochlorothiazide (69.5%, $p = 0.778$). The odds ratio for the difference in the response to treatment (zofenopril plus hydrochlorothiazide versus irbesartan plus hydrochlorothiazide) was 1.066 (95% confidence interval: 0.685–1.659): since the observed lower bound of the confidence interval (0.685) was higher than that estimated for a 10% difference (0.580), the achievement of the noninferiority criterion could be confirmed.

In the patients taking the low drug doses at study end, the proportion of responders did not differ ($p = 0.693$) between zofenopril (76.4%) and irbesartan (78.9%). The odds ratio for treatment differences was estimated at 1.159 (0.456, 2.415): as for the whole study group and also for the low dose subgroup the observed lower bound of the confidence interval (0.456) was higher than that estimated for a 10% difference (0.420), and thus the noninferiority assumption could be satisfied.

The rate of responders for the two low dose drug treatments was similar also in subgroups of patients with mild hypertension (74.6% zofenopril versus 78.8% irbesartan; odds ratio and 95% confidence interval: 1.267 (0.587, 2.736), $p = 0.546$) and moderate hypertension (88.9% versus 80.0%; 0.500 (0.037, 6.683), $p = 0.596$).

```
┌─────────────┐
│ Enrollment  │                    ┌──────────────────────────────────┐
└─────────────┘                    │ Assessed for eligibility (n = 560) │
                                    └──────────────────────────────────┘
                                                    │
                                                    │      ┌──────────────────────┐
                                                    ├─────→│ Excluded (n = 98)     │
                                                    │      └──────────────────────┘
                                                    ▼
                                    ┌──────────────────────────┐
                                    │ Randomized (n = 462)       │
                                    └──────────────────────────┘
```

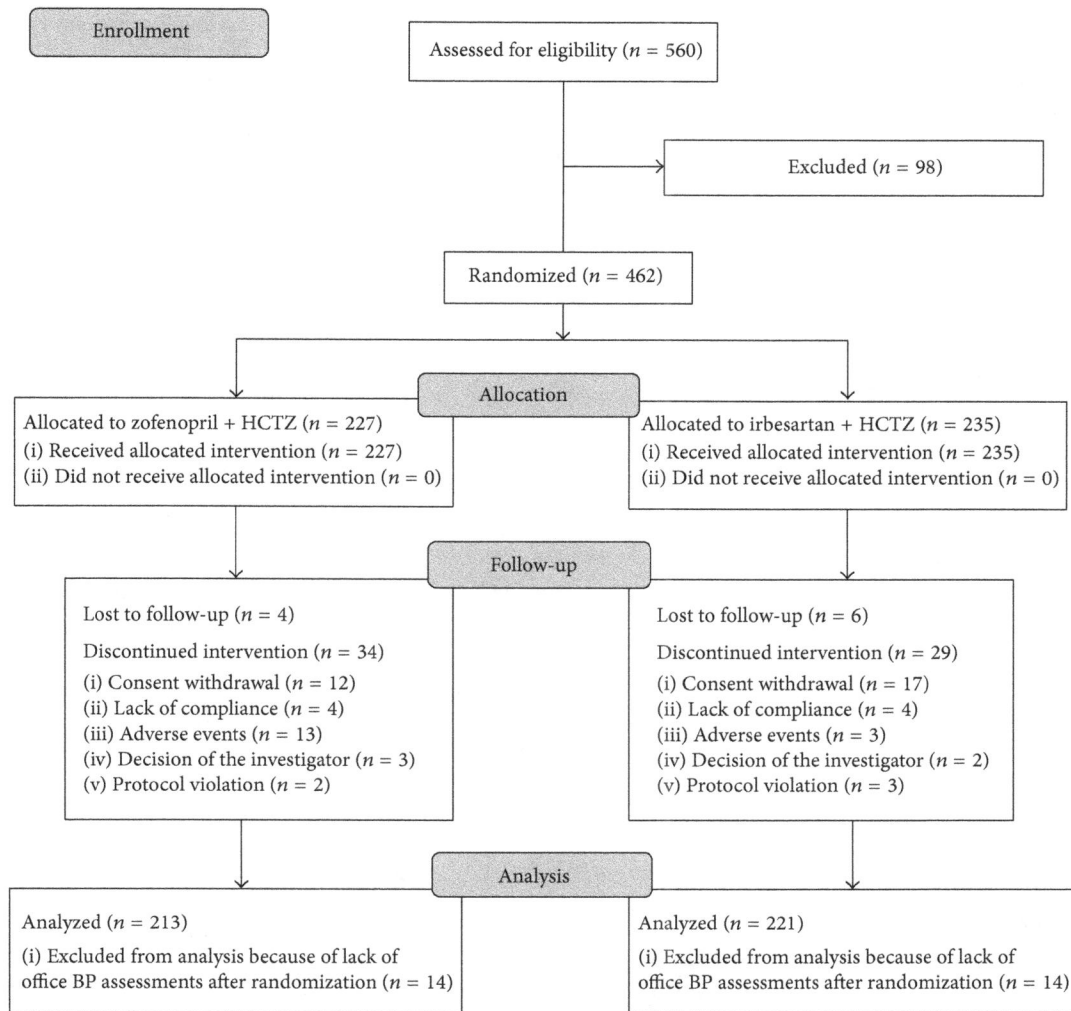

FIGURE 1: Flow diagram of the patients through the different phases of the study.

The flow diagram shows:

Enrollment
- Assessed for eligibility (n = 560)
- Excluded (n = 98)
- Randomized (n = 462)

Allocation
- Allocated to zofenopril + HCTZ (n = 227)
  - (i) Received allocated intervention (n = 227)
  - (ii) Did not receive allocated intervention (n = 0)
- Allocated to irbesartan + HCTZ (n = 235)
  - (i) Received allocated intervention (n = 235)
  - (ii) Did not receive allocated intervention (n = 0)

Follow-up
- Lost to follow-up (n = 4)
- Discontinued intervention (n = 34)
  - (i) Consent withdrawal (n = 12)
  - (ii) Lack of compliance (n = 4)
  - (iii) Adverse events (n = 13)
  - (iv) Decision of the investigator (n = 3)
  - (v) Protocol violation (n = 2)
- Lost to follow-up (n = 6)
- Discontinued intervention (n = 29)
  - (i) Consent withdrawal (n = 17)
  - (ii) Lack of compliance (n = 4)
  - (iii) Adverse events (n = 3)
  - (iv) Decision of the investigator (n = 2)
  - (v) Protocol violation (n = 3)

Analysis
- Analyzed (n = 213)
  - (i) Excluded from analysis because of lack of office BP assessments after randomization (n = 14)
- Analyzed (n = 221)
  - (i) Excluded from analysis because of lack of office BP assessments after randomization (n = 14)

3.4. Sitting Office BP Changes. Sitting office BP values were progressively and significantly ($p < 0.01$) reduced by both treatment regimens during the study (Figure 3). At the final evaluation (week 18), sitting office SBP and DBP were reduced on average (±SD) by 15.7 ± 13.7 and 8.6 ± 9.1 mmHg with zofenopril combined with the diuretic and by 19.3 ± 13.8 and 11.6 ± 9.1 mmHg with irbesartan + hydrochlorothiazide (intertreatment differences: $p < 0.01$ for SBP and $p < 0.001$ for DBP) (Figure 3 and Table 2). In patients taking the low drug dose SBP and DBP reductions were similar between the two treatment groups (Table 2).

3.5. 24-Hour Ambulatory BP Responders. The percentage of responders over the 24 hours (average 24-hour BP <130/80 mmHg or SBP reduction ≥10 mmHg or a DBP reduction ≥5 mmHg at study end) was higher than that of office responders and similar for zofenopril- and irbesartan-treated patients (85.0 versus 83.6%, $p = 0.781$) (Figure 2).

Both treatments effectively reduced ambulatory BP. 24-hour SBP was similarly ($p = 0.050$) reduced by zofenopril + hydrochlorothiazide (from 129.4 ± 10.4 to 122.7 ± 9.4 mmHg;

reduction of 6.4 (8.4, 4.4) mmHg) and irbesartan + hydrochlorothiazide (from 131.8 ± 11.8 to 120.9 ± 10.9 mmHg, 9.2 (11.1, 7.3) mmHg), while for 24-hour DBP significantly ($p = 0.001$) higher reductions were obtained under the irbesartan + hydrochlorothiazide (from 80.2 ± 8.1 to 73.0 ± 6.8 mmHg, reduction of 7.0 (8.2, 5.7) mmHg) than under the zofenopril + hydrochlorothiazide combination (from 81.4 ± 8.1 to 76.8 ± 6.9 mmHg, 3.6 (4.9, 2.3) mmHg).

We did not perform an analysis for 24-hour BPs on the low dose subgroup, since the sample size (34 patients receiving zofenopril and 49 receiving irbesartan) was too small to obtain reliable results.

3.6. Treatment Effect on Target Organ Damage. A summary of the effects of treatment on target organ damage measures is reported in Table 3. Both treatments had a similar positive effect on regression of cardiac and renal damage. A small reduction in the maximal IMT detected at any examined carotid district was also observed, with a significantly ($p = 0.047$) larger chance of carotid plaque regression under zofenopril (31.6%) than under irbesartan (16.1%).

TABLE 1: Demographic and clinical data of the patients of the intention-to-treat population at the time of randomization ($n = 434$). Data are separately shown for the two groups of randomization and reported as mean ($\pm$SD) or absolute (n) and relative frequency (%). BMI: Body Mass Index; LDL: Low Density Lipoprotein; HDL: High Density Lipoprotein; CV: cardiovascular; SBP: systolic blood pressure; DBP: diastolic blood pressure.

	Zofenopril 30–60 mg + HCTZ 12.5 mg ($n = 213$)	Irbesartan 150–300 mg + HCTZ 12.5 mg ($n = 221$)	p value
Age (years, mean ± SD)	56 ± 11	56 ± 11	0.926
Males (n, %)	124 (58)	120 (54)	0.411
BMI (kg/m², mean ± SD)	27 ± 3	27 ± 3	0.415
Waist circumference (cm, mean ± SD)	98 ± 10	98 ± 10	0.674
Age at first diagnosis of hypertension (years, mean ± SD)	49 ± 11	50 ± 11	0.850
Concomitant diseases (n, %)	140 (66)	133 (60)	0.232
Alcohol drinking (n, %)	62 (29)	74 (33)	0.326
Cigarette smoking (n, %)	61 (29)	65 (29)	0.859
Diabetes (n, %)	23 (11)	23 (10)	0.895
Elevated total cholesterol (n, %)	153 (72)	165 (75)	0.506
Elevated LDL cholesterol (n, %)	147 (69)	156 (71)	0.721
Low HDL cholesterol (n, %)	51 (24)	57 (26)	0.656
Abdominal obesity (n, %)	181 (85)	187 (85)	0.917
Family history of premature CV disease (n, %)	35 (16)	32 (15)	0.574
High CV risk (n, %)	197 (93)	204 (92)	0.943
Sitting office SBP (mmHg)	150 ± 11	151 ± 11	0.335
Sitting office DBP (mmHg)	93 ± 7	93 ± 7	0.366

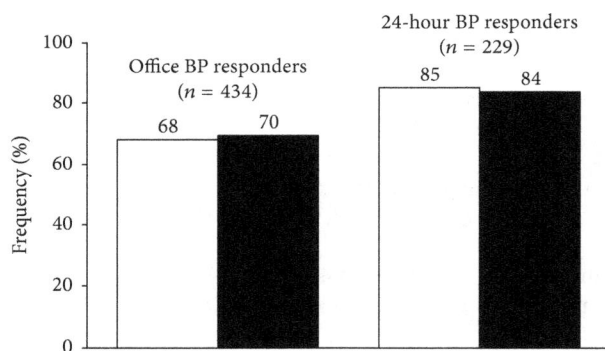

FIGURE 2: Percentage (%) of office blood pressure (BP) responders (<140/90 mmHg in nondiabetics and <130/80 mmHg in diabetics or high-risk patients, or SBP reduction ≥20 mmHg or DBP reduction ≥10 mm) and of 24-hour BP responders (<130/80 mmHg or a SBP reduction ≥10 mmHg or a DBP reduction ≥5 mmHg) after 18 weeks of treatment with zofenopril 30–60 mg plus hydrochlorothiazide 12.5 mg (open bars) and irbesartan 150–300 mg plus hydrochlorothiazide 12.5 mg (full bars). Data are shown for the intention-to-treat population ($n = 434$ office BP set; $n = 229$ ambulatory BP set).

3.7. *Double-Blind Extension Period.* For the 223 patients receiving drug dose uptitration at the end of the 18 weeks of treatment and continuing the study for additional 30 weeks, no differences were observed in office BP response and office and 24-hour BP reductions between the two treatment groups (Table 4). Similarly, the impact of treatment on target organ

damage did not significantly differ between the two study drugs (Table 5).

3.8. *Safety and Tolerability.* Laboratory and safety analyses were carried out in all randomized patients ($n = 462$). A total number of 62 (13.4%) patients (37 in the zofenopril plus hydrochlorothiazide and 25 in the irbesartan plus hydrochlorothiazide treatment group, $p = 0.075$) reported 73 adverse events (43 under zofenopril and 30 under irbesartan). Most of the adverse events (69.9%) were of a mild intensity. Eighteen (3.9%) patients were withdrawn from the study due to adverse events, 14 in the zofenopril and 4 in the irbesartan treatment group; of these patients, 9 (4.0%) receiving zofenopril and 3 receiving irbesartan (1.3%) reported drug-related adverse events ($p = 0.091$).

A total of 29 drug-related adverse events (22 under zofenopril and 7 under irbesartan) occurred in 24 patients (5.1%), of which 17 (7.5%) were treated with zofenopril plus the diuretic and 7 (3.0%) with irbesartan plus the diuretic ($p = 0.052$). The most common drug-related adverse event observed under zofenopril was cough (4 cases), whereas erectile dysfunction was the most prevalent drug adverse reaction in irbesartan-treated patients (2 cases).

In the extension phase 16 patients under high dose zofenopril plus hydrochlorothiazide (12.3%) and 13 patients under high dose irbesartan plus hydrochlorothiazide (11.4%) reported an adverse event ($p = 0.843$). Treatment-related adverse events occurred in 5 (3.8%) and 4 (3.5%) patients under the two study drugs ($p = 0.859$): of these patients,

TABLE 2: Baseline-adjusted office systolic blood pressure (SBP) and diastolic blood pressure (DBP) reductions after 18 weeks of treatment with zofenopril + hydrochlorothiazide (HCTZ) or irbesartan + HCTZ in the whole study group and in the subgroup of patients treated with the low drug dose (zofenopril 30 mg or irbesartan 150 mg). Data are shown for the intention-to-treat population and reported as mean ± SD or as mean and 95% confidence interval. The p value refers to the statistical significance of the intertreatment difference.

Office	SBP		DBP	
	Zofenopril 30–60 mg + HCTZ 12.5 mg	Irbesartan 150–300 mg + HCTZ 12.5 mg	Zofenopril 30–60 mg + HCTZ 12.5 mg	Irbesartan 150–300 mg + HCTZ 12.5 mg
All subjects	$n = 213$	$n = 221$	$n = 213$	$n = 221$
Baseline (mmHg)	148.4 ± 9.6	149.3 ± 10.1	91.6 ± 6.7	91.6 ± 6.8
Reduction with treatment (mmHg)	15.7 (13.9, 17.5)	19.3 (17.5, 21.1)	8.6 (7.4, 9.8)	11.6 (10.4, 12.8)
p value	0.001		<0.001	
Low dose subgroup	$n = 119$	$n = 104$	$n = 119$	$n = 104$
Baseline (mmHg)	147.4 ± 9.5	147.4 ± 8.3	90.4 ± 6.8	91.4 ± 6.7
Reduction with treatment (mmHg)	19.5 (18.0, 21.0)	22.5 (20.7, 24.3)	12.7 (11.0, 14.4)	15.2 (13.8, 16.6)
p value	0.065		0.096	

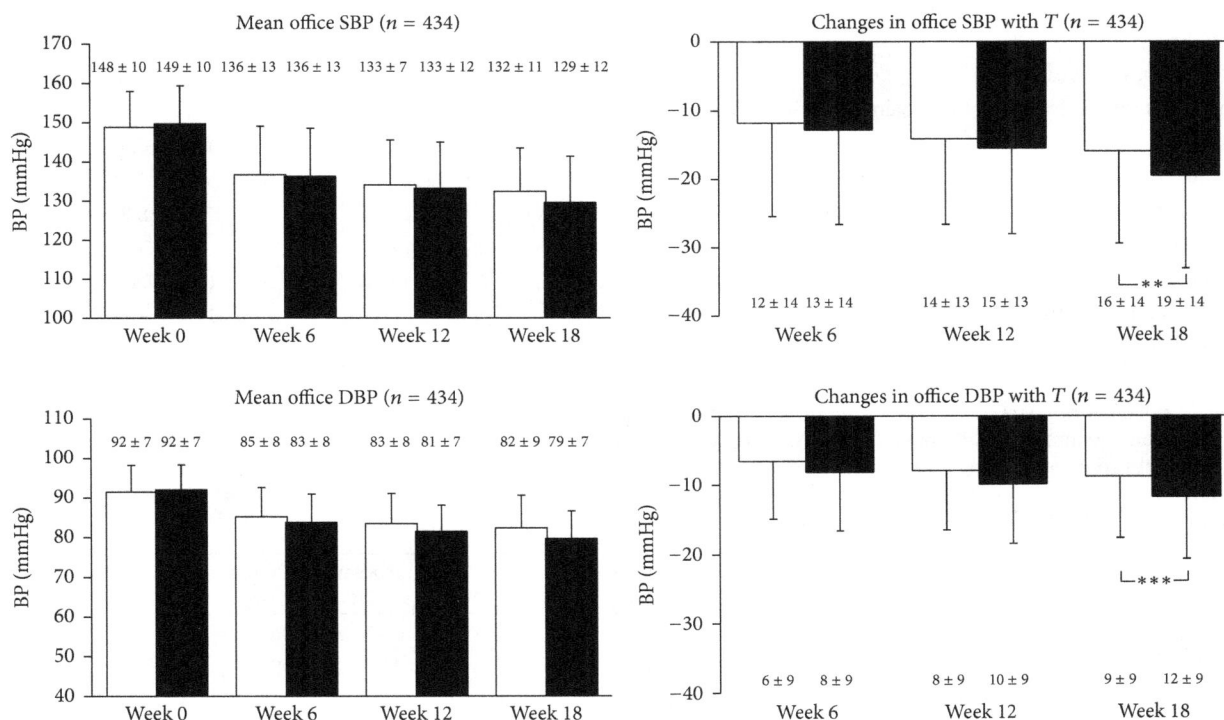

FIGURE 3: Mean office systolic blood pressure (SBP) and diastolic blood pressure (DBP) values and changes with treatment (T) in patients treated with zofenopril 30–60 mg plus hydrochlorothiazide 12.5 mg (open bars) or irbesartan 150–300 mg plus hydrochlorothiazide 12.5 mg (full bars). Data are shown for the intention-to-treat population and as mean values ±SD. Asterisks refer to the statistical significance of the intertreatment differences (** $p < 0.01$; *** $p < 0.001$).

4 were definitely withdrawn from the extension phase (3 zofenopril versus 1 irbesartan, $p = 0.368$).

Treatment was accompanied by either no change or only small and meaningless changes in the laboratory values considered in the study.

4. Discussion

Our study aimed at comparing the efficacy of 18 weeks of treatment with zofenopril 30 or 60 mg plus hydrochlorothiazide 12.5 mg once daily and irbesartan 150 or 300 mg plus hydrochlorothiazide 12.5 mg once daily in hypertensive patients uncontrolled by a previous monotherapy and with additional cardiovascular risk factors. At the end of follow-up the proportion of responders to treatment (<140/90 mmHg in nondiabetics and <130/80 mmHg in diabetics or high-risk patients, or SBP reduction ≥20 mmHg or DBP reduction ≥10 mmHg) was similar in zofenopril- and irbesartan-treated patients (68 versus 70%), with a similar use of the highest drug dose (56% zofenopril versus 47% irbesartan). The good office BP control obtained with either drug was confirmed over the 24 hours by ambulatory monitoring. At study end,

TABLE 3: Summary measures for cardiac (LVMI, left ventricular mass index), renal (urine protein), and vascular (IMT, intima-media thickness) damage for the intention-to-treat population and for the two study treatment groups. For any measure the baseline value (±SD), the adjusted reduction (and 95% confidence interval), and the absolute (n) and relative (%) frequency of patients with damage at baseline showing regression with treatment are reported. Adjustment was made by the baseline value and other potentially confounding variables (age, gender, abdominal obesity, HDL cholesterol, family history for premature cardiovascular disease, baseline blood pressure, and blood pressure changes with treatment). The p value refers to the statistical significance of the intertreatment difference.

	Zofenopril 30–60 mg + HCTZ 12.5 mg	Irbesartan 150–300 mg + HCTZ 12.5 mg	p value
Cardiac damage	$n = 204$	$n = 218$	
Baseline LVMI (g/m^2)	118.3 ± 35.3	124.6 ± 44.9	
LVMI reduction with treatment LVMI (g/m^2)	7.9 (17.4, +1.5)	10.7 (19.7, 1.6)	0.467
Patients with LVH at baseline showing LVH regression at study end (n, %)	20/84 (23.8)	24/86 (27.9)	0.648
Renal damage			
Albumin/creatinine ratio (mg/g)	$n = 38$	$n = 41$	
Baseline	14.0 ± 23.4	10.3 ± 20.3	
Reduction with treatment	3.2 (10.3, +3.9)	5.3 (11.8, +1.2)	0.490
Microalbuminuria over the 24 hours (mg/24 h)	$n = 56$	$n = 62$	
Baseline	21.1 ± 33.0	23.2 ± 37.1	
Reduction with treatment	+0.9 (20.8, +22.6)	+8.2 (14.1, +30.5)	0.387
Semiquantitative assessment of microalbuminuria by dipstick (mg)	$n = 87$	$n = 81$	
Baseline	14.2 ± 23.4	19.3 ± 31.3	
Reduction with treatment	12.3 (20.0, 4.6)	11.6 (18.7, 4.4)	0.801
Patients with renal damage at baseline showing regression at study end (n, %)	9/17 (52.9)	15/22 (68.2)	0.404
Vascular damage (maximum IMT in all districts)	$n = 211$	$n = 220$	
Baseline IMT (mm)	1.22 ± 0.47	1.21 ± 0.47	—
IMT reduction with treatment (mm)	0.07 (0.15, +0.01)	0.03 (0.11, +0.05)	0.143
Patients with carotid plaque at baseline showing regression at study end (n, %)	18/57 (31.6)	9/56 (16.1)	0.047

TABLE 4: Rate of office blood pressure (BP) responders (<140/90 mmHg in nondiabetics and <130/80 mmHg in diabetics or high-risk patients, or SBP reduction ≥20 mmHg or DBP reduction ≥10 mmHg) and baseline-adjusted office and 24-hour SBP and DBP reductions after 48 weeks of treatment with zofenopril 60 mg + hydrochlorothiazide (HCTZ) or irbesartan 300 mg + HCTZ. Data are shown for the intention-to-treat population and reported as absolute (n) and relative (%) frequencies and as mean and 95% confidence interval. The p value refers to the statistical significance of the intertreatment difference.

	Zofenopril 60 mg + HCTZ 12.5 mg	Irbesartan 300 mg + HCTZ 12.5 mg	p value
Office BP responders (n, %)	$n = 119$	$n = 104$	
	34 (28.6)	23 (22.1)	0.178
Office BP reduction with treatment	$n = 119$	$n = 104$	
SBP (mmHg)	17.8 (15.6, 20.0)	21.2 (18.6, 23.8)	0.052
DBP (mmHg)	11.7 (10.3, 13.1)	12.9 (11.3, 14.5)	0.268
24-hour BP reduction with treatment	$n = 50$	$n = 44$	
SBP (mmHg)	7.6 (9.7, 5.6)	7.2 (9.3, 5.1)	0.744
DBP (mmHg)	4.5 (6.1, 2.8)	5.9 (7.5, 4.2)	0.250

both drugs yielded a similarly high percentage of 24-hour responders (<130/80 mmHg or a SBP reduction ≥10 mmHg or a DBP reduction ≥5 mmHg): 85% zofenopril versus 84% irbesartan.

The large proportion of responders in both treatment arms supports the finding of previous studies that, in most patients not responding to a single antihypertensive medication, combination treatment with two drugs may substantially increase the chance of response [8, 9]. Our results also confirm that combination treatment between a drug acting on the angiotensin-renin-aldosterone system and a thiazide diuretic should be among the preferred choices when monotherapies fail to lower BP to or below target levels [36].

It is worth noticing that more than 90% of our subjects displayed multiple risk factors, which placed them in the high- or very high-risk category [3]. In these subjects current guidelines recommend initiation with a low dose

TABLE 5: Summary measures for cardiac (LVMI, left ventricular mass index), renal (urine protein), and vascular (IMT, intima-media thickness) damage after 48 weeks of treatment with zofenopril 60 mg + hydrochlorothiazide (HCTZ) or irbesartan 300 mg + HCTZ. Data are shown for the intention-to-treat population. For any measure the baseline value ($\pm$SD), the adjusted reduction (and 95% confidence interval), and the absolute (n) and relative (%) frequency of patients with damage at baseline showing regression with treatment are reported. Adjustment was made by the baseline value and other potentially confounding variables (age, gender, abdominal obesity, HDL cholesterol, family history for premature cardiovascular disease, baseline blood pressure, and blood pressure changes with treatment). The p value refers to the statistical significance of the intertreatment difference.

	Zofenopril 60 mg + HCTZ 12.5 mg	Irbesartan 300 mg + HCTZ 12.5 mg	p value
Cardiac damage	$n = 115$	$n = 104$	
Baseline LVMI (g/m^2)	118.8 $\pm$ 40.3	132.0 $\pm$ 50.3	
LVMI reduction with treatment LVMI (g/m^2)	23.3 (40.6, 6.0)	27.0 (44.3, 9.6)	0.445
Patients with LVH at baseline showing LVH regression at study end (n, %)	35/44 (79.5)	39/49 (79.6)	0.989
Renal damage			
Albumin/creatinine ratio (mg/g)	$n = 17$	$n = 12$	
Baseline	12.2 $\pm$ 16.7	2.3 $\pm$ 3.6	
Reduction with treatment	+9.0 (+2.1, +15.9)	+11.7 (+3.9, +19.5)	0.348
Microalbuminuria over the 24 hours (mg/24 h)	$n = 29$	$n = 34$	
Baseline	25.5 $\pm$ 41.2	19.4 $\pm$ 32.3	
Reduction with treatment	24.8 (72.8, +23.2)	0.22 (50.6, +50.1)	0.191
Semiquantitative assessment of microalbuminuria by dipstick (mg)	$n = 36$	$n = 27$	
Baseline	10.2 $\pm$ 11.3	24.7 $\pm$ 42.9	
Reduction with treatment	6.1 (15.1, +2.9)	6.5 (15.0, +2.0)	0.924
Patients with renal damage at baseline showing regression at study end (n, %)	1/8 (12.5)	2/9 (22.2)	0.617
Vascular damage (maximum IMT in all districts)	$n = 119$	$n = 104$	
Baseline IMT (mm)	1.27 $\pm$ 0.53	1.23 $\pm$ 0.49	
IMT reduction with treatment (mm)	+0.24 (0.05, +0.52)	+0.28 (0.01, +0.57)	0.693
Patients with carotid plaque at baseline showing regression at study end (n, %)	6/32 (18.8)	8/26 (30.8)	0.190

two-drug combination, which may offer the advantage of a prompter response and a greater probability of achieving the target BP [3]. As a matter of fact in the relatively small subset of patients taking the low drug dose at study end (30 mg for zofenopril and 150 mg for irbesartan) the rate of responders was high and did not significantly differ between the two groups (76% versus 79%). This means that even the low dose combination treatment has a high chance of success in patients previously classified as nonresponders to monotherapy and thus might represent a reasonable initial approach for treating these patients. This also strengthens the evidence from previous large randomized studies in patients with mild-moderate hypertension, in which treatment with the low dose of zofenopril (30 mg) combined with hydrochlorothiazide 12.5 mg once daily showed a greater efficacy than the monotherapy with either agent, with an increase in the response rate up to 55–65% [22, 23].

We also explored the effect of both treatments on target organ damage but could not find any relevant difference between the two study drugs. Likely, this was due to the fact that the study was not designed to assess this objective and the study sample was not adequate to detect a clinically plausible difference. A specific, adequately designed study in a large sample of patients and over a longer follow-up period might address this aspect.

This is the first study assessing the antihypertensive efficacy of high dose zofenopril (60 mg) plus hydrochlorothiazide 12.5 mg. In a previous dose-finding multifactorial study after 12 weeks of treatment with zofenopril 30 or 60 mg plus hydrochlorothiazide 12.5 mg the overall proportion of DBP responders to zofenopril plus hydrochlorothiazide was 86% and that of SBP responders was 60% [32]. As far as the benefits of the irbesartan and hydrochlorothiazide combination therapy are regarded, these have been documented in a number of trials in patients with mild hypertension, including those failing to achieve BP control with monotherapy, showing normalization rates up to 80–85% [37–40].

This is also the first study comparing zofenopril in combination with a thiazide diuretic with an ARB combined with a diuretic: previous direct comparative studies based on zofenopril monotherapy did not show any relevant difference in treatment efficacy versus an ARB-based monotherapy regimen [20, 21]. The combination between irbesartan and a thiazide diuretic has also never been directly compared against that of an ACE-inhibitor plus a diuretic, while evidence from comparative trials versus an ACE-inhibitor monotherapy is available, showing better BP response than enalapril [41–44] and fosinopril [45].

Both combination treatments were well tolerated, with a very limited number of drug-related adverse events. As expected, the combination containing zofenopril was associated with more cases of cough (6 versus none with irbesartan), but only for one patient cough led to study drug discontinuation. Other adverse drug reactions were well balanced between the two groups and the overall tolerability profile of zofenopril and irbesartan, including metabolic adverse effects, was comparable with that of previous reports [22, 46, 47].

5. Study Limitations

Finally, some limitations of the present study deserve to be discussed. The number of subjects included in the intention-to-treat analysis halved when the subgroup of patients undergoing ambulatory BP monitoring was considered. This occurred because many recordings were missing or qualitatively inadequate. However, in the ambulatory BP monitoring subgroup the percentage of responders was still comparable between the two treatment groups, indicating that the two populations were homogeneous. Evaluation of hypertension organ damage was done locally at each site and no centralized reading or specific quality control of original examinations (including ultrasound scans, serum creatinine, and urinary albumin) was planned. The fact that the measurements were done manually makes it highly unlikely to have enough sensitivity and reproducibility to detect reliable intertreatment changes in the short period of follow-up, particularly for segments such as the internal and external carotid artery which are very difficult to visualize and cannot clearly be detected in all patients. Additionally, urinary albumin excretion was assessed with different methodologies in the various investigating centers, with this potentially leading to inaccuracy and high variability in the estimates. We cannot exclude that our results might have been biased in this sense. We used separate BP targets for nondiabetic (<140/90 mmHg) and diabetic (<130/80 mmHg) patients, which are no longer required by current hypertension guidelines [3]. However, at the time the study was planned, designed, and then started, guidelines required separate BP goals for these two populations [31]. Since the investigators adjusted treatment doses on the basis of such thresholds during the study we could not change such limits when analyzing the data, in order to avoid any possible bias on the final results. Finally, the fact that we did not observe any difference between the two treatment groups in the rate of response but we documented a significant difference in the BP drop in favor of irbesartan, even after adjustment for baseline values, might simply be the result of chance and has a limited clinical value. As a matter of fact, the primary study objective and the investigator's reference for drug titration were the BP response and not the BP reduction with treatment.

6. Conclusions

The present pharmacological trial demonstrated that the combination of zofenopril and hydrochlorothiazide and that of irbesartan and hydrochlorothiazide both provide similarly effective and well tolerated control of BP in hypertensive patients not responders to a previous monotherapy and with a high or very high cardiovascular risk profile. Both antihypertensive regimens effectively retarded the progression of cardiovascular, renal, and vascular damage of hypertension.

Authors' Contribution

All named authors meet the ICMJE criteria for authorship for this paper, take responsibility for the integrity of the work as a whole, and have given final approval to the version to be published.

Acknowledgments

Ettore Malacco (Milano), Stefano Omboni (Varese), and Gianfranco Parati (Milano) are the study coordinators. List of study sites and investigators is as follows: Gianfranco Parati (Milano), Francesco Locatelli (Lecco), Silvano Perotti (Esine), Giancarlo Antonucci (Genova), Calogero Minneci (Firenze), Giambattista Desideri (Pescina), Vincenzo Capuano (Mercato San Severino), Roberto Pedrinelli (Pisa), Anna Gargiulo (Caserta), Giuseppe Licata (Palermo), Saverio Leone (Torino), Antonino Granatelli (Tivoli), Salvatore Felis (Catania), Michele Gulizia (Catania), Vitaliano Spagnuolo (Cosenza), Guglielmo De Curtis (S. Benedetto Del Tronto), Paolo Dessì-Fulgheri (Torrette Ancona), Mauro Campanini (Novara), Luciano Bardazzi (Prato), Gianfranco Clemenzia, Amalia Mariotti (Roma), Daniele Bertoli (Sarzana), Maria D'avino (Napoli), Andrea Maria Maresca (Varese), Gaetano Mottola (Mercogliano), Anna Belfiore (Bari), Pio Caso (Napoli), Enrica Rovero (Orbassano), Roberto Frediani (Domodossola), Roberto Sega (Vimercate), Giuseppe Alfio Caruso (Catania), Giuseppe Villa (Pavia), Colomba Falcone (Pavia), Giuseppe Lembo (Pozzilli), Stefano Taddei (Pisa), Luigi Anastasio (Vibo Valentia), Nicola Glorioso (Sassari), Antonio D'ospina (Stradella), Piero Luigi Caroli (Lecce), Ferdinando D'amico (Patti), and Francesco Portaluppi (Ferrara).

References

[1] C. M. Lawes, S. V. Hoorn, and A. Rodgers, "Global burden of blood-pressure-related disease, 2001," *The Lancet*, vol. 371, no. 9623, pp. 1513–1518, 2008.

[2] F. Turnbull and Blood Pressure Lowering Treatment Trialists' Collaboration, "Effects of different blood-pressure-lowering regimens on major cardiovascular events: results of prospectively-designed overviews of randomised trials," *The Lancet*, vol. 362, no. 9395, pp. 1527–1535, 2003.

[3] G. Mancia, R. Fagard, K. Narkiewicz et al., "2013 ESH/ESC Guidelines for the management of arterial hypertension: the task force for the management of arterial hypertension of the European Society of Hypertension (ESH) and of the European Society of Cardiology (ESC)," *Blood Pressure*, vol. 23, no. 1, pp. 3–16, 2014.

[4] The Heart Outcome Prevention Evaluation Study Investigators, "Effects of an angiotensin-converting-enzyme inhibitor, ramipril, on cardiovascular events in high-risk patients," *The New England Journal of Medicine*, vol. 342, pp. 145–153, 2000.

[5] PROGRESS Collaborative Study Group, "Randomised trial of a perindopril-based blood-pressure-lowering regimen among 6105 individuals with previous stroke or transient ischaemic attack," *The Lancet*, vol. 358, no. 9287, pp. 1033–1041, 2001.

[6] The ALLHAT Officers and Coordinators for the ALLHAT Collaborative Research Group, "Major outcomes in high-risk hypertensive patients randomized to angiotensin-converting enzyme inhibitor or calcium canne blocker vs diuretic: the Antihypertensive and Lipid-Lowering treatment to prevent Heart Attack Trial (ALLHAT)," *The Journal of the American Medical Association*, vol. 288, no. 23, pp. 2981–2997, 2002.

[7] B. Dahlöf, P. S. Sever, N. R. Poulter et al., "Prevention of cardiovascular events with an antihypertensive regimen of amlodipine adding perindopril as required versus atenolol adding bendroflumethiazide as required, in the Anglo-Scandinavian Cardiac Outcomes Trial-Blood Pressure Lowering Arm (ASCOT-BPLA): a multicentre randomised controlled trial," *The Lancet*, vol. 366, no. 9489, pp. 895–906, 2005.

[8] D. S. Wald, M. Law, J. K. Morris, J. P. Bestwick, and N. J. Wald, "Combination therapy versus monotherapy in reducing blood pressure: meta-analysis on 11,000 participants from 42 trials," *The American Journal of Medicine*, vol. 122, no. 3, pp. 290–300, 2009.

[9] M. R. Law, N. J. Wald, J. K. Morris, and R. E. Jordan, "Value of low dose combination treatment with blood pressure lowering drugs: analysis of 354 randomised trials," *British Medical Journal*, vol. 326, no. 7404, article 1427, 2003.

[10] B. Waeber, "Combination therapy with ACE inhibitors/angiotensin II receptor antagonists and diuretics in hypertension." *Expert Review of Cardiovascular Therapy*, vol. 1, no. 1, pp. 43–50, 2003.

[11] E. Ambrosioni, "Defining the role of zofenopril in the management of hypertension and ischemic heart disorders," *American Journal of Cardiovascular Drugs*, vol. 7, no. 1, pp. 17–24, 2007.

[12] C. Borghi, S. Bacchelli, and D. D. Esposti, "Long-term clinical experience with zofenopril," *Expert Review of Cardiovascular Therapy*, vol. 10, no. 8, pp. 973–982, 2012.

[13] C. Borghi, E. Ambrosioni, S. Omboni et al., "Zofenopril and ramipril and acetylsalicylic acid in postmyocardial infarction patients with left ventricular systolic dysfunction: a retrospective analysis in hypertensive patients of the SMILE-4 study," *Journal of Hypertension*, vol. 31, no. 6, pp. 1256–1264, 2013.

[14] C. Borghi, S. Bacchelli, D. D. Esposti, A. Bignamini, B. Magnani, and E. Ambrosioni, "Effects of the administration of an angiotensin-converting enzyme inhibitor during the acute phase of myocardial infarction in patients with arterial hypertension," *American Journal of Hypertension*, vol. 12, no. 7, pp. 665–672, 1999.

[15] P. Nilsson, "Antihypertensive efficacy of zofenopril compared with atenolol in patients with mild to moderate hypertension," *Blood Pressure*, vol. 2, pp. 25–30, 2007.

[16] Y. Lacourciere and P. Provencher, "Comparative effects of zofenopril and hydrochlorothiazide on office and ambulatory blood pressures in mild to moderate essential hypertension," *British Journal of Clinical Pharmacology*, vol. 27, no. 3, pp. 371–376, 1989.

[17] C. Farsang, "Blood pressure control and response rates with zofenopril compared with amlodipine in hypertensive patients," *Blood Pressure*, vol. 16, supplement 2, pp. 19–24, 2007.

[18] J.-M. Mallion, "An evaluation of the initial and long-term antihypertensive efficacy of zofenopril compared with enalapril in mild to moderate hypertension," *Blood Pressure*, vol. 16, no. 2, supplement, pp. 13–18, 2007.

[19] E. Malacco, S. Piazza, and S. Omboni, "Zofenopril versus lisinopril in the treatment of essential hypertension in elderly patients: a randomised, double-blind, multicentre study," *Clinical Drug Investigation*, vol. 25, no. 3, pp. 175–182, 2005.

[20] K. Narkiewicz, "Comparison of home and office blood pressure in hypertensive patients treated with zofenopril or losartan," *Blood Pressure*, vol. 2, supplement, pp. 7–12, 2007.

[21] G. Leonetti, A. Rappelli, and S. Omboni, "A similar 24-h blood pressure control is obtained by zofenopril and candesartan in primary hypertensive patients," *Blood Press*, vol. 15, supplement 1, pp. 18–26, 2006.

[22] S. Omboni, E. Malacco, and G. Parati, "Zofenopril plus hydrochlorothiazide fixed combination in the treatment of hypertension and associated clinical conditions," *Cardiovascular Therapeutics*, vol. 27, no. 4, pp. 275–288, 2009.

[23] A. Zanchetti, G. Parati, and E. Malacco, "Zofenopril plus hydrochlorothiazide: combination therapy for the treatment of mild to moderate hypertension," *Drugs*, vol. 66, no. 8, pp. 1107–1115, 2006.

[24] A. N. Rogoza, T. S. Pavlova, and M. V. Sergeeva, "Validation of A and D UA-767 device for the self-measurement of blood pressure," *Blood Pressure Monitoring*, vol. 5, no. 4, pp. 227–231, 2000.

[25] P. Palatini, G. Frigo, O. Bertolo, E. Roman, R. Da Cortà, and M. Winnicki, "Validation of the A&D TM-2430 device for ambulatory blood pressure monitoring and evaluation of performance according to subjects' characteristics," *Blood Pressure Monitoring*, vol. 3, no. 4, pp. 255–260, 1998.

[26] MOREPRESS website, MOnitoring REmotely blood PRESSure, http://www.morepress.net/.

[27] S. T. Reeves, K. E. Glas, H. Eltzschig et al., "Guidelines for performing a comprehensive epicardial echocardiography examination: recommendations of the American Society of Echocardiography and the Society of Cardiovascular Anesthesiologists," *Journal of the American Society of Echocardiography*, vol. 20, no. 4, pp. 427–437, 2007.

[28] R. B. Devereux, P. N. Casale, P. Kligfield et al., "Performance of primary and derived M-mode echocardiographic measurements for detection of left ventricular hypertrophy in necropsied subjects and in patients with systemic hypertension, mitral regurgitation and dilated cardiomyopathy," *The American Journal of Cardiology*, vol. 57, no. 15, pp. 1388–1393, 1986.

[29] D. Du Bois and E. F. Du Bois, "A formula to estimate the approximate surface area if height and weight be known. 1916," *Nutrition*, vol. 5, no. 5, pp. 303–311, 1989.

[30] J. H. Stein, C. E. Korcarz, and W. S. Post, "Use of carotid ultrasound to identify subclinical vascular disease and evaluate cardiovascular disease risk: summary and discussion of the american society of echocardiography consensus statement," *Preventive Cardiology*, vol. 12, no. 1, pp. 34–38, 2009.

[31] G. Mancia, G. De Backer, A. Dominiczak et al., "2007 guidelines for the management of arterial hypertension: the task force for the management of arterial hypertension of the European Society of Hypertension (ESH) and of the European Society of Cardiology (ESC)," *Journal of Hypertension*, vol. 25, pp. 1105–1187, 2007.

[32] G. Parati, S. Omboni, E. Malacco et al., "Antihypertensive efficacy of zofenopril and hydrochlorothiazide combination on ambulatory blood pressure," *Blood Pressure*, vol. 15, supplement 1, pp. 7–17, 2006.

[33] P. Bramlage, "Fixed combination of irbesartan and hydro-chlorothiazide in the management of hypertension," *Vascular Health and Risk Management*, vol. 5, pp. 213–224, 2009.

[34] E. Agabiti-Rosei, A. Manolis, D. Zava, and S. Omboni, "Zofenopril plus hydrochlorothiazide and irbesartan plus hydrochlorothiazide in previously treated and uncontrolled diabetic and non-diabetic essential hypertensive patients," *Advances in Therapy*, vol. 31, no. 2, pp. 217–233, 2014.

[35] G. Parati, S. Omboni, P. Palatini et al., "Italian society of hypertension guidelines for conventional and automated blood pressure measurement in the office, at home and over 24 hours," *High Blood Pressure & Cardiovascular Prevention*, vol. 15, no. 4, pp. 283–310, 2008.

[36] D. A. Sica, "Rationale for fixed-dose combinations in the treatment of hypertension: the cycle repeats," *Drugs*, vol. 62, no. 3, pp. 443–462, 2002.

[37] J. Schrader, P. Bramlage, S. Lüders, M. Thoenes, A. Schirmer, and D. W. Paar, "BP goal achievement in patients with uncontrolled hypertension: results of the treat-to-target post-marketing survey with irbesartan," *Clinical Drug Investigation* vol. 27, no. 11, pp. 783–796, 2007.

[38] N.-L. Sun, S. Jing, and J. Chen, "The control rate of irbesar-tan/hydrochlorothiazide combination regimen in the treatment of Chinese patients with mild to moderate hypertension," *Zhonghua Xin Xue Guan Bing Za Zhi*, vol. 33, no. 7, pp. 618–621, 2005.

[39] G. Bobrie, J. Delonca, C. Moulin, A. Giacomino, N. Postel-Vinay, and R. Asmar, "A home blood pressure monitoring study comparing the antihypertensive efficacy of two angiotensin II receptor antagonist fixed combinations," *American Journal of Hypertension*, vol. 18, no. 11, pp. 1482–1488, 2005.

[40] J. M. Neutel, E. Saunders, G. L. Bakris et al., "The efficacy and safety of low- and high-dose fixed combinations of irbesar-tan/hydrochlorothiazide in patients with uncontrolled systolic blood pressure on monotherapy: the INCLUSIVE trial," *Journal of Clinical Hypertension*, vol. 7, no. 10, pp. 578–586, 2005.

[41] A. Coca, C. Calvo, J. García-Puig et al., "A multicenter, ran-domized, double-blind comparison of the efficacy and safety of irbesartan and enalapril in adults with mild to moderate essential hypertension, as assessed by ambulatory blood pres-sure monitoring: the MAPAVEL study," *Clinical Therapeutics* vol. 24, no. 1, pp. 126–138, 2002.

[42] Y. Lacourcière, "A multicenter, randomized, double-blind study of the antihypertensive efficacy and tolerability of irbesartan in patients aged ≥65 years with mild to moderate hypertension," *Clinical Therapeutics*, vol. 22, no. 10, pp. 1213–1224, 2000.

[43] K. R. Chiou, C. H. Chen, P. Y. Ding et al., "Randomized, double-blind comparison of irbesartan and enalapril for treatment of mild to moderate hypertension," *Zhonghua Yi Xue Za Zhi*, vol. 63, pp. 368–376, 2000.

[44] A. Mimran, L. Ruilope, L. Kerwin et al., "A randomised, double-blind comparison of the angiotensin II receptor antagonist, irbesartan, with the full dose range of enalapril for the treatment of mild-to-moderate hypertension," *Journal of Human Hyper-tension*, vol. 12, no. 3, pp. 203–208, 1998.

[45] E. Angulo, N. R. Robles, J. Grois, A. Barquero, and M. Pérez Miranda, "Comparison of the antihypertensive activity of fos-inopril and irbesartan," *Anales de Medicina Interna*, vol. 19, pp. 571–575, 2002.

[46] R. Kunz, C. Friedrich, M. Wolbers, and J. F. E. Mann, "Meta-analysis: effect of monotherapy and combination therapy with inhibitors of the renin-angiotensin system on proteinuria in renal disease," *Annals of Internal Medicine*, vol. 148, no. 1, pp. 30–48, 2008.

[47] V. Forni, G. Wuerzner, M. Pruijm, and M. Burnier, "Long-term use and tolerability of irbesartan for control of hypertension," *Integrated Blood Pressure Control*, vol. 4, pp. 17–26, 2011.

Prevalence, Treatment, and Associated Factors of Hypertension

Arturo Corbatón-Anchuelo [iD],[1,2] María Teresa Martínez-Larrad,[1,2]
Náyade del Prado-González,[1] Cristina Fernández-Pérez,[1,2]
Rafael Gabriel,[3] and Manuel Serrano-Ríos [iD][1,2]

[1]*Instituto de Investigación Sanitaria, Hospital Clínico San Carlos (IdISSC), Madrid, Spain*
[2]*Spanish Biomedical Research Centre in Diabetes and Associated Metabolic Disorders (CIBERDEM), Madrid, Spain*
[3]*Escuela Nacional de Salud, ISCIII, Spain*

Correspondence should be addressed to Manuel Serrano-Ríos; manuel.serrano@salud.madrid.org

Academic Editor: Markus P. Schlaich

The prevalence and related factors of hypertensive subjects according to the resident area (rural versus urban) were investigated in two population-based studies from Spain. Medical questionnaires were administered and anthropometrics were measured, using standardized protocols. Hypertension was diagnosed in pharmacology treated subjects or those with blood pressure (BP) ≥140/90 mm Hg. Regarding BP control, it was defined as under control if BP was <140/90 or <140/85 mm Hg in type 2 diabetic subjects. Information on educational status, social class, smoking habit, and alcohol intake was obtained. 3,816 subjects (54.38 % women) were included. Prevalence of diagnosed hypertension was higher in women and showed no differences according to the living area (men: urban 21.88 versus rural 21.92 %, p = 0.986; women: urban 28.73 versus rural 30.01 %, p = 0.540). Women living in rural areas and men with secondary or tertiary education levels had a lower probability of being BP uncontrolled (OR (95 % CI): 0.501 (0.258–0.970)/p=0.040, 0.245 (0.092–0.654)/p=0.005, and 0.156 (0.044–0.549)/p=0.004, respectively). Urban young men (31-45 years) and medium aged women (46-60 years) were less BP controlled than their rural counterparts (41.30 versus 65.79 %/p=0.025 and 35.24 versus 53.27 %/p=0.002, respectively).

1. Introduction

Hypertension is one of the most important risk factors for cardiovascular, cerebrovascular, and peripheral vascular diseases as well as end-stage renal disease, together with diabetes mellitus, dyslipidemia, and smoking. These factors are significant contributors to deaths and disability in the developed countries [1]. In a recently published study in Catalonia (Spain), hypertension and lipid disorders were the most prevalent founded pair of chronic disorders in subjects older than 45 years old [2]. Regional differences and a gradient from northwest to southeast in adiposity and cardiovascular morbidity and mortality have been widely demonstrated in previous studies in Spain [3], but oppositely to other ethnic populations and countries [4–6], we lack studies on cardiovascular risk factors, specifically hypertension, comparing rural

and urban areas. In fact, some recently described strategies on healthy lifestyle have shown to lower blood pressure (BP), reducing the risk of complications associated with hypertension [7–9]. Differences on diet and physical activities have also been found and described in rural and urban areas across Spain [10–12], and, therefore, we believe that there are differences in the prevalence and characteristics of hypertension as well as in the associated factors.

The *Spanish Insulin Resistance (SIRS)* and the *Segovia Insulin Resistance* population-based studies were carried out by well-trained personnel in rural and urban areas of six autonomous communities in Spain, with the aim of knowing the prevalence of Metabolic Syndrome (MetS) and its associated cardiovascular risk factors. The prevalence of glucose tolerance categories and MetS was recently reported [13]. In conclusion, we found that MetS prevalence according to the most recent Harmonized Criteria remained stable in the last decade in Spanish females but slightly increased in males, with about one out of three men affected. Moreover, one out of four subjects had prediabetes. Thus, in this study our aim was to describe the prevalence and characteristics of hypertensive subjects as well as blood pressure control, according to the resident area.

2. Materials and Methods

We studied two Spanish cohorts focused on cardiovascular risk factors, whose recruitment procedures have been previously reported [13]: (A) The *Spanish Insulin Resistance Study (SIRS)* [14] is a cross-sectional population-based study carried out in 7 small and middle-size towns across Spain. It was estimated that it would be necessary to recruit a random sample of 3,000 individuals from a targeted population of 348,980 inhabitants aged 35 to 69 years old to get a precision lower than 2 % for a 20 % MetS prevalence [15]. To get this appropriate sample size, we selected 5,363 subjects from the census with the following result: 1,177 (21.9 %) census errors, 1,014 (18.9 %) refused, 3,172 accepted (response rate, 75.8 %), 147 met exclusion criteria, and 92 did not complete the study for diverse reasons. Finally, 4 subjects missed some clinical data, so 2,929 men and nonpregnant women were included in the current analysis. (B) The *Segovia Insulin Resistance Study* [12, 16], cross-sectional population-based study in the Spanish province of Segovia (Autonomous Community of Castilla-León), included subjects from 14 small and middle-sized towns. Assuming a prevalence of MetS of 20 % according to previous data [16], it was calculated that it would be necessary to recruit from the census a random sample of 2,992 individuals aged 35 to 74 years old (target population of 63,417 inhabitants, 62 % rural). Nevertheless, individuals who agreed to participate were 1,166 (response rate, 39 %), and, from those, only 900 completed the survey. For the final analysis, 13 cases were excluded as blood pressure was not obtained accurately. In summary, 7,115 males and nonpregnant females aged 35 to 74 years old were invited to participate from a targeted population of 412,397 subjects from 21 small and middle-sized towns across Spain, and 3,816 (1,741 males and 2,075 females) were finally included (overall response rate 53.8 %). In both studies, subjects with type 1 diabetes mellitus, heart failure or hepatic insufficiency, surgery in the previous year, abdominal wall hernias, weight loss or gain $\geq$ 5 kg in the previous six months, or institutionalized were excluded. All subjects were sent a personalized letter signed by the principal investigator and the Regional Public Authorities, explaining the purpose of the study and requesting volunteering for participation. In case of no response, people were again contacted by telephone up to three times. The standard procedures were adapted from the WHO MONICA protocol (WHO, 1990) [17] and approved by the respective ethics committees. All participants were given written information and signed the informed consent. A medical questionnaire was obtained by trained interviewers, requesting from each participant data related to demographic characteristics, including age, sex, education status, socioeconomic status, physical activity,

cigarette smoking, alcohol consumption, family history of diabetes and its treatment, hypertension, and other selected chronic diseases.

Anthropometrics measurements were performed using standardized protocols and included weight, height, and waist circumference (in cm). The waist circumference (WC) was measured three times using an anthropometric tape while study participants were standing erect in a relaxed position with both feet together on a flat surface at the smallest horizontal girth between the costal margins and the iliac crests at minimal respiration and averaged for analysis. Body mass index (BMI) was defined as weight (kg) divided by the square of height (m^2). Blood pressure (BP) was averaged from three attended measures performed in a resting and sitting position by own subjects' primary care physicians, or alternatively trained technicians, after a 10-minute seated rest. A minimum interval of 5 minutes was observed within the three measures, carried out with a random-zero mercury sphygmomanometer with an appropriate sized cuff, and following a standard protocol. Systolic BP and diastolic BP were defined as the points of the appearance and disappearance of Korotkoff sounds, respectively.

Information on pharmacological treatment of hypertension and elevated glucose was based on the participant's reported use of any medication and the transcription and coding of all medication names.

Educational status was estimated as the highest number of completed schooling years [18]. Social class classification was estimated according to the type of job or professional activity as described [18]. Alcohol intake was categorized in the following intervals: no alcohol intake 0 g alcohol/day, 1–14.99 g/day, $\geq$ 15–29.99 g/day, and $\geq$ 30 g/day [19, 20]. Smoking was grouped in three categories: current (at least one cigarette per day); never (those who had never smoked); and former (people who quit smoking >1 year ago at the time of the study) [21].

2.1. Procedures and Laboratory Studies. Hypertension was diagnosed in those subjects treated with blood pressure medication and/or had a mean systolic BP $\geq$ 140 mm Hg or alternatively equal or higher of diastolic BP $\geq$ 90 mm Hg, according to the guidelines of the European Hypertension Society [22]. BP control was defined as < 140/90 mm Hg in nondiabetic subjects and < 140/85 mm Hg in type 2 diabetic subjects [22]. Individuals with a history of hyperlipidemia, hypertension, or diabetes mellitus were deemed to have their respective risk factors, regardless of the biochemical values. Subjects were considered obese if their BMI was $\geq$ 30 kg/m^2.

After an overnight period, 20 ml of blood were obtained from an antecubital vein without compression. Plasma glucose concentration was determined twice by a glucose-oxidase method adapted to an Autoanalyzer (Hitachi 704, Boehringer Mannheim, Germany). Total cholesterol, triglycerides, and high-density lipoprotein (HDL-C) cholesterol were determined by enzymatic methods using commercial kits (Boehringer Mannheim, Germany). Low-density lipoprotein (LDL-C) cholesterol was calculated by the Friedewald formula. A 75 g oral glucose tolerance test (OGTT) was performed and interpreted according to the 2003 criteria of the

American Diabetes Association [23] after excluding clinically diagnosed diabetic patients. DM was analytically diagnosed when fasting plasma glucose (FPG) was ≥ 7.0 mmol/l (≥ 126 mg/dl) or 2-h glucose ≥ 11.1 mmol/l (≥ 200 mg/dl). Subjects on antidiabetic medications were also considered to have diabetes. In nondiabetic subjects, prediabetes was diagnosed in any of the following cases: IFG was defined as FPG 5.6–6.9 mmol/l (100–125 mg/dl), IGT as 2-h glucose 7.8–11.0 mmol/l (140–199 mg/dl), and IFG/IGT as FPG 5.6–6.9 mmol/l (100–125 mg/dl) and 2-h glucose 7.8–11.0 mmol/l (140–199 mg/dl).

2.2. Statistical Methods. Student t-test or analysis of variance ANOVA test were used to compare continuous variables expressed as means ± standard deviation (SD). The level of significance was set at 0.05 for all analyses. Linear regression was used to calculate quantitative variables adjusted for age and sex and their 95 % confidence intervals (CI). Age-standardized rates were based on direct standardization using the Spanish Population Census obtained from the Spanish Statistic Institute (www.ine.es). Otherwise, multivariate logistic regression analyses were performed to evaluate associations of age, body mass index, diabetes, cardiovascular disease, hypercholesterolemia, education level, alcohol, and smoking habits with being hypertensive and with the risk of being blood pressure uncontrolled. Adjusted Odds Ratios (ORs) and their 95 % CI were calculated. All analyses were performed using STATA software (version 11.0; StataCorp, College Station, TX, USA).

3. Results

We included 3,816 subjects (Table 1(a)) with no differences in the mean age between sexes, but subjects from rural areas were close to 2 years older (men p=.006, women p<.001). No differences between areas were found in both sexes for BMI, microalbuminuria, number of obesity subjects, known and unknown type 2 DM, known hypertension, and coronary and cerebrovascular diseases. WC was higher in urban versus rural men (um 95.45 versus rm 93.99 cm, p=.003). Diastolic blood pressure was different according to areas for both sexes (um 80.81 versus rm 78.82 mm Hg, p<.001; uw 79.24 versus rw 78.15, p=.035), as well as systolic blood pressure in women (uw 127.97 versus rw 126.05, p=.043). Rural diabetic women were more aware of suffering the disease than their urban counterparts (uw 3.01 versus rw 5.07 %, p=.024). More prediabetic men were found in the rural area (30 versus 24.4 %, p=.041). Known dyslipidemia was more prevalent in the urban area in both sexes (um 61.97 versus rm 52.28 %, p<.001; uw 60.00 versus rw 52.57 %, p=.001). Regarding habits (Table 1(b)), there was a higher alcohol intake in the rural area in both sexes [men: moderate (um 30.36 versus rm 33.59 %) and heavy drinkers (um 24.68 versus rm 30.42 %), p=.001; women: moderate (uw 13.27 versus rw 17.51 %), and heavy drinkers (uw 1.42 versus rw 2.10 %), p=.030], but more current smokers in the urban setting [men: um 43.62 versus rm 39.77 %, p<.001; women: (uw 20.32 versus rw 11.79 %), p<.001]. A higher degree of achieved studies was also found for both sexes in urban areas [men: secondary studies

(um 53.51 versus rm 58.12 %) and third degree studies (um 22.11 versus rm 7.36 %), p=.001; women: secondary studies (uw 43.56 versus rw 57.78 %) and third degree studies (uw 16.21 versus rw 10.12 %), p<.001], as well as a higher number of unemployed and lower number of manual workers in both sexes in the urban area (p<.001).

3.1. Hypertension (Diagnosed and Undiagnosed) and Blood Pressure Control. The age-standardized prevalence of hypertension was 25.45 % (CI 95 %: 23.76 – 27.14). According to sex, the age-standardized prevalence of hypertension was 21.39 % (CI 95 %: 19.13 – 23.65) in men and 29.10 % (CI 95 %: 26.59 – 31.62) in women. The prevalence of hypertension (Table 2(a)) increased with age (13.66, 25.92, 28.74 % / p<.001 in men and 12.64, 35.18, 45.81 % / p<.001 in women, aged 31-45, 46-60, and 61-77 years old, respectively) with no differences between areas in the age's groups considered. Regarding the prevalence of undiagnosed hypertension (Table 2(b)), we found a 16.68 % (CI 95 %: 14.98 – 18.39) of age-standardized prevalence. According to sex, the age-standardized prevalence of undiagnosed hypertension was 17.29 % (CI 95 %: 14.91 – 19.68) in men and 16.38 % (CI 95 %: 13.87 – 18.88) in women. The prevalence of undiagnosed hypertension also increased with age (11.39, 17.50, and 27.00 %/ p<.001 in men and 6,02, 17.88, and 29.41 %/ p<.001 in women aged 31-45, 46-60, and 61-77 years old, respectively). Interestingly, there was a 5 % higher prevalence of undiagnosed hypertension in urban versus rural women aged 46-60 years old (uw 19.85 versus rw 14.18 %, p=.018).

The prevalence of BP control (Figure 1) decreased significantly with age in rural but not urban men [um 41.30, 42.45, and 42.22 % (p >.05), rm 65.79, 45.59, and 26.92 % (p<.001) aged 31-45, 46-60, and 61-77 years old, respectively] and for urban and rural women [uw 64.00, 35.24, and 28.89 % (p<.001); rw 75.00, 53.27, and 37.04 % (p<.001) aged 31-45, 46-60, and 61-77 years old, respectively]. The BP control was higher in younger (aged 31 to 45 old) hypertensive rural men as compared to urban (uw 65.79 versus rw 41.30 %, p=.025). Similarly occurred with medium aged (46 to 60 years old) rural women (uw 35.24 versus rw 53.27 %, p=.002). No differences were found regarding the BP control in urban versus rural area populations at other age's categories.

Multivariate-adjusted logistic regression analyses showed that the probability of being hypertensive is higher in older and obese men and women, women with prediabetes or history of cardiovascular disease, nonsmoker women, and hypercholesteraemic men and women (Table 3). Women with secondary studies were less frequently diagnosed with hypertension [OR 0.486 (0.310-0.761), p <.001], oppositely to nonsmoker women [OR 3.703 (1.866-7.349), p<.001]. Uncontrolled blood pressure (Table 4) was most frequent in men with diabetes [OR 6.460 (1.260-33.125), p=.025] or nonsmokers [OR 3.126 (1.012-9.655), p=.048], while women living in rural areas [OR 0.501 (0.258-0.970), p=.040] and men with secondary or tertiary education levels [OR 0.245 (0.092-0.654), p=.005, and OR 0.156 (0.044-0.549), p=.004, respectively] were more prone to be controlled. Women with secondary or tertiary education levels had a trend towards better BP control [OR 0.467 (0.211–1.038), p=.060, and OR 0.337 (0.108–1.046), p=.060].

TABLE 1

(a) Clinical characteristics of the study population according to sex and living area.

	Men				Women			
	Urban	Rural	p	Total	Urban	Rural	p	Total
N (%)	952 (54.68)	789 (45.32)		1,741 (45.62)	1,265 (60.96)	810 (39.04)		2,075 (54.38)
Age (years), mean ± SD	49.96 ± 9.51	51.27 ± 10.50	0.006	50.55 ± 9.99	49.97 ± 9.33	51.92 ± 10.54	< 0.001	50.73 ± 9.87
Age ranges (years)								
31-45 n (%)	371 (38.97)	288 (36.50)		659 (37.85)	470 (37.15)	279 (34.44)		749 (36.10)
46-60 n (%)	420 (44.12)	309 (39.16)	0.001	729 (41.87)	604 (47.75)	329 (40.62)	< 0.001	933 (44.96)
61-77 n (%)	161 (16.91)	192 (24.33)		353 (20.28)	191 (15.10)	202 (24.94)		393 (18.94)
BMI (kg/m2), mean ± SD	27.65 ± 3.58	27.45 ± 3.62	0.230	27.56 ± 3.60	28.04 ± 4.86	27.96 ± 4.99	0.720	28.01 ± 4.91
Waist circumference (cm), mean ± SD	95.45 ± 10.12	93.99 ± 9.79	0.003	94.79 ± 10.00	85.85 ± 11.50	85.87 ± 10.83	0.965	85.86 ± 10.83
SBP (mm Hg), mean ± SD	127.89 ± 18.61	126.39 ± 8.33	0.093	127.21 ± 18.50	127.97 ± 21.63	126.05 ± 20.17	0.043	127.22 ± 21.09
DBP (mm Hg), mean ± SD	80.61 ± 11.20	78.82 ± 10.88	< 0.001	79.81 ± 11.09	79.24 ± 11.64	78.15 ± 11.12	0.035	78.82 ± 11.45
Microalbuminuria (mg/l), median (p25-p75).	5.9 (3.9 - 9.0)	5.3 (3.5 - 10.2)	0.146	5.55 (3.5 - 9.6)	4.0 (2.5 - 7.3)	4.2 (2.5 - 7.9)	0.804	4.2 (2.5 - 7.7)
Obesity (%) (BMI ≥ 30 kg/m2)	23.63	22.59	0.609	23.16	30.70	32.13	0.494	31.26
Diabetes Mellitus (%) (unknown + known)	8.93	8.08	0.546	8.54	6.72	7.48	0.526	7.02
Diabetes Mellitus (%) (known)	5.08	4.93	0.744	5.02	3.01	5.07	0.024	3.82
Diabetes Mellitus (%) (unknown)	3.84	3.15		3.53	3.70	2.40		3.19
Prediabetes (%) (IFG + IGT)	24.41	30.00	0.041	26.93	20.59	22.43	0.465	21.31
Coronary disease (%)	3.36	2.53	0.311	2.98	1.19	1.11	0.868	1.16
Cerebrovascular disease (%)	1.47	1.52	0.934	1.49	0.71	0.86	0.704	0.77
Peripheral artery disease (%)	0.10	0.38	0.232	0.23	--	--	--	-- (*)
Known hypertension (%)	21.88	21.92	0.986	21.90	28.73	30.01	0.540	29.23
Known dyslipidemia (%)	61.97	52.28	< 0.001	57.57	60.00	52.57	0.001	57.08

(∗) No cases were reported. IFG: Impaired Fasting Glucose. IGT: Impaired Glucose Tolerance. Statistically significant values (p< 0.05) are highlighted in bold letters.

(b) Habits, education, and socioeconomic status of the study population according to sex and living area.

	Men				Women			
	Urban	Rural	p	Total	Urban	Rural	p	Total
Alcohol intake (%)								
Never	19.96	17.74		18.95	56.16	53.88		55.27
Occasionally	25.00	18.25	0.001	21.94	29.15	26.51	0.030	28.12
Moderate	30.36	33.59		31.82	13.27	17.51		14.93
Heavy drinker	24.68	30.42		27.28	1.42	2.10		1.69
Smoking habit (%)								
Smoker	43.62	39.77		41.87	20.32	11.79		16.97
Non smoker	19.07	28.16	< 0.001	23.21	67.79	79.16	< 0.001	72.26
Formersmoker	37.30	32.07		34.92	11.89	9.06		10.78
Education level (%)								
Illiterate	21.23	32.74		25.93	31.55	27.41		30.02
Primary studies	3.16	1.78	< 0.001	2.59	8.68	4.69	< 0.001	7.21
Secondary studies	53.51	58.12		55.39	43.56	57.78		48.81
Third degree studies	22.11	7.36		16.08	16.21	10.12		13.96
Socioeconomic status (%)								
Student	0.11	-- (*)		0.06	-- (*)	0.13		0.06
Retired	23.31	25.16		24.17	41.17	38.58		40.08
Unemployed	10.29	4.08	< 0.001	7.41	10.65	4.86	< 0.001	8.20
Manual worker	36.46	43.74		39.84	28.69	36.09		31.82
Other jobs	29.83	27.01		28.52	19.48	20.34		19.84

(*): no cases were reported. Statistically significant values (p< 0.05) are highlighted in bold letters.

TABLE 2

(a) Prevalence of diagnosed hypertension by age groups and living area in the sample.

%				Age groups (years)								
	31 – 45				46 – 60				61-77			
	Urban	Rural	p	Total (95 % CI)	Urban	Rural	p	Total (95 % CI)	Urban	Rural	p	Total (95 % CI)
Men	13.26	14.18	0.741	13.66 (11.04 – 16.63) [*]	26.60	24.91	0.620	25.92 (22.67 – 29.37) [*]	29.11	28.42	0.887	28.74 (23.99 – 33.86) [*]
Women	11.11	15.27	0.108	12.64 (10.29 – 15.31) [+]	35.59	34.39	0.719	35.18 (32.06 – 38.39) [+]	49.20	42.56	0.193	45.81(40.73 – 50.95) [+]
Total	12.05	14.72	0.158	13.11 (11.34 – 15.05)	31.93	29.95	0.411	31.19 (28.92 – 33.53)	40.00	35.71	0.235	37.76 (34.21 – 41.41)

[*] p < 0.001 for the comparison of the three age categories in men. [+] p < 0.001 for the comparison of the three age categories in women.

(b) Prevalence of undiagnosed hypertension by age groups and living area in the sample.

%				Age groups (years)								
	31 – 45				46 – 60				61-77			
	Urban	Rural	p	Total (95 % CI)	Urban	Rural	p	Total (95 % CI)	Urban	Rural	p	Total (95 % CI)
Men	11.37	11.40	0.991	11.39 (8.95 – 14.38) [*]	19.87	14.08	0.093	17.50 (14.42 – 21.06) [*]	29.36	25.00	0.451	27.00 (21.75 – 32.99) [*]
Women	6.09	5.88	0.917	6.02 (4.40 – 8.18) [+]	19.84	14.29	0.097	17.88 (14.97 – 21.22) [+]	25.53	32.73	0.261	29.41 (23.59 – 36.00) [+]
Total	8.37	8.69	0.851	8.49 (7.01 – 10.25)	19.85	14.18	0.018	17.70 (15.54 – 20.09)	27.59	28.57	0.819	28.12 (24.12 – 32.49)

(*) p < 0.001 for the comparison of the three age categories in men. (+) p < 0.001 for the comparison of the three age categories in women. The statistical significance is highlighted in bold letters.

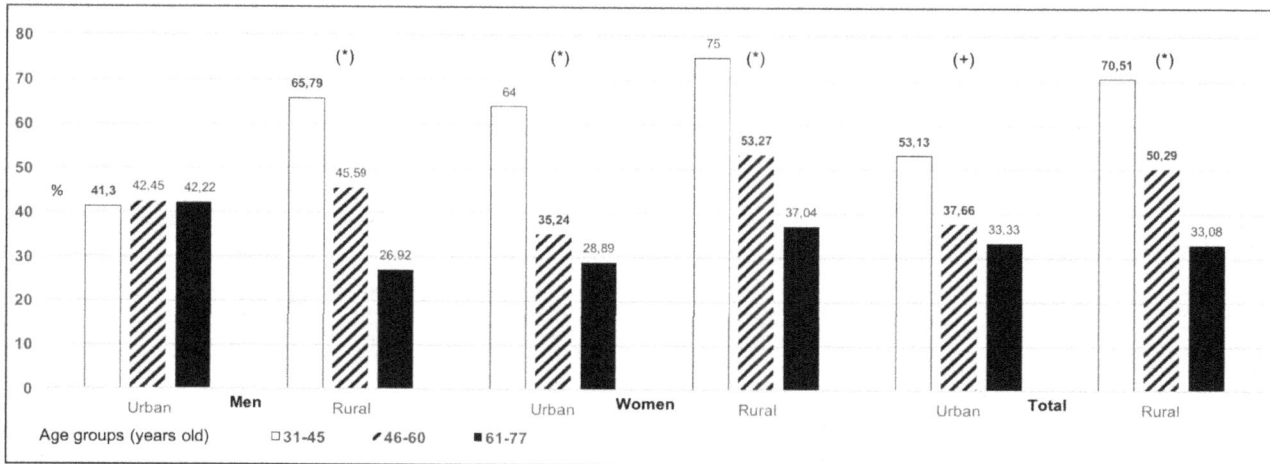

FIGURE 1: **Prevalence of controlled blood pressure in hypertensive subjects according to the age group and living area.** (∗) Overall age categories comparison p<.001 (+). Overall age categories comparison p=.004. Comparatives: **31 to 45 year-old urban versus rural men (41.30 versus 65.79 %, p=.025)**, 31 to 45 year-old urban versus rural women (64.00 versus 75.00 %, p=.263), **31 to 45 year-old urban versus rural subjects (53.13 versus 70.51 %, p=.019)**, 46 to 60 year-old urban versus rural men (42.45 versus 45.59 %, p=.684), **46 to 60 year-old urban versus rural women (35.24 versus 53.27 %, p=.002)**, **46 to 60 year-old urban versus rural subjects (37.66 versus 50.29 %, p=.002)**, 61 to 77 year-old urban versus rural men (42.22 versus 26.92 %, p=.113), 61 to 77 year-old urban versus rural women (28.89 versus 37.04 %, p=.257), 61 to 77 year-old urban versus rural subjects (33.33 versus 33.08 %, p=.965). Statistically significant values are highlighted in bold letters.

3.2. Pharmacological Therapy. Most of pharmacologically treated subjects were on monotherapy (data shown in Supplementary Table 1). Most frequent used drugs were diuretics and angiotensin converting enzyme inhibitors (32.1 and 30.3 % of subjects, respectively). The most frequent combined therapy was a diuretic with an inhibitor of the angiotensin converting enzyme (30 %).

4. Discussion

In this adult population from Spain, the prevalence of known hypertension is higher in women than men (29.23 versus 21.90 %) without differences between areas. In contrast, in a recent nationwide population-based study from Spain [24], the prevalence of known and unknown hypertension in subjects of similar mean age was significantly high (42.6 and 37.4 %, respectively). Nevertheless, that study was designed to report on the prevalence of diabetes mellitus type 2 (DM2) and had a higher proportion of DM2 subjects than our study. Another important study [25] included prevalence data on hypertension from 6 European countries. The hypertension prevalence in Spain was 49.0 % in men and 44.6 % in women (age range 35 to 65 years old), that together with other European countries represented a 60 % higher prevalence than the reported in United States and Canada. Other representative study of the Spanish Population [26], the *ENRICA* study, found a prevalence of hypertension of 33.3 %, more in accordance with our findings. Interesting from this study was that only 59.4 % of the subjects were aware of their condition and only 48.5 % of them were blood pressure (BP) controlled. Authors reported that education level was influencing BP control, in correlation to our finding that men with secondary or tertiary education levels had a lower probability of being BP uncontrolled.

In the northeast of Spain, prevalence of hypertension was higher to the herein reported, with one out of three subjects diagnosed with hypertension and, interestingly, near 1 of 2 subjects suffering from unknown hypertension [27]. There was a significant correlation with alcohol intake, obesity, and family history of hypertension or cardiovascular disease, and no correlation with professional level, education, or hypertension in the spouse. Probably, the main limitation of this study was the number of participating subjects (n = 670), too low for a comprehensive study of hypertension associated variables. On the other hand, a larger study with near 3,000 subjects in the northwest of Spain [10] found that prevalence of hypertension was higher in subjects with low educational level in which close association was observed with cardiovascular diseases. The authors reported that one up to four subjects had a diagnosis of hypertension, in accordance with our study results, and as in the previously mentioned ENRICA study [26], only 1 of 2 subjects was aware of its hypertensive status. Another population-based study in subjects aged ≥ 60 years old found that BP control was related to living in rural areas, as we have found in rural women, being uncoupled or doing moderate physical activity in men, as well as drinking moderate alcohol in women [11]. Relevant of this study is that it is one of the few studies in Spain that clearly defines and addresses the living area, a factor that in our opinion should be considered in the study of hypertension prevalence and incidence, as a consequence of the different ways of live [10–12, 16]. In fact, the type of diet and the physical activity are two of the seven defined factors involving cardiovascular health according to the *American Heart Association* [28]. On the other hand, it

TABLE 3: Multiple logistic regression analysis of subjects' probability of being hypertensive after adjusting for age, body mass index, diabetes, cardiovascular disease, hypercholesterolemia, education level, alcohol, and smoking habits.

	Men		Women	
	OR (95 % CI)	p	OR (95 % CI)	p
Living area				
Urban area	1		1	
Rural area	0.905 (0.614 – 1.334)	0.614	1.017 (0.703 – 1.472)	0.927
Age categories (years)				
31 – 45	1		1	
46 - 60	**1.863** (1.212 – 2.862)	**0.005**	**1.679** (1.078 – 2.616)	**0.022**
61 - 77	**2.717** (1.473 – 5.010)	**0.001**	1.635 (0.895 – 2.986)	0.110
BMI (kg/m2)				
< 30	1		1	
≥ 30	**1.943** (1.281 – 2.949)	**0.002**	**3.219** (2.228 – 4.650)	**< 0.001**
Diabetes Mellitus				
No	1		1	
Prediabetes	1.041 (0.685 – 1.582)	0.852	**1.823** (1.228 – 2.706)	**0.003**
Diabetes	**0.799** (0.400 – 1.598)	**< 0.001**	1.040 (0.529 – 2.043)	0.910
Cardiovascular disease				
No	1		1	
Yes	2.129 (0.978 – 4.638)	0.057	**4.029** (1.369 – 11.862)	**0.008**
Hypercholesterolemia				
No	1		1	
Yes	**1.670** (1.148 – 2.525)	**0.008**	**1.651** (1.151 – 2.369)	**0.007**
Education level				
None	1		1	
Primary	1.084 (0.311 – 3.780)	0.863	1.076 (0.555 – 2.085)	0.828
Secondary	0.984 (0.601 – 1.611)	0.950	**0.486** (0.310 – 0.761)	**0.002**
Tertiary	0.798 (0.419 – 1.519)	0.550	0.802 (0.428 – 1.505)	0.493
Alcohol intake				
No	1		1	
Occasionally	0.881 (0.491 – 1.579)	0.669	0.855 (0.555 – 1.315)	0.475
Low-Moderate	0.840 (0.486 – 1.453)	0.533	0.982 (0.595 – 1.622)	0.945
Heavy	1.143 (0.661 – 1.976)	0.631	0.836 (0.193 – 3.627)	0.810
Smoking habit				
Yes	1		1	
No	0.795 (0.471– 1.342)	0.391	**3.703** (1.866 – 7.349)	**< 0.001**
Former	0.961 (0.632 – 1.464)	0.857	2.126 (0.929 – 4.868)	0.074

Statistically significant values (p< 0.05) are highlighted in bold letters.

has been reported that underserved rural areas had higher rates of hypertension diagnosis as well as other cardiovascular risk factors, but also high rates of uncontrolled BP [4]. For this reason, achieving a similar degree of BP control in rural versus urban areas could be an indicator of a better and more widespread healthcare system. Thus, it is noticeable that we have found a better BP control in rural women but not men after adjusting for multiple confounders. The reason for this finding is not clear and could be a consequence of differences in lifestyle across areas in women, such as diet or exercise, rather than differences in the access to the healthcare system.

More recently, a large study in Italy, including ten thousand subjects with a mean age of 56 years old, confirmed a high prevalence of hypertension (between 55.4 and 59.0 %) in the real life setting for the period of 2004 to 2014, with a slight tendency over a better BP control over the 10-year period (from 50 to 57.6 %). In contrast, we found a lower proportion of patients with an adequate BP control, higher in women than men and lowering with increasing age. Moreover, less than one in three patients achieves optimal BP control after the age of 60 in our study. Also in Italy, in a recent study with near 10,000 outpatients from 1,666 primary care physicians'

TABLE 4: Multiple logistic regression analysis of hypertensive treated subjects of being blood pressure uncontrolled after adjusting for age, body mass index, diabetes, cardiovascular disease, hypercholesterolemia, education level, alcohol, and smoking habits.

	Men		Women	
	OR (95 % CI)	p	OR (95 % CI)	p
Living area				
Urban area	1		1	
Rural area	0.819 (0.380 – 1.765)	0.610	**0.501** (0.258 – 0.970)	**0.040**
Age categories (years)				
31 – 45	1		1	
46 - 60	0.933 (0.392 – 2.220)	0.876	1.595 (0.650 – 3.917)	0.308
61 - 77	1.187 (0.387 – 3.642)	0.765	2.045 (0.651 – 6.424)	0.220
BMI (kg/m2)				
< 30	1		1	
≥ 30	0.757 (0.342 – 1.675)	0.492	1.403 (0.752 – 2.617)	0.287
Diabetes Mellitus				
No	1		1	
Prediabetes	0.769 (0.345 – 1.714)	0.520	1.898 (0.990 – 3.642)	0.054
Diabetes	**6.460** (1.260 – 33.125)	**0.025**	1.799 (0.554 – 5.839)	0.329
Cardiovascular disease				
No	1		1	
Yes	1.376 (0.360 – 5.270)	0.641	0.967 (0.241 – 3.881)	0.963
Hypercholesterolemia				
No	1		1	
Yes	0.819 (0.350 – 1.918)	0.646	0.596 (0.305 – 1.166)	0.131
Education level				
None	1		1	
Primary	0.855 (0.685 – 10.666)	0.903	1.180 (0.425 – 3.277)	0.751
Secondary	**0.245** (0.092 – 0.654)	**0.005**	0.467 (0.211 – 1.038)	0.062
Tertiary	**0.156** (0.044 – 0.549)	**0.004**	0.337 (0.108 – 1.046)	0.060
Alcohol intake				
No	1		1	
Occasionally	1.181 (0.356 – 3.917)	0.785	0.560 (0.250 – 1.255)	0.159
Low-Moderate	1.760 (0.562 – 5.512)	0.332	0.531 (0.221 – 1.272)	0.155
Heavy	2.258 (0.720 – 7.08)	0.163	1.082 (0.069 – 16.989)	0.955
Smoking habit				
Yes	1		1	
No	**3.126** (1.012 – 9.655)	**0.048**	1.237 (0.282 – 5.430)	0.778
Former	1.828 (0.789 – 4.234)	0.159	0.914 (0.153 – 5.473)	0.922

Statistically significant values (p< 0.05) are highlighted in bold letters.

consultations, Tocci et al. [29] found 72.5 % of hypertension diagnosed subjects. The main reported result was that less than a third of hypertensive subjects (30 %) achieved the recommended BP target levels in Italy, results in accordance with our study and other studies in Spain [30].

Our findings in the prescribed pharmacologic therapy differ with other studies, as we have found a significant high prescription of diuretics in the monotherapy group. The reason could be related to the years of recruitment of our study, as diuretics were highly prescribed as a first line therapy in the 80s and 90s of the past century and our subjects were recruited at the end of the 90s and 2001-2002. In fact, diuretics occupied the fourth hypertension treatment position in the

PRESCAP study in 2002 (prescribed in 10.6 % of men and 18.8 % of women), while eight years later, in the PRESCAP 2010 study, a downward trend in the prescription of diuretics as monotherapy was highlighted (7.3 % in men and 17.2 % in women) [31]. Angiotensin converting enzyme drugs were the second more prescribed pharmacologic group class after diuretics in our population, although these drugs are already the first therapeutic prescribed class in other studies [24, 29].

5. Study Limitations

Causal inferences from our data are not possible because of the cross-sectional design. Otherwise, the reduction in the initial sample size could have conducted to a nonrepresentative population study. Due to this fact, we compared our cohorts (age, sex distribution, and area frequencies of subjects finally included in the study) to the Census of the National Institute of Statistics of Spain (www.ine.es) for the same years and found that they were nearly identical. We did not assess physical exercise and nutrient intake story through dietary standardized questionnaire, missing important information as, for example, the degree of adherence to Mediterranean diet, that is associated with a higher prevalence of hypertension and related factors. Other potential biases are as follows: first, estimated prevalence of hypertension might be too high because healthy population could have declined to participate; second, alcohol consumption was self-reported so it could be underestimated; and third, information on ambulatory BP or at least a second day BP measurement was not available; thus we cannot provide data on proportions of patients achieving sustained BP control.

6. Conclusions

The prevalence of diagnosed hypertension in a Caucasian population of Spain was higher in women and showed no differences according to the living area (urban versus rural) in both sexes. Women living in rural areas and men with secondary or tertiary education levels have a lower probability of being blood pressure uncontrolled. Urban young men (31-45 years old) and medium aged women (46-60 years old) are less blood pressure controlled than their rural counterparts.

Disclosure

The funders had no role in study design, data collection and analysis, decision to publish, or preparation of the manuscript. This study was presented in an oral session at the 28th European Meeting on Hypertension and Cardiovascular Protection of the European Society of Hypertension, Barcelona, Spain, 8-11th June, 2018. The abstract form can be read in the Journal of Hypertension [32].

Authors' Contributions

The first author (Arturo Corbatón-Anchuelo) is responsible for the design of the study and preparation of the first draft of the manuscript. The second, fourth, fifth, and corresponding author (María Teresa Martínez-Larrad, Cristina Fernández-Pérez, Rafael Gabriel, and Manuel Serrano-Ríos) participated actively in the design and development of the field studies. First and third authors (Arturo Corbatón-Anchuelo, Náyade del Prado-González) extracted the data and take responsibility for the integrity of the analyses. The corresponding author (Manuel Serrano-Ríos) substantially contributed to the interpretation of data, critical revision of the manuscript, and final approval of the manuscript to be published.

Acknowledgments

This work was supported by Grants FEDER 2FD 1997/2309 from the Fondo Europeo para el Desarrollo Regional, Red de Centros RCMN (C03/08), FIS 03/1618 from Instituto de Salud Carlos III-RETIC RD06/0015/0012, Madrid, Spain. The authors also acknowledge CIBER in Diabetes and Associated Metabolic Disorders (ISCIII, Ministerio de Ciencia e Innovación) and Madrid Autonomous Community (MOIR S2010/BMD-2423). Partial support also came from Educational Grants from Eli Lilly Lab, Spain, Bayer Pharmaceutical Co., Spain and Fundación Mutua Madrileña 2008, Spain. Members of the Segovia Insulin Resistance Study Group are acknowledged. The authors also acknowledge Milagros Pérez-Barba for dedicated and careful technical assistance.

References

[1] M. Ezzati, A. D. Lopez, A. Rodgers, S. Vander Hoorn, and C. J. L. Murray, Comparative Risk Assessment Collaborating Group, "Selected major risk factors and global and regional burden of disease," The Lancet, vol. 360, pp. 1347–1360, 2002.

[2] Q. Foguet-Boreu, C. Violan, A. Roso-Llorach et al., "Impact of multimorbidity: acute morbidity, area of residency, and use of health services across life span in a region of South Europe," BMC Family Practice, vol. 15, no. 1, article no. 55, 2014.

[3] Plan Integral de Cardiopatía Isquémica 2004-2007, Health plans, Spanish Ministry of Health, 2003.

[4] B. Bale, "Optimizing hypertension management in underserved rural populations," Journal of the National Medical Association, vol. 102, no. 1, pp. 10–17, 2010.

[5] K. A. Moser, S. Agrawal, G. D. Smith, and S. Ebrahim, "Socio-demographic inequalities in the prevalence, diagnosis and management of hypertension in India: Analysis of nationally-representative survey data," PLoS ONE, vol. 9, no. 1, Article ID e86043, 2014.

[6] J. Li, L. Shi, S. Li, L. Xu, W. Qin, and H. Wang, "Urban-rural disparities in hypertension prevalence, detection, and medication use among Chinese Adults from 1993 to 2011," International Journal for Equity in Health, vol. 16, no. 1, article no. 50, 2017.

[7] H. Y. Zhao, X. X. Liu, A. X. Wang et al., "Ideal cardiovascular health and incident hypertension. The longitudinal community-based Kailuan study," Medicine (Baltimore), vol. 95, no. 50, p. e5415, 2016.

[8] L. J. Appel, M. W. Brands, S. R. Daniels, N. Karanja, P. J. Elmer, and F. M. Sacks, "Dietary approaches to prevent and treat hypertension: a scientific statement from the American Heart Association," Hypertension, vol. 47, no. 2, pp. 296–308, 2006.

[9] J. Gao, H. Sun, X. Liang et al., "Ideal cardiovascular health behaviors and factors prevent the development of hypertension in prehypertensive subjects," Clinical and Experimental Hypertension, vol. 37, no. 8, pp. 650–655, 2015.

[10] R. Perez-Fernandez, A. F. Mariño, C. Cadarso-Suarez et al., "Prevalence, awareness, treatment and control of hypertension in Galicia (Spain) and association with related diseases," Journal of Human Hypertension, vol. 21, no. 5, pp. 366–373, 2007.

[11] R. Tuesca-Molina, P. Guallar-Castillón, J. R. Banegas-Banegas, and A. Graciani-Pérez Regadera, "Factores asociados al control de la hipertensión arterial en personas mayores de 60 años en España," Revista Española de Salud Pública, vol. 80, pp. 233–242, 2006.

[12] A. Corbatón-Anchuelo, M. T. Martínez-Larrad, C. Fernández-Pérez et al., "Metabolic syndrome, adiponectin, and cardiovascular risk in Spain (The Segovia Study): Impact of consensus societies criteria," *Metabolic Syndrome and Related Disorders*, vol. 11, no. 5, pp. 309–318, 2013.

[13] M. T. Martínez-Larrad, A. Corbatón-Anchuelo, C. Fernández-Pérez, Y. Lazcano-Redondo, F. Escobar-Jiménez, and M. Serrano-Ríos, "Metabolic syndrome, glucose tolerance categories and the cardiovascular risk in Spanish population," *Diabetes Research and Clinical Practice*, vol. 114, pp. 23–31, 2016.

[14] C. Lorenzo, M. Serrano-Rios, M. T. Martinez-Larrad et al., "Prevalence of hypertension in Hispanic and non-Hispanic white populations," *Hypertension*, vol. 39, no. 2 I, pp. 203–208, 2002.

[15] B. Balkau, M. A. Charles, T. Drivsholm, European Group for the Study of Insulin Resistance (EGIR) et al., "Frequency of the WHO metabolic syndrome in European cohorts, and an alternative definition of an insulin resistance syndrome," *Diabetes & Metabolism*, vol. 28, pp. 364–376, 2002.

[16] M. T. Martínez-Larrad, C. Fernández-Pérez, J. L. González-Sánchez et al., "Prevalence of the metabolic syndrome [ATP-III criteria]. Population-based study of rural and urban areas in the Spanish Province of Segovia," *Medicina Clínica*, vol. 125, no. 13, Article ID 99.763, pp. 481–486, 2005.

[17] World Health Organization, "WHO MONICA project: part III: population survey. Section 1: population survey data component," in *MONICA Manual*, World Health Organization, Geneva, Switzerland, 1990.

[18] D. C. Álvarez, J. Alonso, A. Domingo, and E. Regidor, "La medición de la clase social en Ciencias de la Salud," in *Informe de un grupo de trabajo de la Sociedad Española de Epidemiología*, pp. 63–74, SG Editors, Barcelona, Spain, 1995.

[19] A. Buja, E. Scafato, G. Sergi et al., "Alcohol consumption and metabolic syndrome in the elderly: results from the Italian longitudinal study on aging," *European Journal of Clinical Nutrition*, vol. 64, no. 3, pp. 297–307, 2010.

[20] Y. S. Yoon, S. W. Oh, H. W. Baik, H. S. Park, and W. Y. Kim, "Alcohol consumption and the metabolic syndrome in Korean adults: the 1998 Korean National Health and Nutrition Examination Survey," *American Journal of Clinical Nutrition*, vol. 80, no. 1, pp. 217–224, 2004.

[21] World Health Organization [WHO], *Guidelines for controlling and monitoring the tobacco epidemic*, WHO Tobacco or Health Programme, Geneva, Switzerland, 1997.

[22] The Task Force for the management of arterial hypertension of the European Society of Hypertension (ESH) and of the European Society of Cardiology, "ESC 2013 ESH/ESC Guidelines for the management of arterial hypertension," *European Heart Journal*, vol. 34, pp. 2159–2219, 2013.

[23] Expert Committee on the Diagnosis and Classification of Diabetes Mellitus, "Follow up Report on the Diagnosis of Diabetes Mellitus," *Diabetes Care*, vol. 26, no. 3, pp. 160–167, 2003.

[24] E. Menéndez, E. Delgado, F. Fernández-Vega, MA. Prieto, E. Bordiú, A. Calle et al., "Prevalence, diagnosis, treatment and grade control of hypertension in Spain. Results from the *Di@betes study*," *Revista Española de Cardiología*, vol. 69, pp. 572–578, 2016.

[25] K. Wolf-Maier, R. S. Cooper, J. R. Banegas et al., "Hypertension prevalence and blood pressure levels in 6 European countries, Canada, and the United States," *The Journal of the American Medical Association*, vol. 289, no. 18, pp. 2363–2369, 2003.

[26] J. R. Banegas, A. Graciani, J. J. De La Cruz-Troca et al., "Achievement of cardiometabolic goals in aware hypertensive patients in Spain: A nationwide population-based study," *Hypertension*, vol. 60, no. 4, pp. 898–905, 2012.

[27] J. Custodi, J. L. Llor, M. Farrús et al., "Arterial hypertension in the Baix Ebre region (Tarragona)," *Atencion Primaria*, vol. 6, no. 3, pp. 151–158, 1989.

[28] D. M. Lloyd-Jones, Y. Hong, D. Labarthe et al., "Defining and setting national goals for cardiovascular health promotion and disease reduction: the American heart association's strategic impact goal through 2020 and beyond," *Circulation*, vol. 121, no. 4, pp. 586–613, 2010.

[29] G. Tocci, A. Battistoni, M. D'Agostino et al., "Impact of hypertension on global cardiovascular risk stratification: Analysis of a large cohort of outpatient population in Italy," *Clinical Cardiology*, vol. 38, no. 1, pp. 39–47, 2015.

[30] F. Catalá-López, G. Sanfélix-Gimeno, C. García-Torres, M. Ridao, and S. Peiró, "Control of arterial hypertension in Spain: A systematic review and meta-analysis of 76 epidemiological studies on 341,632 participants," *Journal of Hypertension*, vol. 30, pp. 168–176, 2011.

[31] V. Barrios, C. Escobar, F. J. Alonso-Moreno et al., "Evolution of clinical profile, treatment and blood pressure control in treated hypertensive patients according to the sex from 2002 to 2010 in Spain," *Journal of Hypertension*, vol. 33, no. 5, pp. 1098–1107, 2015.

[32] A. Corbatón Anchuelo, M. T. Martínez Larrad, N. Del Prado González, C. Fernández Pérez, R. Gabriel Sánchez, and M. Serrano Ríos, "Prevalence, treatment and associated factors of hypertension in urban and rural areas of Spain," *Journal of Hypertension*, vol. 36, p. e228, 2018.

3

Renin-Angiotensin System Genes Polymorphisms and Essential Hypertension

Daméhan Tchelougou,[1,2,3] Jonas K. Kologo,[4,5] Simplice D. Karou,[1,2,3]
Valentin N. Yaméogo,[4,5] Cyrille Bisseye,[1,2,6] Florencia W. Djigma,[1,2,5]
Djeneba Ouermi,[1,2,5] Tegwindé R. Compaoré,[1,2] Maléki Assih,[1,2,3]
Virginio Pietra,[1,2,3] Patrice Zabsonré,[4] and Jacques Simpore[1,2,5]

[1] Centre de Recherche Biomoléculaire Pietro Annigoni (CERBA), BP 364, Ouagadougou 01, Burkina Faso
[2] Laboratoire de Biologie et Génétique Moléculaires (LABIOGENE), Université de Ouagadougou, BP 7021,
 Ouagadougou 03, Burkina Faso
[3] Ecole Supérieure des Techniques Biologiques et Alimentaires (ESTBA-UL), Université de Lomé, BP 1515, Togo
[4] Service de Cardiologie, CHU-Yalgado Ouédraogo, BP 7022, Ouagadougou 03, Burkina Faso
[5] Centre Médical Saint Camille (CMSC), BP 444, Ouagadougou 09, Burkina Faso
[6] Laboratoire de Biologie Moléculaire et Cellulaire (LABMC), Université des Sciences et Techniques de Masuku (USTM),
 BP 943, Franceville, Gabon

Correspondence should be addressed to Simplice D. Karou; simplicekarou@hotmail.com

Academic Editor: Tomohiro Katsuya

Objective. This study aimed to investigate the association between three polymorphisms of renin-angiotensin system and the essential hypertension in the population of Burkina Faso. *Methodology.* This was a case-control study including 202 cases and 204 matched controls subjects. The polymorphisms were identified by a classical and a real-time PCR. *Results.* The AGT 235M/T and AT1R 1166A/C polymorphisms were not associated with the hypertension while the genotype frequencies of the ACE I/D polymorphism between patients and controls (DD: 66.83% and 35.78%, ID: 28.22% and 50.98%, II: 4.95% and 13.24%, resp.) were significantly different ($p < 10^{-4}$). The genotype DD of ACE gene (OR = 3.40, $p < 0.0001$), the increasing age (OR = 3.83, $p < 0.0001$), obesity (OR = 4.84, $p < 0.0001$), dyslipidemia (OR = 3.43, $p = 0.021$), and alcohol intake (OR = 2.76, $p < 0.0001$) were identified as the independent risk factors for hypertension by multinomial logistic regression. *Conclusion.* The DD genotype of the ACE gene is involved in susceptibility to hypertension. Further investigations are needed to better monitor and provide individualized care for hypertensive patients.

1. Introduction

The arterial hypertension is a great public health concern in both industrialized and developing countries. It affects 972 million persons over the world, around one-quarter of the adult population. Among the affected persons, 639 million are living in the developing countries [1]. The arterial hypertension is a multifactorial disease with genetic, environmental, and behavioral determinants [2]. Genetic contribution to blood pressure (BP) variations ranges from 25 to 50% [3].

Among the genetic markers commonly involved, the polymorphisms of several genes, including those encoding vasoactive metabolites such as the components of the renin-angiotensin system (RAS), have been proposed as candidates in association with essential hypertension. The special attention given to the RAS gene polymorphisms is not only due to the fact that its components play an important role in regulation of vascular homeostasis, but also because of the place of angiotensin I converting enzyme (ACE) inhibitors in the therapeutic management of the hypertension.

The polymorphism in exon 2 of the angiotensinogen (AGT) gene, on chromosome 1q42, consists of a substitution of threonine by methionine at position 235 (235M/T). The insertion/deletion polymorphism of the gene encoding the angiotensin I converting enzyme (ACE) consists in the presence (I) or the absence (D) of a 287 bp Alu sequence in intron 16 of this gene on chromosome 17q2. The 1166A/C polymorphism was identified in the 3' UTR (chromosome 3) of angiotensin II type 1 receptor (AT1R) gene and consists of a substitution of adenosine by cytosine in the messenger RNA. Previous studies focused on the relationship between these polymorphisms and cardiovascular diseases such as hypertension have reported conflicting data [4–7]. In addition, no gene has yet been definitively established to date as responsible for changes in blood pressure, or as a predisposing gene for the hypertension. Thus, the aim of this study was to evaluate the relation between the RAS genes polymorphisms (AGT 235M/T, ACE I/D, and AT1R 1166A/C) and the essential hypertension in the population of Burkina Faso and to determine hypertension main risk factors.

2. Materials and Methods

2.1. Study Population. The study focused on a population of Burkina Faso (West Africa). This study was approved by the Saint-Camille/CERBA ethical committee. All study participants gave their informed consent and were between 20 and 79 years old. A manual aneroid sphygmomanometer, with armbands adapted to patients and controls morphotypes, was used to measure blood pressure values (systolic and diastolic) by the auscultation method for each subject in a sitting or lying position after at least 10 minutes of rest.

Hypertensive subjects (202) were recruited from the cardiology services in four medical centers of the city of Ouagadougou. The recommendations of scientific societies were used to define and classify the hypertension [8, 9]. A total of 204 matched controls subjects with no cardiovascular disease antecedent were recruited.

Two measurements were made during the same visit, and the retained value was the mean value in the arm with the highest arterial pressure. A standardized questionnaire and clinical examination allowed the collection of data and excluded secondary hypertension and subjects under hormonal treatment to avoid the bias related to the hypertension definition.

Hypertension was defined as BP ≥ 140/90 mmHg. The body mass index (BMI) was determined for each subject by dividing the weight in kg by the square of the height in m^2. This allowed classifying the subjects into four different groups: subjects of low weight (BMI < 18.5 kg/m^2), subjects of normal weight (BMI between 18.5 and 24.99 kg/m^2), overweight subjects (BMI between 25 and 29.99 kg/m^2), and obese subjects (BMI ≥ 30 kg/m^2).

The venous peripheral blood was collected from each fasting subject for biochemical and molecular tests. Plasma levels of the following parameters including glucose, total cholesterol, HDL-cholesterol, LDL-cholesterol, and triglycerides were detected using an enzymatic method by the COBAS C311 (Roche-Hitachi, France) automated analyzer.

2.2. DNA Extraction and Genotyping. The genomic DNA was extracted from leucocytes using the "DNA Rapid Salting-Out" as described by Miller et al. [10].

2.3. Detection of RAS Genes Polymorphisms. The ACE I/D polymorphism (rs4646994) genotyping was performed according to the method described by Rigat et al. [11]. A first PCR was performed with 10 pmol of each primer (sense: 5'-CTG-GAG-ACC-ACT-CCC-ATC-ATT-TCT-3'; antisense: 5'-GTG-GTC-GCC-ATC-ACA-TTG-GTC-AGA-T-3') in a final volume of 25 μL. Amplification was carried out in 30 cycles with a denaturation phase (94°C for 1 minute), annealing (58°C for 1 minute), and elongation (72°C for 2 minutes) for each cycle and a final extension of 10 minutes at 72°C. Given the fact that the D allele is preferably genotyped with respect to the I allele [12], DD homozygotes were reamplified using the previous protocol [11], with specific primers to the insertion sequence (sense: 5'-TGG-GAC-CAC-AGC-GCC-CGC-CAC-TAC-3'; antisense: 5'-TCG-CCA-GCC-CTC-CCA-TGC-CCA-TAA-3') [13]. PCR products were electrophoresed on a 2% agarose gel, stained with ethidium bromide, and digitally photographed using a GenFlash instrument.

The AGT 235M/T (rs699) and AT1R 1166A/C (rs5186) polymorphisms were detected by real-time PCR using Taq-Man probes on the 7500 Fast Real-Time PCR Systems (Life Technologies, California, USA).

2.4. Statistical Analysis. SPSS version 20.0 was used for data analysis. The PowerMarker software Version 3.25 was used for the determination of the Hardy-Weinberg equilibrium and the calculation of allele and genotype frequencies. The Chi-square test (χ^2) allowed us to compare the differences in the distribution of genotypes and other study variables. Changes were considered statistically significant at $p < 0.05$. Odds ratio (OR) and confidence intervals (CI) at 95% were calculated to estimate the relative risk of hypertension for AGT 235M/T, ACE I/D, and AT1R 1166A/C polymorphisms associated with the continuous categorical variables (age < 50 or ≥50 years, BMI < 25 or ≥25 kg/m^2, glucose < 6.11 or ≥6.11 mmol/L, total cholesterol < 5.17 or ≥5.17 mmol/L, HDL-cholesterol < 1.68 or ≥1.68 mmol/L, LDL-cholesterol < 2.58 or ≥2.58 mmol/L, and triglycerides < 1.53 or ≥1.53 mmol/L) and discrete variables (sex (M/F), alcohol consumption (yes/no), tobacco consumption (yes/no), lack of physical activity (yes/no), and taking stimulants (yes/no)). The independent predictors of hypertension risk were determined by a multiple logistic regression analysis (forward stepwise method) using HTA status as dependent variable.

3. Results

3.1. General Characteristics of the Study Population. Table 1 shows the general characteristics of the study population. This population was predominantly female (58.56%). When

TABLE 1: General characteristics of study population (cases versus controls).

Characteristics	Controls	Cases	p value
Total	**204**	**202**	
Sex ratio (M/F)	85/119	84/118	0.99
Age, years$^{\#}$	49.50 ± 13.54 (20–78)	51 ± 10.01 (21–76)	0.205
BMI, Kg/m$^{2\#}$	23 ± 4.90	27 ± 6.48	<0.00001
SBP, mmHg$^{\#}$	120 ± 11.47	160 ± 20.66	<0.00001
DBP, mmHg$^{\#}$	70 ± 8.24	95 ± 11.87	<0.00001
PP, mmHg$^{\#}$	40 ± 10.29	70 ± 16.75	<0.00001
Glycemia, mmol/L$^{\#}$	3 ± 1.70	5 ± 2.34	<0.00001
Total-C, mmol/L$^{\#}$	4 ± 1.54	5 ± 1.29	<0.00001
HDL-C, mmol/L$^{\#}$	1 ± 0.43	1 ± 0.59	NA
LDL-C, mmol/L$^{\#}$	2 ± 1.17	3 ± 1.13	<0.00001
Triglycerides, mmol/L$^{\#}$	1 ± 0.74	1 ± 0.61	NA
Hyperglycemia, %	8.51	21.05	0.000236
Dyslipidemia, %	51.06	77.27	<0.00001
Obesity, %	11.76	30.69	0.000003
Alcohol intake, %	22.55	46.53	<0.00001
Smoking, %	6.37	11.39	0.07559
Excitant intake, %	42.16	46.53	0.3746
Sedentary, %	14.22	17.82	0.3218

$^{\#}$Median ± SD for continuous variables; NA: not applicable.
BMI: body mass index; SBP: systolic blood pressure; DBP: diastolic blood pressure; PP: pulse pressure; Total-C: total cholesterol; HDL-C: high density lipoprotein cholesterol; LDL-C: low density lipoprotein cholesterol; Trigly: triglycerides.

compared to controls, hypertensive subjects had a similar sex ratio and age but with some significant difference. They were more sedentary, a lot more obese, more hyperglycemic, and more dyslipidemic. Furthermore, they consumed more alcohol, tobacco, and caffeine (coffee, tea, and cola). As it might be expected, their blood pressure values were also high relative to those of controls ($p < 0.05$).

3.2. Distribution of Genotypes between Cases and Controls. For each of the three polymorphisms studied (AGT 235M/T, ACE I/D, and AT1R 1166A/C), the genotypes distribution was in Hardy-Weinberg equilibrium for both patients and controls. Allelic and genotypic frequencies of these polymorphisms are presented in Table 2. We had a high frequency for TT genotype (AGT 235M/T), but there were no significant differences in distribution between cases and controls (84.65% versus 86.76%, resp.). The DD genotype and D allele of ACE I/D polymorphism were significantly more frequent in patients than in controls (DD: OR = 3.62, 95% CI = 2.35 to 5.56, $p < 0.00001$; D: OR = 2.68, 95% CI = 1.93 to 3.74, $p < 0.00001$). No homozygous genotype was obtained for the C allele (AT1R 1166A/C), which justifies the null frequencies reported in cases and in controls for this genotype.

We then conducted a stratified analysis to assess the distribution of genotypes of each polymorphism in the different study groups. These results are shown in Table 3. Overall, the same trends as those mentioned in Table 2 emerged. For AGT 235M/T and AT1R 1166A/C polymorphisms, no significant differences were observed between cases and controls. Similarly, difference was observed for the ACE I/D polymorphism between cases and controls.

3.3. Risk Factors for Hypertension. Multiple logistic regression analysis (forward stepwise method), using the hypertension status as the dependent variable, including the conventional cardiovascular disease risk factors (sex, smoking, diabetes, obesity, total cholesterol, LDL, HDL, and triglycerides) and new risk factor, such as DD genotype, showed that obesity, increasing age, dyslipidemia, DD genotype, and alcohol intake are independent risk factors for HTA, in decreasing order (Table 4).

4. Discussion

The main purpose of this study was to investigate the existence of a possible association between RAS genes polymorphisms and the hypertension and also to identify the main risk factors for this chronic condition in the Burkinabe population. Strong female predominance (58.56%) was found in our study. Yaméogo et al. and Baragou et al. also found similar frequencies in their studies, 56.8% of the hypertensive patients in Burkina Faso [14] and 55.1% of the hypertensive population in urban population in Togo [15], respectively. This dominance could be a simple mass effect or reflect greater susceptibility of the female gender to hypertension among adults. In this study, the median age for a hypertensive was 51 ± 10.01 years. This age is close to the 48.96 ± 12.99 years reported by Yayehd et al. in Togo [16] but was higher than the 33.1 ± 13.3 years reported by Niakara et al. in Burkina Faso [17].

The age of study population varied from 20 to 79 years. This is because there was an important proportion of young subjects (under 50 years) among hypertensives, and so we needed to have young subjects in controls group to match cases. However, the young age of some controls may constitute a limitation of this study. Indeed, among the young controls, some may be hypertensive in the future skewing the selection of controls subjects.

The different approaches used in studies focused on genetic susceptibility to disease in African populations have been previously described by Sirugo et al. [18]. Among the approaches used for searching for hypertension loci, few are linkage studies and most often are association studies [19]. The use of candidate gene approach includes the renin-angiotensin system genes but given the ethnic diversity and the selection bias, the results from these studies are often faced with interpretation difficulties [20–23]. The uniqueness of this study lies in the fact that it is the first of its kind in the Burkinabe population that combines the RAS genes polymorphisms and the hypertension. Furthermore, selection bias was minimized by overlapping controls to cases for sex and age variable, which are nonmodifiable risk factors.

Jeunemaitre et al. reported an association between the TT genotype of the AGT gene and the risk of hypertension

TABLE 2: Frequencies of renin-angiotensin system genes polymorphisms (cases versus controls).

Polymorphisms	Controls	Cases	OR	95% CI	p value
Total	**204**	**202**			
AGT 235M/T					
TT versus MT + MM, n (%)	177 (86.76)	171 (84.65)	0.84	0.46–1.53	0.57
MT versus TT + MM, n (%)	24 (11.77)	29 (14.36)	1.26	0.68–2.35	0.46
MM versus TT + MT, n (%)	3 (1.47)	2 (0.99)	0.67	0.06–5.92	1
T versus M, n (%)	378 (0.93)	371 (0.92)	0.89	0.51–1.54	0.70
HWE p value	**0.15**	**0.83**			
ACE I/D					
DD versus ID + II, n (%)	73 (35.78)	135 (66.83)	3.62	2.35–5.56	**<0.00001**
ID versus II + DD, n (%)	104 (50.98)	57 (28.22)	0.38	0.25–0.58	**<0.00001**
II versus DD + ID, n (%)	27 (13.24)	10 (4.95)	0.34	0.14–0.76	**0.005**
D versus I, n (%)	250 (0.61)	327 (0.81)	2.68	1.93–3.74	**<0.00001**
HWE p value	**0.57**	**0.48**			
AT1R 1166 A/C					
CC versus AC + AA, n (%)	0 (0.00)	0 (0.00)	0	0–4.21	0.19
AC versus AA + CC, n (%)	7 (3.43)	7 (3.47)	1.01	0.30–3.44	1.00
AA versus CC + AC, n (%)	197 (96.57)	195 (96.53)	0.99	0.29–3.38	1.00
C versus A, n (%)	7 (0.02)	7 (0.02)	1.01	0.30–3.41	1.00
HWE p value	**0.97**	**0.97**			

OR: odds ratio; CI: confidence intervals; HWE: Hardy-Weinberg equilibrium; AGT: angiotensinogen; ACE: angiotensin converting enzyme; AT1R: angiotensin II type 1 receptor.

in Utah and France [24]. Subsequently, cases of associations between the same genotype TT and the risk of hypertension in other populations have been reported [20, 21, 25, 26]. Nevertheless, we did not find any evidence of association between AGT 235M/T polymorphism and the incidence of hypertension in our study population. Similarly, Rotimi et al. [6] and Tiago et al. [23] found no association between AGT 235M/T polymorphism and the hypertension in their study. But compared to the previous work, we obtained a higher frequency of the TT genotype in this study.

The DD genotype of the ACE gene was present in 35.78% of controls, compared to 66.83% of hypertensive patients. This result showed a strong association between the ACE I/D polymorphism and the risk of hypertension in the Burkinabe population ($p < 0.0001$). Mehri et al. [26] and Jiménez et al. [27] also reported strong associations between the DD genotype and the risk of hypertension in their study populations. However, Castellano et al. [28] did not find any evidence of association between the D allele and the risk of hypertension in the Italian population. Thus, the DD homozygous persons have an increased risk, almost four times, of developing hypertension in the Burkinabe population compared with homozygous I allele carriers. In other studies, a positive association between the ACE I/D polymorphism and obesity is also reported [26]. However, in this work, we had found no association between the ACE I/D polymorphism and obesity (data not shown), suggesting that this polymorphism is independent of the body mass levels as it is related to the risk of hypertension. The logistic regression analysis confirmed that the DD genotype of the ACE gene is a risk factor that would increase by nearly 4 times the

incidence of hypertension among patients, regardless of other environmental risk factors. Moreover, Kato et al. [29] had found that the DD genotype of the ACE I/D polymorphism is a major risk factor for cerebral and cardiovascular events like stroke in Japanese hypertensive patients.

The potential effects of AT1R 1166 A/C polymorphism in the predisposition to hypertension are not well understood. Bonnardeaux et al. had initially found high prevalence of the allele 1166C in hypertensive subjects compared to what they found in normotensive subjects [5]. Recently, Mehri et al. reported an association between this polymorphism and hypertension in Tunisian patients with type 2 diabetes [26]. In our study, not only was there no association observed between the AT1R 1166C allele and hypertension, but we did not find homozygous genotype for this allele, both in cases and controls. The lack of association has also been reported in other populations [30]. These observations should be therefore interpreted with some caution.

Our results showed a strong association between the ACE I/D polymorphism and the development of hypertension. Thus, DD genotype is a predictor of hypertension risk, independent of other environmental factors. This work has also shown that obesity prevalence was 11% among controls and was the major risk factor of hypertension among the Burkinabe population (OR = 4.84, 95% CI = 2.96 to 7.92; $p < 0.0001$). This obesity frequency was twice as high in women as in men ($p < 0.001$; data not shown). The high prevalence of obesity in developing countries is related to the socioeconomic level of the population [31], along with the adoption of harmful eating behaviors, including snacking, a diet low in fiber and high in fat. In addition, the high

TABLE 3: Genotypes distribution among study population groups.

Groups	AGT 235M/T			ACE I/D			AT1R 1166A/C			Total
	TT	MT	MM	DD	ID	II	CC	AC	AA	
Males										
Controls	91.8%	7.1%	1.2%	36.5%	51.8%**	11.8%	0.0%	2.4%	97.6%	**85**
Cases	82.1%	16.7%	1.2%	69.0%**	25.0%	6.0%	0.0%	4.8%	95.2%	**84**
Females										
Controls	83.2%	15.1%	1.7%	35.3%	50.4%*	14.3%*	0.0%	4.2%	95.8%	**119**
Cases	86.4%	12.7%	0.9%	65.3%**	30.5%	4.2%	0.0%	2.5%	97.5%	**118**
<50 years										
Controls	87.1%	10.9%	2.0%	34.0%	53.1%**	12.9%	0.0%	3.4%	96.6%	**147**
Cases	83.5%	15.2%	1.3%	67.1%**	26.6%	6.3%	0.0%	3.8%	96.2%	**79**
≥50 years										
Controls	86.0%	14.0%	0.0%	40.4%	45.6%*	14.0%*	0.0%	3.5%	96.5%	**57**
Cases	85.4%	13.8%	0.8%	66.6%**	29.3%	4.1%	0.0%	3.3%	96.7%	**123**
<25 kg/m^2										
Controls	87.1%	11.6%	1.3%	36.7%	49.0%*	14.3%*	0.0%	4.1%	95.9%	**147**
Cases	86.7%	12.0%	1.3%	66.7%**	29.3%	4.0%	0.0%	2.7%	97.3%	**75**
≥25 kg/m^2										
Controls	86.0%	12.3%	1.7%	33.3%	56.2%**	10.5%	0.0%	1.8%	98.2%	**57**
Cases	83.5%	15.7%	0.8%	66.9%**	27.6%	5.5%	0.0%	3.9%	96.1%	**127**

$^* p < 0.05$; $^{**} p < 0.001$.

TABLE 4: Multinomial logistic regression analysis for hypertension risk factors.

	OR	95% CI	p value
Age	**3.83**	**2.32–6.32**	**<0.0001**
Sex	1.19	0.55–2.59	0.664
Obesity	**4.84**	**2.96–7.92**	**<0.0001**
DD	**3.40**	**2.1–5.5**	**<0.0001**
Smoking	0.52	0.108–2.48	0.410
Alcohol intake	**2.76**	**1.65–4.61**	**<0.0001**
Sedentary	0.15	0.017–1.23	0.077
Excitant intake	0.48	0.27–0.85	0.012
Hyperglycemia	1.52	0.34–6.87	0.586
Dyslipidemia	**3.43**	**1.21–9.79**	**0.021**

OR: odds ratio; CI: confidence intervals; DD: DD genotype of ACE I/D polymorphism.

prevalence of overweight in women is due to their physical inactivity and cultural conceptions [32].

For the three polymorphisms studied, we find evidence of the association with hypertension risk only for the ACE I/D polymorphism. However, Niu et al. [20] and Mehri et al. [26] had reported, respectively, in Chinese and Tunisian populations, a positive association between all the three polymorphisms and hypertension.

The reported discrepancies reflect genetic, cultural, and ethnic diversity within populations of study, people who mostly live in different environmental contexts, and are therefore exposed to various problems. Thus, the negative associations reported may be due to these differences and possible sampling bias [33]. In addition, the markers studied could be linked to other genes with which they have an impact on hypertension incidence in the population or on other disease events. This reinforces the idea of studying several polymorphisms in different ethnic groups to have good appreciation [34].

5. Conclusion

AGT 235M/T and AT1R 1166A/C polymorphisms showed no association with the risk of developing hypertension. However, the ACE gene DD genotype predisposes to the occurrence of hypertension in the Burkinabe population. Other major risk factors identified are obesity, advancing age, dyslipidemia, and alcohol consumption. ACE I/D polymorphism can serve as a marker for early diagnosis of hypertension if we have similar findings elsewhere. More studies involving ACE I/D polymorphism with hypertension therapeutic responses are still needed to better monitor and provide individualized care for hypertensive patients.

Authors' Contribution

Daméhan Tchelougou and Jonas K. Kologo equally contributed to this paper.

Acknowledgments

The authors thank all the staff of St. Camille Medical Center, the CERBA, the Medical Center "Chandelier d'or," and the Camp General Lamizana Medical Center. They would also like to thank the Italian Episcopal Conference (CEI) and the WAEMU Commission through the PACER-II program for their financial support.

References

[1] P. M. Kearney, M. Whelton, K. Reynolds, P. Muntner, P. K. Whelton, and J. He, "Global burden of hypertension: analysis of worldwide data," *The Lancet*, vol. 365, no. 9455, pp. 217–223, 2005.

[2] R. P. Lifton, "Molecular genetics of human blood pressure variation," *Science*, vol. 272, no. 5262, pp. 676–680, 1996.

[3] R. S. Levine, C. H. Hennekens, A. Perry, J. Cassady, H. Gelband, and M. J. Jesse, "Genetic variance of blood pressure levels in infant twins," *American Journal of Epidemiology*, vol. 116, no. 5, pp. 759–764, 1982.

[4] M. Caulfield, P. Lavender, M. Farrall et al., "Linkage of the angiotensinogen gene to essential hypertension," *The New England Journal of Medicine*, vol. 330, no. 23, pp. 1629–1633, 1994.

[5] A. Bonnardeaux, E. Davies, X. Jeunemaitre et al., "Angiotensin II type 1 receptor gene polymorphisms in human essential hypertension," *Hypertension*, vol. 24, no. 1, pp. 63–69, 1994.

[6] C. Rotimi, L. Morrison, R. Cooper et al., "Angiotensinogen gene in human hypertension: lack of an association of the 235T allele among African Americans," *Hypertension*, vol. 24, no. 5, pp. 591–594, 1994.

[7] X. Jeunemaitre, R. P. Lifton, S. C. Hunt, R. R. Williams, and J.-M. Lalouel, "Absence of linkage between the angiotensin converting enzyme locus and human essential hypertension," *Nature Genetics*, vol. 1, no. 1, pp. 72–75, 1992.

[8] C. Lenfant, A. V. Chobanian, D. W. Jones, and E. J. Roccella, "Seventh report of the Joint National Committee on the Prevention, Detection, Evaluation, and Treatment of High Blood Pressure (JNC 7) resetting the hypertension sails," *Circulation*, vol. 107, no. 24, pp. 2993–2994, 2003.

[9] G. Mancia, R. Fagard, K. Narkiewicz et al., "2013 ESH/ESC guidelines for the management of arterial hypertension: the Task Force for the management of arterial hypertension of the European Society of Hypertension (ESH) and of the European Society of Cardiology (ESC)," *European Heart Journal*, vol. 34, no. 28, pp. 2159–2219, 2013.

[10] S. A. Miller, D. D. Dykes, and H. F. Polesky, "A simple salting out procedure for extracting DNA from human nucleated cells," *Nucleic Acids Research*, vol. 16, no. 3, article 1215, 1988.

[11] B. Rigat, C. Hubert, P. Corvol, and F. Soubrier, "PCR detection of the insertion/deletion polymorphism of the human angiotensin converting enzyme gene (DCP1) (dipeptidyl carboxypeptidase 1)," *Nucleic Acids Research*, vol. 20, no. 6, article 1433, 1992.

[12] M.-H. Lin, C.-H. Tseng, C.-C. Tseng, C.-H. Huang, C.-K. Chong, and C.-P. Tseng, "Real-time PCR for rapid genotyping of angiotensin-converting enzyme insertion/deletion polymorphism," *Clinical Biochemistry*, vol. 34, no. 8, pp. 661–666, 2001.

[13] V. Shanmugam, K. W. Sell, and B. K. Saha, "Mistyping ACE heterozygotes," *Genome Research*, vol. 3, no. 2, pp. 120–121, 1993.

[14] N. V. Yaméogo, A. K. Samadoulougou, L. J. Kagambèga et al., "Epidemiological characteristics and clinical features of black African subject's resistant hypertension," *Annales de Cardiologie et d'Angeiologie*, vol. 63, no. 2, pp. 83–88, 2014.

[15] S. Baragou, M. Djibril, B. Atta, F. Damorou, M. Pio, and A. Balogou, "Prevalence of cardiovascular risk factors in an urban area of Togo: a WHO STEPS-wise approach in Lome, Togo," *Cardiovascular Journal of Africa*, vol. 23, no. 6, pp. 309–311, 2012.

[16] K. Yayehd, F. Damorou, R. Akakpo et al., "Prevalence and determinants of hypertension in Lomé (Togo): results of a screening in May 2011," *Annales de Cardiologie et d'Angéiologie*, vol. 62, no. 1, pp. 43–50, 2013.

[17] A. Niakara, F. Fournet, J. Gary, M. Harang, L. V. A. Nébié, and G. Salem, "Hypertension, urbanization, social and spatial disparities: a cross-sectional population-based survey in a West African urban environment (Ouagadougou, Burkina Faso)," *Transactions of the Royal Society of Tropical Medicine and Hygiene*, vol. 101, no. 11, pp. 1136–1142, 2007.

[18] G. Sirugo, B. J. Hennig, A. A. Adeyemo et al., "Genetic studies of African populations: an overview on disease susceptibility and response to vaccines and therapeutics," *Human Genetics*, vol. 123, no. 6, pp. 557–598, 2008.

[19] R. S. Cooper, A. Luke, X. Zhu et al., "Genome scan among Nigerians linking blood pressure to chromosomes 2, 3, and 19," *Hypertension*, vol. 40, no. 5, pp. 629–633, 2002.

[20] W. Niu, Y. Qi, S. Hou, X. Zhai, W. Zhou, and C. Qiu, "Haplotype-based association of the renin-angiotensin-aldosterone system genes polymorphisms with essential hypertension among Han Chinese: the Fangshan study," *Journal of Hypertension*, vol. 27, no. 7, pp. 1384–1391, 2009.

[21] Y.-H. Say, K.-H. Ling, G. Duraisamy, S. Isaac, and R. Rosli, "Angiotensinogen M235T gene variants and its association with essential hypertension and plasma renin activity in Malaysian subjects: a case control study," *BMC Cardiovascular Disorders*, vol. 5, article 7, 2005.

[22] J. Beige, O. Zilch, H. Hohenbleicher et al., "Genetic variants of the renin-angiotensin system and ambulatory blood pressure in essential hypertension," *Journal of Hypertension*, vol. 15, no. 5, pp. 503–508, 1997.

[23] A. D. Tiago, D. Badenhorst, B. Nkeh et al., "Impact of renin-angiotensin-aldosterone system gene variants on the severity of hypertension in patients with newly diagnosed hypertension," *American Journal of Hypertension*, vol. 16, no. 12, pp. 1006–1010, 2003.

[24] X. Jeunemaitre, F. Soubrier, Y. V. Kotelevtsev et al., "Molecular basis of human hypertension: role of angiotensinogen," *Cell*, vol. 71, no. 1, pp. 169–180, 1992.

[25] R. Kunz, R. Kreutz, J. Beige, A. Distler, and A. M. Sharma, "Association between the angiotensinogen 235T-variant and essential hypertension in whites: a systematic review and methodological appraisal," *Hypertension*, vol. 30, no. 6, pp. 1331–1337, 1997.

[26] S. Mehri, S. Mahjoub, S. Hammami et al., "Renin-angiotensin system polymorphisms in relation to hypertension status and obesity in a Tunisian population," *Molecular Biology Reports*, vol. 39, no. 4, pp. 4059–4065, 2012.

[27] P. M. Jiménez, C. Conde, A. Casanegra, C. Romero, A. H. Tabares, and M. Orías, "Association of ACE genotype and predominantly diastolic hypertension: a preliminary study," *Journal of the Renin-Angiotensin-Aldosterone System*, vol. 8, no. 1, pp. 42–44, 2007.

[28] M. Castellano, N. Glorioso, D. Cusi et al., "Genetic polymorphism of the renin–angiotensin–aldosterone system and arterial hypertension in the Italian population: the GENIPER Project," *Journal of Hypertension*, vol. 21, no. 10, pp. 1853–1860, 2003.

[29] N. Kato, Y. Tatara, M. Ohishi et al., "Angiotensin-converting enzyme single nucleotide polymorphism is a genetic risk factor for cardiovascular disease: a cohort study of hypertensive patients," *Hypertension Research*, vol. 34, no. 6, pp. 728–734, 2011.

[30] S. Schmidt, J. Beige, M. Walla-Friedel, M. C. Michel, A. M. Sharma, and E. Ritz, "A polymorphism in the gene for the angiotensin II type 1 receptor is not associated with hypertension," *Journal of Hypertension*, vol. 15, no. 12, pp. 1385–1388, 1997.

[31] J. A. Poterico, S. Stanojevic, P. Ruiz-Grosso, A. Bernabe-Ortiz, and J. J. Miranda, "The association between socioeconomic status and obesity in Peruvian women," *Obesity*, vol. 20, no. 11, pp. 2283–2289, 2012.

[32] P. S. Yusuf, S. Hawken, S. Ôunpuu et al., "Effect of potentially modifiable risk factors associated with myocardial infarction in 52 countries (the INTERHEART study): case-control study," *The Lancet*, vol. 364, no. 9438, pp. 937–952, 2004.

[33] A. Persu, "Candidate gene studies: accepting negative results," *Journal of Hypertension*, vol. 24, no. 3, pp. 443–445, 2006.

[34] R. Cooper and C. Rotimi, "Hypertension in populations of West African origin: is there a genetic predisposition?" *Journal of Hypertension*, vol. 12, no. 3, pp. 215–227, 1994.

4

Hypertension in Non-Type 2 Diabetes in Isfahan, Iran: Incidence and Risk Factors

Mohsen Janghorbani, Ashraf Aminorroaya, and Masoud Amini

Isfahan Endocrine and Metabolism Research Center, Isfahan University of Medical Sciences, Isfahan, Iran

Correspondence should be addressed to Mohsen Janghorbani; janghorbani@hlth.mui.ac.ir

Academic Editor: Tomohiro Katsuya

Objective. To estimate the incidence of and risk factors for the development of hypertension (HTN) in people with T1D using routinely collected data. *Method.* The mean 16-year incidence of HTN was measured among 1,167 (557 men and 610 women) nonhypertensive patients with T1D from Isfahan Endocrine and Metabolism Research Center outpatient clinics, Iran. HTN was defined as a systolic blood pressure (BP) of 140 mm Hg or higher and/or a diastolic BP 90 mm Hg or higher and/or use of antihypertensive medications. The mean (standard deviation [SD]) age of participants was 20.6 years (10.5 years) with a mean (SD) duration of diabetes of 3.6 years (4.8 years) at registration. *Results.* The prevalence of HTN at baseline was 9.7% (95% CI: 8.2, 11.5). Among the 1,167 patients free of HTN at registration who attended the clinic at least twice in the period 1992–2016, the incidence of HTN was 9.6 (8.0 women and 11.3 men) per 1000 person-years based on 18,870 person-years of follow-up. Multivariate analyses showed that male gender, older age, higher triglyceride, and higher systolic BP were significantly and independently associated with the development of HTN in this population. *Conclusion.* These findings will help the identification of those patients with T1D at particular risk of HTN and strongly support the case for vigorous control of BP in patients with T1D.

1. Introduction

Hypertension (HTN) is the most important risk factor for cardiovascular disease and associated with increased risk of nephropathy [1, 2] and retinopathy [3–5] and is estimated to affect about one-third of patients with T1D [6] and is one of the well-established modifiable risk factors for cardiovascular disease mortality and morbidity [7–9]. Although some studies have examined the prevalence of HTN in patients with T1D in cross-sectional reports, mostly in developed countries, only a few studies have reported the results of a longitudinal analysis on the incidence of HTN in the clinical practice settings and none of them were undertaken in Middle-East countries and in Iranian patients with T1D receiving routine care [10–19]. Earlier studies on the association between patient's characteristics and a higher incidence of HTN have evaluated nondiabetic populations or people with T2D, but rarely patients with T1D [20–26]. Accurate information regarding the incidence of HTN and associated risk factors in people with T1D is important in the prevention or delaying

of its development and of the cardiovascular damage caused by this complication. Information on risk factors of incident HTN can lead to the identification of patients with T1D who may have more difficulty controlling their HTN.

The objective of this report, therefore, was to estimate the incidence of and risk factors of HTN in patients with T1D in routine clinical care. This study could also serve as a platform for future comparison with other studies and with the results obtained in other parts of Iran.

2. Patients and Methods

2.1. Study Population and Data Collection. This was a prospective registry analysis that used data from the clinical information system at Isfahan Endocrine and Metabolism Research Center, Iran, a continuing data collection program in central Iran to collect, analyze, and disseminate data in a standardized manner. Clinical data were collected for all consecutive patients at the first attendance and at review consultations using standard encounter forms. These included an assessment of the ocular fundus, lens, limbs, and blood pressure (BP) and creation of a problem list by the clinician. The following variables were examined at the time of each examination: age, age at diagnosis, duration of diabetes, height, weight, fasting plasma glucose (FPG), glycosylated hemoglobin (HbA1c), urine protein, triglyceride, cholesterol, low-density lipoprotein cholesterol (LDLC), high-density lipoprotein cholesterol (HDLC) and serum creatinine, and reporting of smoking as part of a completed questionnaire on demography, family history and smoking by the patient, and BP.

All patients were referred for the diabetes education program after the start of the therapy by trained nutritionists. The diabetes education classes included six 2 h classes emphasizing the importance of carbohydrate counting, exercise, oral and injectable medications, and microvascular and macrovascular complications of diabetes. The mechanisms of actions of diabetes medications along with proper dosing and use were reviewed, the definition and proper treatment for hypoglycemia were described, and the importance of exercise and proper foot care was explained. A computerized patient registry provided data on patient characteristics, medications, and laboratory values.

The detailed data collection methods of the Isfahan Endocrine and Metabolism Research Center outpatient clinics have been described previously [27].

3. Ethics Statement

The study protocol followed the Iranian government's ethical guidelines for epidemiological studies in accordance with the current version of the Declaration of Helsinki. Isfahan Endocrine and Metabolism Research Center ethical committee approval was granted. This study was based on a routine medical procedure, and additional written consent was not required. The data was processed and analyzed by authorized medical personnel only, the patients remained anonymous, and the information was deidentified prior to analysis.

4. Measurements

Height and weight were measured with subjects in light clothes and without shoes using standard apparatus. Weight was measured to the nearest 0.1 kg on a calibrated beam scale. Height was measured to the nearest 0.5 cm with a measuring tape. Resting systolic (phase I) and diastolic (Phase V) BP were recorded at each examination by a physician with the participants in a sitting position with their legs not crossed and the feet placed firmly on the floor, upon resting in this position for at least 10 min using a mercury column sphygmomanometer and appropriately sized cuffs. Average BP was calculated from the two consecutive measurements. FPG was measured using the glucose oxidase method. The estimated glomerular filtration rate (eGFR) was calculated using the Modification of Diet in Renal Disease (MDRD) formula [28]: eGFR = $186.3 \times$ serum creatinine in mg/dl$^{-1.154} \times$ age$^{-0.203} \times$ 0.742 (if women). The physician defined the type of diabetes using the problem list. All blood sampling procedures were performed in the central laboratory of the Isfahan Endocrine, and Metabolism Research Center.

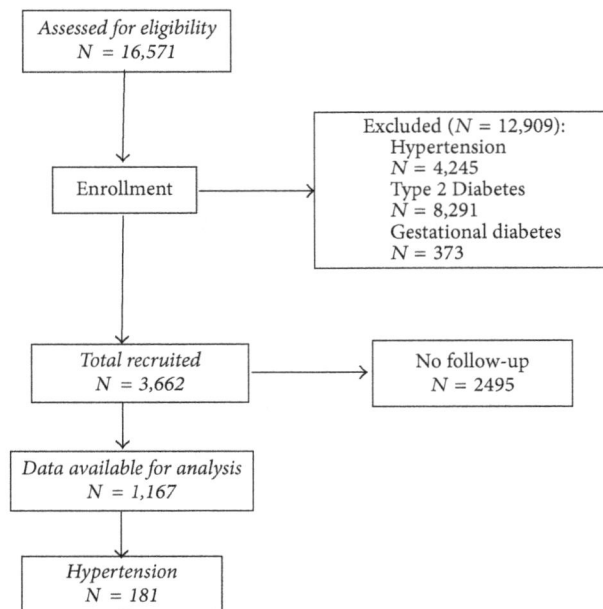

FIGURE 1: Schematic diagram of the study population.

Predictors of HTN were assessed using the following data from the patient's registration consultation: gender, age at diagnosis, age, educational level, time since diagnosis of diabetes, BMI (weight/height^2 [kg/m^2]), smoking status (never, current), FPG, serum creatinine, triglyceride, cholesterol, HDLC (measured using standardized procedures), LDLC (calculated by the Friedewald equation [29]), and BP (systolic and diastolic) at initial registration and number of follow-up visits and follow-up duration.

5. Follow-Up and Diagnosis of HTN

Between 1992 and 2016, a total of 16,571 patients with gestational diabetes, T1D and T2D, were registered in the system. Women with diabetes diagnosed only during pregnancy and T2D were excluded. In order to be included in the analyses, a patient had to have at least one subsequent review during a mean (standard deviation (SD)) follow-up period of 16.2 (6.4) (range 1–25) years. However, this study uses data only for 1,167 (557 (47.7%) men and 610 (52.3%) women) HTN-free patients with T1D at baseline for whom complete data were available (Figure 1). The participants had a mean age of 20.6 (10.5) (range 1–73) years. The guidelines published by the JNC8 [30] were used as definitions for HTN and defined as a systolic BP ≥ 140 mm Hg, and/or a diastolic BP ≥ 90 mm Hg, and/or the current use of antihypertensive medication. Participants were asked as part of the medical interview whether they had ever been told by a physician that they have high or elevated BP and whether they are taking antihypertensive medication.

6. Analysis

Participants were followed until the occurrence of HTN, the date of the last completed follow-up, death, or end of follow-up on October 1, 2016, whichever event occurred first.

Statistical methods included the two-sided Student's *t*-test or Mann–Whitney *U* test, one-way analysis of variance (ANOVA) with Scheffe's method as the post hoc analysis or the Kruskal-Wallis test with the Dunn procedure for continuous variables, the chi-squared test for categorical variables, and multiple logistic regression. Because we had no HTN events registered in between examination cycles, crude and multivariate binary logistic regression were performed to calculate the odds ratios (ORs) with 95% confidence intervals (CI) and *P* values for new-onset HTN as the dependent variable (yes/no) using the SPSS version 18 for Windows (SPSS Inc., Chicago, IL, USA). When a new case of HTN was identified we used the examination visit date as a new case of HTN. A general linear model was used to examine the significance of trends in potential predictors of HTN and compared age- and gender-adjusted means. *P* value < 0.05 was required to confer statistical significance.

7. Results

7.1. Baseline Characteristics. The mean (SD) age of the patients included in this study was 20.6 (10.5) years, mean (SD) diabetes duration was 3.6 (4.8) years, mean (SD) BMI was 20.6 (4.8) kg/m^2, mean (SD) HbA1c was 8.9% (2.6), mean (SD) systolic and diastolic BP were 106.3 (11.5) and 67.6 (9.8) mm Hg at baseline, and 52.3% were women. The women had significantly higher BMI than men (21.0 versus 20.3, $P <$ 0.05). Age, duration of diabetes, HbA1c, age at diagnosis of diabetes, FPG, cholesterol, triglyceride, LDLC, and HDLC did not differ between the genders.

7.2. Prevalence and Incidence of HTN. Of the 1,293 T1D patients, 126 (70 men and 56 women) had HTN at baseline. The overall prevalence of HTN was 9.7% (95% CI: 8.2, 11.5). Prevalence of HTN was higher in men (11.2%; 95% CI: 8.7, 13.6) than women (8.4%; 95% CI: 6.4, 10.8).

During a mean of 16-year follow-up, of the 1,167 patients without HTN at baseline, 181 (15.5%) (101 men and 80 women) developed HTN in a total of 18,870 (8,922 men and 9,948 women) person-years of follow-up. The other 986 patients with T1D had not developed HTN by the end of this study period. The overall incidence of subsequent HTN was 9.6 per 1000 person-years (95% CI: 8.2, 11.0). There was a statistically increasing incidence of HTN with increasing age ($P <$ 0.001): 4.9 per 1000 person-year for those aged ≤ 10 years, 8.5 for those aged 11 through 20 years, 11.5 for those aged 21 through 30 years, and 13.3 for those aged >30 years. Incidence rates were higher in men (11.3 (95% CI: 9.1, 13.5) per 1000 person-years) than women (8.0 (95% CI: 6.3, 9.8)).

7.3. Risk Factors. Table 1 shows the group means (SD) and proportions for those participants who did and did not develop HTN. Those who developed HTN had higher systolic (108.0 versus 106.7 mm Hg; $P <$ 0.05) and diastolic (69.5 versus 67.3 mm Hg; $P <$ 0.01) BP, follow-up duration (18.7 versus 15.8 yr.; $P <$ 0.001), and number of follow-up visits (30.7 versus 16.9 times; $P <$ 0.001) and were diagnosed with diabetes at older ages (19.3 versus 16.5 yr.; $P <$ 0.001) and were older at registration (23.7 versus 20.0; $P <$ 0.001). They had

higher triglyceride (169.4 versus 128.1 mg/dl; $P <$ 0.01) and HbA1c (9.3% versus 8.8%; $P <$ 0.05) at the baseline examination. A lower proportion of those who developed HTN were the normal weight (77.3% versus 84.6%; $P <$ 0.05), but higher proportion were overweight (18.2% versus 10.8%; $P <$ 0.05) and were men (55.8 versus 46.2; $P <$ 0.05).

To determine the influence of potential factors on HTN, univariate analysis was first performed (Table 2). Crude OR showed that those who had HTN were more likely to be older at registration and diagnosis of diabetes and had a higher duration of diabetes, HbA1c, BMI, cholesterol, and triglyceride. Age- and gender-adjusted multiple logistic regression coefficients among those free of HTN at registration showed that significant risk factors for developing HTN were male gender, older age, higher HbA1c, and triglyceride.

To determine the independent predictors of the incidence of HTN a forward (likelihood ratio) multiple logistic regression was performed. Sequential adjustment showed that only male (OR 1.48 (95% CI: 1.07, 2.05)), older age at registration (OR per SD increment, 1.03 (95% CI: 1.02, 1.04)), higher triglyceride (OR per SD increment, 1.002 (95% CI: 1.001, 1.003)), and higher systolic BP (OR per SD increment, 1.02 (95% CI: 1.003, 1.03)), significantly increased the risk of developing HTN. No other variables were significant when other covariates were considered (Table 3).

8. Discussion

This follow-up study of 1,167 HTN-free T1D clinic attendees found an overall incidence of HTN of 9.6 per 1000 person-years (181 patients) over an average follow-up of 16.3 years. HTN was associated with male gender, older age, higher triglycerides, and higher systolic BP. To the best of our knowledge, no other incidence rates for HTN among Iranian T1D population have been reported. Previously, many studies have examined the prevalence and incidence of HTN in the nondiabetic population [20, 21] or T2D patients [22–26] whereas information for patients with T1D are limited and reported a prevalence of 20 to 43% [10–18]. Estimates of the prevalence of HTN will depend upon the definition of the HTN used and the composition of the community examined by age, diabetes duration, and social class, making comparisons between studies of limited values. The Coronary Artery Calcification in Type 1 Diabetes Study [10] with a mean age of 37 years and duration of diabetes of 23.2 years demonstrated a higher prevalence rate of HTN among patients with T1D (43%) compared to individuals without diabetes (15%). The EURODIAB study (a prospective cohort study of people with T1D from 16 European countries) demonstrates an HTN prevalence of 24% among 3,250 patients with T1D [11] with a mean age of 32.7 years and duration of diabetes of 14.7. The prevalence of HTN in Brazil in patients with T1D with a mean age of 21.2 years and duration of diabetes of 9.6 years was 19.2% [12]. The prevalence of HTN in Pittsburgh in patients with T1D with a mean age of 29.1 years and duration of diabetes of 20.4 years at baseline was 29.0% [31]. Several possible explanations exist for our lower prevalence of HTN in patients with T1D (9.7%) compared with earlier reports. These include age and duration of diabetes (the Pittsburgh

TABLE 1: Age and age-adjusted means (SD) and proportions of selected baseline characteristics in 181 type 1 diabetes patients who did and 986 who did not develop hypertension at baseline.

Variables	Developed hypertension	Not developed hypertension	P value
	Mean (SD)	Mean (SD)	
Age (yr.)	23.7 (12.3)	20.0 (10.1)	<0.001
Age at diagnosis (yr.)	19.3 (10.6)	16.5 (9.0)	<0.001
Years since diabetes diagnosis	3.6 (0.33)	3.6 (0.14)	0.981
Number of follow-up visits	28.9 (24.8)	17.3 (18.6)	<0.001
Height (cm)	155.1 (15.5)	155.2 (18.6)	0.989
Weight (kg)	50.8 (16.3)	51.2 (18.0)	0.781
Body mass index (kg/m^2)	20.4 (4.6)	20.6 (4.9)	0.651
Follow-up duration (yr.)	18.7 (5.5)	15.8 (6.4)	<0.001
Estimated glomerular filtration rate (eGFR) (mL/min)	120.3 (38.7)	117.7 (44.6)	0.442
Glomerular filtration rate (GFR) (mL/min)	82.6 (30.1)	82.1 (42.8)	0.884
Systolic BP (mmHg)	108.0 (11.8)	106.8 (11.3)	0.018
Diastolic BP (mmHg)	69.5 (9.7)	67.3 (9.8)	0.006
Baseline fasting glucose (mg/dl)	198.3 (98.7)	198.7 (100.5)	0.952
Creatinine (μM/l)	0.83 (0.24)	0.86 (0.47)	0.428
HbA1c (%)	9.3 (2.5)	8.8 (2.6)	0.021
Triglyceride (mg/dl)	169.4 (198.8)	128.1 (105.2)	<0.001
Cholesterol (mg/dl)	186.9 (46.9)	182.8 (43.6)	0.254
HDL cholesterol (mg/dl)	47.5 (11.4)	47.1 (11.9)	0.819
LDL cholesterol (mg/dl)	111.7 (37.1)	107.7 (38.8)	0.472
	Number (%)	Number (%)	
Men	101 (55.8)	456 (46.2)	0.019
Therapeutic regimen %			
Noninsulin	31 (17.1)	128 (12.9)	0.449
Insulin	150 (82.9)	862 (87.0)	-
Education %			
Less than high school	106 (62.0)	551 (60.3)	0.636
High school	42 (24.6)	253 (27.5)	-
College graduate	23 (13.5)	112 (12.2)	-
Glycated hemoglobin %			
<7%	27 (19.7)	177 (26.7)	0.117
7%–9.5%	47 (34.3)	236 (35.6)	-
>9.5%	63 (46.0)	249 (37.6)	-
Weight category %			
Normal weight (BMI < 25.0 kg/m^2)	136 (77.3)	805 (84.6)	0.022
Overweight (BMI 25–29.9 kg/m^2)	32 (18.2)	103 (10.8)	-
Obese (BMI ≥ 30.0 kg/m^2)	8 (4.5)	44 (4.6)	-

Note. Total of each variable may vary because of missing value. Differences in the mean or percentage values of variables between participants who developed and did not develop hypertension.

cohort had a mean age of 28 years with 20 years of duration, whereas the EURODIAB cohort had a mean age of 33 years with mean duration of 15 years at baseline; the Brazil study had a mean age of 21 years and mean duration of diabetes of 10 years compared with our mean age of 20 years and 3.6 years of duration). In addition, differences of ethnicity, clinical practice, and medical care access could also contribute to differences.

The 10-year incidence of HTN in Wisconsin Epidemiological Study of Diabetic Retinopathy in T1D was 25.9% [19]. In black persons with T1D, the 6-year incidence of HTN

was 29.3% [13]. Our clinic-based incidence is lower than the values reported in Wisconsin Epidemiological Study of Diabetic Retinopathy. Lower rates in our study could have been due to a different definition of HTN, age, and duration of diabetes, and differences in medical care access and therapy might be one reason.

Klein et al. [19] reported a positive relationship between HbA1c and the incidence of HTN in T1D and suggested that glycemic control may be an effective approach for preventing the development of HTN in T1D. De Boer et al. [32] in Diabetes Control and Complications Trial

TABLE 2: Incidence rates of hypertension by baseline variables.

Variables	At risk (number)	Cases (number)	Person-year	Incidence per 1000 person-year	Crude Odds ratio (95% CI)	Age- and gender-adjusted odds ratio (95% CI)[†]
Gender						
Female	610	80	9948	8.0	1.00	1.00
Male	557	101	8922	11.3	1.47 (1.07, 2.02)[*]	1.48 (1.07, 2.05)[*]
Age at registration (yr.)						
≤10	160	14	2865	4.9	1.00	-
11–20	496	69	8150	8.5	1.69 (0.92, 3.08)	-
21–30	342	57	4951	11.5	2.09 (1.13, 3.87)[*]	-
>30	163	39	2928	13.3	3.28 (1.70, 6.73)[***]	-
Age at diagnosis (yr.)						
≤10	280	35	4969	7.0	1.00	1.00
11–20	534	72	8468	8.5	1.09 (0.71, 1.68)	0.84 (0.53, 1.36)
21–30	250	48	3722	12.9	1.66 (1.04, 2.67)[*]	0.95 (0.50, 1.80)
>30	84	21	1527	13.8	2.33 (1.27, 4.29)[**]	0.84 (0.30, 2.36)
Duration of diabetes (yr.)						
≤1	659	90	10198	8.8	1.00	1.00
2-3	179	29	2991	9.7	1.22 (0.78, 1.93)	1.13 (0.71, 1.80)
4-5	90	14	1654	8.5	1.16 (0.63, 2.15)	0.94 (0.50, 1.79)
6–10	119	22	2114	10.4	1.43 (0.86, 2.40)	1.23 (0.72, 2.10)
>10	110	23	1787	12.9	1.87 (1.09, 3.19)[*]	1.13 (0.64, 2.01)
Fasting blood glucose (mg/dl)						
<100	201	33	3294	10.0	1.00	1.00
100–126	141	22	2185	10.1	0.94 (0.52, 1.70)	0.92 (0.51, 1.66)
≥126	813	126	13267	9.5	0.93 (0.61, 1.42)	0.89 (0.58, 1.36)
HbA1 (%)						
<7.0	204	27	2430	11.1	1.00	1.00
7.0–9.5	283	47	4065	11.6	1.30 (0.78, 2.19)	1.30 (0.77, 2.18)
≥9.5	312	63	4665	13.5	1.66 (1.02, 2.71)[*]	1.72 (1.04, 2.82)[*]
BMI (Kg/m^2)						
<25	941	136	15509	8.8	1.00	1.00
25–30	135	32	2077	14.4	1.84 (1.19, 2.85)[**]	1.54 (0.96, 2.45)
>30	52	8	650	12.3	1.08 (0.50, 2.34)	0.92 (0.40, 2.17)
Creatinine (μM/l)						
≤1.2	914	156	14291	10.9	1.00	1.00
>1.2	47	11	800	13.8	1.49 (0.74, 2.98)	1.12 (0.54, 2.30)
Cholesterol (mg/dl)						
<200	732	106	11297	9.4	1.00	1.00
≥200	355	73	6442	11.3	1.53 (1.10, 2.13)[*]	1.37 (0.98, 1.93)
Triglyceride (mg/dl)						
<150	806	118	13048	9.0	1.00	1.00
≥150	275	61	4581	13.3	1.66 (1.18, 2.35)[**]	1.45 (1.01, 2.08)[*]

Total number of person-years and at risk is not the same for each variable because of missing values. [*]$P < 0.5$, [**]$P < 0.01$, [***]$P < 0.001$. [†]Odds ratios (with 95% CI) calculated by multiple logistic regression.

TABLE 3: Impact of sequential adjusted risk factors related to mean 16-year incidence of hypertension for patients with type 1 diabetes.

Variables	Odds ratio (95% confidence interval)	P value
Age (yr.)	1.03 (1.02, 1.04)	<0.001
Adjusted for age and gender		
Female	1.00	
Male	1.48 (1.07, 2.05)	0.017
Adjusted for all above and systolic BP (mm Hg)	1.02 (1.003, 1.03)	0.021
Adjusted for all above and triglyceride (mg/dl)	1.002 (1.001, 1.003)	0.001

(DCCT)/Epidemiology of Diabetes Interventions and Complications (EDIC) Study Research Group also reported a positive relationship between hyperglycemia and the incidence of HTN in T1D, and intensive insulin therapy reduces the long-term risk of developing HTN. In univariate analysis, the level of HbA1c $\geq$ 9.5%, as measured by one HbA1c determination at baseline, was associated with the development of HTN. After age- and gender-adjustment, the level of HbA1c $\geq$ 9.5% was found to be a predictor of incidence of HTN. After adjustment for other covariates in the multivariate analysis, the level of HbA1c was nonsignificant. Although these data have failed to confirm a relationship between metabolic control and the incidence of HTN, they in no way diminish the need for optimal glycemic control for the prevention of T1D complications, which has been well demonstrated both epidemiologically and interventionally.

Previous studies differ in relation to the importance of obesity as a risk factor. BMI but not HbA1c was significantly associated with the systolic BP in children with T1D participating in the Oxford Regional Prospective Study [33]. By multivariate analysis, however, we found no association between BMI and HTN.

While our real-life data has strengths, including its large cohort size and long-term follow-up, frequent measurement of relevant covariates, a well-characterized cohort of people with T1D, and the use of standardized protocols to measure risk factors and HTN, it also has some limitations. Because of the single center and nonrandom selection of patients, we cannot exclude the possibility of selection bias in the registry and the results may not apply to area/country groups. The study was a clinic, rather than population, based and so may not contain a clinical spectrum representative of patients with T1D in the community. Clinic-based estimates of the incidence or prevalence of complications are most likely to be affected by referral patterns. Selection bias is less likely to affect incidence rates and associations between risk factors and complications as investigated in this study. Our diagnosis of HTN is not based on a single examination but continuing examination during follow-up, using a problem list as the basis for further clinical decisions. Nevertheless, several observers made observations over the years, and problems of observer error need to be considered. It seems reasonable to assume that observer error is independent of such variables as age, gender, and duration of diabetes. If this is so, misclassification resulting from observer error will tend to reduce rather than increase the significance of differences between groups of patients. If therefore a significant difference is found between two otherwise comparable groups of patients, it is reasonable to infer that it is not due to observer error but must reflect a true difference. We could not rule out the possibility of residual confounding because of unmeasured or inaccurately measured covariates. We used a clinical definition of T1D that was assigned by clinicians and was applicable to all patients. However, autoantibody and C-peptide levels were not measured. Therefore, some patients with other types of diabetes may have been included. Nevertheless, it is important to emphasize that 86% of our patients were diagnosed before the age of 30, which supports the high probability that these patients had T1D. This is the first report of incident HTN in people with T1D in routine care in a Middle-East country and provides new data from Iran which has been underrepresented in past studies.

The results of this study highlight the need for increased attention to diagnosing HTN and vigorous blood pressure control in patients with T1D.

Authors' Contributions

Mohsen Janghorbani developed the original idea for the study and designed the study, performed statistical analyses, and interpreted the data and wrote the manuscript; Ashraf Aminorroaya and Masoud Amini found samples, contributed to interpretation of results, and revised the manuscript. All authors approved the final version submitted for publication.

Acknowledgments

The authors thank M. Abyar for technical computer assistance. This study was supported by Isfahan Endocrine and Metabolism Research Center Grant Committee, Iran.

References

[1] A. R. Christlieb, J. H. Warram, A. S. Królewski et al., "Hypertension: the major risk factor in juvenile-onset insulin-dependent diabetics." Diabetes, vol. 30, no. 2, pp. 90–96, 1981.

[2] H.-H. Parving, A. Andersen, U. Smidt, and P. Svendsen, "Early aggressive antihypertensive treatment reduces rate of decline in kidney function in diabetic nephropathy," The Lancet, vol. 1, no. 8335, pp. 1175–1179, 1983.

[3] C. E. Mogensen, "Long-term antihypertensive treatment inhibiting progression of diabetic nephropathy," BMJ, vol. 285, no. 6343, pp. 685–688, 1982.

[4] A. Teuscher, H. Schnell, and P. W. F. Wilson, "Incidence of diabetic retinopathy and relationship to baseline plasma glucose and blood pressure," Diabetes Care, vol. 11, no. 3, pp. 246–251, 1988.

[5] R. Klein, B. E. K. Klein, S. E. Moss, M. D. Davis, and D. L. DeMets, "Is blood pressure a predictor of the incidence or progression of diabetic retinopathy?" *JAMA Internal Medicine*, vol. 149, no. 11, pp. 2427–2432, 1989.

[6] C. Arauz-Pacheco, M. A. Parrott, and P. Raskin, "The treatment of hypertension in adult patients with diabetes.," *Diabetes Care*, vol. 25, no. 1, pp. 134–147, 2002.

[7] A. V. Chobanian, G. L. Bakris, H. R. Black et al., "The seventh report of the joint national committee on prevention, detection, evaluation, and treatment of high blood pressure: the JNC 7 report," *The Journal of the American Medical Association*, vol. 289, no. 19, pp. 2560–2572, 2003.

[8] P. Rossing, P. Hougaard, K. Borch-Johnsen, and H.-H. Parving, "Predictors of mortality in insulin dependent diabetes; 10 year observational follow up study," *British Medical Journal*, vol. 313, no. 7060, pp. 779–784, 1996.

[9] K. Y.-Z. Forrest, D. J. Becker, L. H. Kuller, S. K. Wolfson, and T. J. Orchard, "Are predictors of coronary heart disease and lower-extremity arterial disease in type 1 diabetes the same?: A prospective study," *Atherosclerosis*, vol. 148, no. 1, pp. 159–169, 2000.

[10] D. M. Maahs, G. L. Kinney, P. Wadwa et al., "Hypertension prevalence, awareness, treatment, and control in an adult type 1 diabetes population and a comparable general population," *Diabetes Care*, vol. 28, no. 2, pp. 301–306, 2005.

[11] F. Collado-Mesa, H. M. Colhoun, L. K. Stevens et al., "Prevalence and management of hypertension in type 1 diabetes mellitus in Europe: the EURODIAB IDDM complications study," *Diabetic Medicine*, vol. 16, no. 1, pp. 41–48, 1999.

[12] M. B. Gomes, L. R. M. Tannus, A. S. D. M. Matheus et al., "Prevalence, awareness, and treatment of hypertension in patients with type 1 diabetes: a nationwide multicenter study in Brazil," *International Journal of Hypertension*, vol. 2013, Article ID 565263, 8 pages, 2013.

[13] M. S. Roy, M. N. Janal, and A. Roy, "Medical and psychological risk factors for incident hypertension in type 1 diabetic African-Americans," *International Journal of Hypertension*, vol. 2011, Article ID 856067, 10 pages, 2011.

[14] K. Dahl-Jørgensen, J. R. Larsen, and K. F. Hanssen, "Atherosclerosis in childhood and adolescent type 1 diabetes: early disease, early treatment?" *Diabetologia*, vol. 48, no. 8, pp. 1445–1453, 2005.

[15] B. L. Rodriguez, D. Dabelea, A. D. Liese et al., "Prevalence and correlates of elevated blood pressure in youth with diabetes mellitus: The search for diabetes in youth study," *Journal of Pediatrics*, vol. 157, no. 2, pp. 245.e1–251, 2010.

[16] K. O. Schwab, J. Doerfer, W. Marg, E. Schober, and R. W. Holl, "Characterization of 33 488 children and adolescents with type 1 diabetes based on the gender-specific increase of cardiovascular risk factors," *Pediatric Diabetes*, vol. 11, no. 5, pp. 357–363, 2010.

[17] M. van Vliet, J. C. Van der Heyden, M. Diamant et al., "Overweight is highly prevalent in children with type 1 diabetes and associates with cardiometabolic risk," *Journal of Pediatrics*, vol. 156, no. 6, pp. 923–929, 2010.

[18] H. D. Margeirsdottir, J. R. Larsen, C. Brunborg, N. C. Øverby, and K. Dahl-Jørgensen, "High prevalence of cardiovascular risk factors in children and adolescents with type 1 diabetes: A population-based study," *Diabetologia*, vol. 51, no. 4, pp. 554–561, 2008.

[19] R. Klein, B. E. K. Klein, K. E. Lee, K. J. Cruickshanks, and S. E. Moss, "The incidence of hypertension in insulin-dependent diabetes," *JAMA Internal Medicine*, vol. 156, no. 6, pp. 622–627, 1996.

[20] I. Hajjar and T. A. Kotchen, "Trends in prevalence, awareness, treatment, and control of hypertension in the United States, 1988–2000," *Journal of the American Medical Association*, vol. 290, no. 2, pp. 199–206, 2003.

[21] K. Wolf-Maier, R. S. Cooper, H. Kramer et al., "Hypertension treatment and control in five european countries, Canada, and the United States," *Hypertension*, vol. 43, no. 1, pp. 10–17, 2004.

[22] L. S. Geiss, D. B. Rolka, and M. M. Engelgau, "Elevated blood pressure among U.S. adults with diabetes, 1988-1994," *American Journal of Preventive Medicine*, vol. 22, no. 1, pp. 42–48, 2002.

[23] J. I. Barzilay, C. L. Jones, B. R. Davis et al., "Baseline characteristics of the diabetic participants in the antihypertensive and lipid-lowering treatment to prevent heart attack trial (ALLHAT)," *Diabetes Care*, vol. 24, no. 4, pp. 654–658, 2001.

[24] A. Gnasso, M. C. Calindro, C. Carallo et al., "Awareness, treatment and control of hyperlipidaemia, hypertension and diabetes mellitus in a selected population of southern Italy," *European Journal of Epidemiology*, vol. 13, no. 4, pp. 421–428, 1997.

[25] R. Donnelly, L. Molyneaux, M. McGill, and D. K. Yue, "Detection and treatment of hypertension in patients with non-insulin-dependent diabetes mellitus: does the 'rule of halves' apply to a diabetic population?" *Diabetes Research and Clinical Practice*, vol. 37, no. 1, pp. 35–40, 1997.

[26] D. R. Berlowitz, A. S. Ash, E. C. Hickey, M. Glickman, R. Friedman, and B. Kader, "Hypertension management in patients with diabetes: The need for more aggressive therapy," *Diabetes Care*, vol. 26, no. 2, pp. 355–359, 2003.

[27] M. Janghorbani, M. Amini, H. Ghanbari, and H. Safaiee, "Incidence of and risk factors for diabetic retinopathy in Isfahan, Iran," *Ophthalmic Epidemiology*, vol. 10, no. 2, pp. 81–95, 2003.

[28] A. S. Levey, J. Coresh, T. Greene et al., "Using standardized serum creatinine values in the modification of diet in renal disease study equation for estimating glomerular filtration rate," *Annals of Internal Medicine*, vol. 145, pp. 247–254, 2006.

[29] W. T. Friedewald, R. I. Levy, and D. S. Fredrickson, "Estimation of the concentration of low-density lipoprotein cholesterol in plasma, without use of the preparative ultracentrifuge," *Clinical Chemistry*, vol. 18, no. 6, pp. 499–502, 1972.

[30] P. A. James, S. Oparil, B. L. Carter et al., "2014 Evidence-based guideline for the management of high blood pressure in adults: report from the panel members appointed to the Eighth Joint National Committee (JNC 8)," *Journal of the American Medical Association*, vol. 311, no. 5, pp. 507–520, 2014.

[31] J. C. Zgibor, R. R. Wilson, and T. J. Orchard, "Has control of hypercholesterolemia and hypertension in type 1 diabetes improved over time?" *Diabetes Care*, vol. 28, no. 3, pp. 521–526, 2005.

[32] I. H. De Boer, B. Kestenbaum, T. C. Rue et al., "Insulin therapy, hyperglycemia, and hypertension in type 1 diabetes mellitus," *JAMA Internal Medicine*, vol. 168, no. 17, pp. 1867–1873, 2008.

[33] C. J. Schultz, H. A. Neil, R. N. Dalton, T. Konopelska Bahu, and D. B. Dunger, "Blood pressure does not rise before the onset of microalbuminuria in children followed from diagnosis of type 1 diabetes. Oxford Regional Prospective Study Group," *Diabetes Care*, vol. 24, pp. 555–560, 2001.

5

A Theory-Based Self-Care Intervention with the Application of Health Literacy Strategies in Patients with High Blood Pressure and Limited Health Literacy

Homamodin Javadzade [ID],[1] Azam Larki [ID],[1] Rahim Tahmasebi,[2] and Mahnoush Reisi [ID][1]

[1]Department of Health Education and Health Promotion, Bushehr University of Medical Sciences, Bushehr, Iran
[2]Department of Biostatistics, Bushehr University of Medical Sciences, Bushehr, Iran

Correspondence should be addressed to Mahnoush Reisi; reisi_mr@yahoo.com

Academic Editor: Srinivas Nammi

The purpose of this study is to assess the effectiveness of a theory-based self-care intervention with the application of health literacy strategies in patients with high blood pressure and limited health literacy. This is a randomized controlled trial, with measurements at baseline and 1 and 3 months follow-up. 100 patients with high blood pressure and limited health literacy will be randomly allocated to either an intervention group or a usual care control group. We will mainly establish the intervention model based on the principal health belief model components. Patients randomized to the intervention group will receive four educational sessions during four weeks. Considering the limited health literacy level of the patients of the study, health literacy strategies will be used in educational material design for enhancing the quality of the intervention. In order to cover these strategies, we will design four standard animated comics and fact sheets with illustrations and photos consistent with the health belief model constructs and educational sessions' topics. Data will be collected using some questionnaires and will be analyzed using the SPSS software. The findings of this study may assist with the development of a theoretical model for self-care intervention in patients with high blood pressure and limited health literacy.

1. Introduction

Hypertension is a chronic condition affecting approximately one billion individuals worldwide [1]. A 24% increase in developed and 80% in developing countries are predicted for the year 2025 and the increase is expected to be much higher than these predictions [2]. In this regard, it was reported to be 14 to 34 percent in Iran [3] and a systematically review study reported high rates of hypertension among males and females globally [4]. This chronic disease can lead to very serious consequences such as cardiovascular and kidney disease [5]. Due to the high prevalence of hypertension and its serious complications, the World Health Organization (WHO) assigned the theme of World Health Day 2013 to hypertension as a "silent killer, global public health crisis" [6].

Despite the benefits of evidence-based hypertension self-care behaviors in improving blood pressure, hypertensive patients usually have low compliance with the recommended self-care behaviors. Various studies all over the world suggest a high prevalence of uncontrolled blood pressure among people with hypertension [7, 8]. One approach that may advance blood pressure control and be practicable for the most of hypertensive patients is patient compliance with self-care behaviors [9]. The findings of a meta-analysis that examined the results of 87 studies indicated that optimal self-care in hypertensive patients could reduce systolic and diastolic blood pressure by 5 and 4.3 mmHg, respectively [10]. Self-care for people with high blood pressure includes a diet rich in fruits and vegetables, cessation of smoking, sufficient physical activity, antihypertensive medication, reduction in weight, saturated and total fat, and sodium, and moderate alcohol consumption [11]. Despite the benefits of evidence-based hypertension self-care behaviors in improving blood pressure, hypertensive patients generally do not follow medical or lifestyle recommendations and compliance with self-care behaviors in these patients is not desirable [12].

The WHO has emphasized patient education as an important strategy to improve the active participation of patients in their disease management process [13]. Self-care behaviors are influenced by demographic variables and modifiable psychological variables such as self-efficacy, perceived threats, perceived benefits and barriers [11, 14]. Although some studies have examined educational interventions in patients with high blood pressure, they often lack a theoretical framework describing how the educational emphasis on social, psychological, and cognitive variables can affect self-care behaviors in these patients.

Health Belief Model (HBM) is one of the most important theories of behavior change that have been widely considered in behavioral health sciences and successfully applied in the design of health interventions. This model has emphasized the role of moderating factors (demographic, social, and structural factors) and individual perceptions (perceived sensitivity, perceived severity, perceived benefits, perceived barriers, guidance for action, and self-efficacy) in determining the likelihood of performing a behavior [15]. According to this model, a person's decision and motivation to perform a particular behavior included items such as person's perception of being at risk (perceived susceptibility) and its seriousness (perceived severity), belief in the perceived action of usefulness to reduce the risk of disease, and understanding of the health benefits (perceived benefits) due to obstacles and moderating factors such as demographic and psychosocial variables (awareness) and people's judgments of their capabilities to execute given level of performance (self-efficacy)[16, 17]. The results of a cross-sectional study carried out in an earlier study showed that the HBM and its related structures, especially self-efficacy, perceived susceptibility, and severity of complications, are important determinants of self-care behaviors in hypertensive patients with limited health literacy [18].

Although education and especially the theory or model-based education are effective in controlling the blood pressure of patients, there is some evidence suggesting that limited health literacy of patients could act as a barrier in the result of the interventions [19]. Evidence suggests that limited health literacy patients may understand less than half of what is told to them during medical communication [20] Moreover, patients with low health literacy may be ashamed by their condition and hide their low level of literacy from healthcare providers who could possibly help [21]. In this regard, the results of a study on diabetic patients showed that despite the fact that 73% of patients with inadequate health literacy participated in diabetes education classes, 50% of them did not know the signs and symptoms of low blood sugar and 62% of them were unaware of the treatment methods for reducing blood glucose [22].

Choosing proper strategies, based on deeper understanding of needs and capabilities of patients with limited health literacy may help healthcare providers to communicate more efficiently with these patients [23]. Although low health literacy patients regularly rely on verbal instructions, they may have difficulty remembering and comprehending information [24]. Health literacy experts recommend incorporating a few effective and feasible strategies to advance communication and patients' understanding during the communication. Strategies such as plain language and using pictorial media in education will be used in this study.

Regarding high prevalence of hypertension in Iran and limited health literacy among a large population of these patients, it is indispensable to evaluate the effectiveness of an educational intervention based on influencing psychological factors using HBM applying health literacy strategies to promote self-care behaviors in patients with high blood pressure.

2. Material and Methods

2.1. Design. This randomized control trial (RCT) will be conducted with the high blood pressure patients attending to Haft-e-Tir comprehensive health services center of Bushehr, south of Iran. The trial was registered at the Iranian Registry of Clinical Trials with the IRCT code: IRCT2017011731999N1. The participants will be invited to the study to measure their health literacy level at first. Patients who have limited health literacy level according to S-TOFHLA result will be assigned to the two groups: HBM and health literacy strategies-based self-care intervention (trial) and usual care group (control).

2.2. Setting. All patients recruited are those diagnosed with high blood pressure who are referred to Haft-e-Tir comprehensive health services center in Bushehr city (south of Iran) between July 2017 and August 2017.

2.3. Patient Eligibility. The patients will be entered into the study if they are diagnosed with high blood pressure. Inclusion criteria for this study are as follows: (a) passing at least 6 months since the definitive diagnosis of the disease, (b) being able to read, write, and speak Persian, (c) being 30 years old and over, (d) having no severe complications caused by hypertension, including cardiovascular disease, kidney disease, retinal disease, and stroke, and (e) having the desire to participate in the study. Exclusion criteria for the study consist of (a) causing severe complications from hypertension, including cardiovascular disease, kidney disease, retina, and stroke during the study and (b) missing attending educational classes more than once.

2.4. Ethical Consideration. The study protocol will follow the principals of the "Declaration of Helsinki." The participants will be told that they can withdraw from the study at any time and all information will be kept secret and anonymous. This study was approved by Bushehr University of Medical Sciences Ethics Committee (Number IR.BPUMS.REC.1395.128). Informed consent will be obtained from all the participants who will agree to participate in the study.

2.5. Sample Size. According to the study performed by Eftekhar Ardebili et al., 2014 [25], the effect size for the study has obtained based on 90% power, 5 % type one error level, and 1 unit difference between the mean score of knowledge before and, after the intervention, 40 patient per group have been estimated. Considering a dropout rate of 10% during the study, we aim to recruit 50 patients per group.

2.6. Measurement and Procedure. After checking the medical records file in the Haft-e-Tir comprehensive health services center and invitation of patients who meet the inclusion criteria for the study, invited participants will undergo a screening test by Test of Functional Health Literacy in Adults (S-TOFHLA) [26] for selecting those who have limited health literacy. S-TOFHLA is a valid and widely used measure which takes 12 minutes or less to administer. The S-TOFHLA includes reading comprehension and numeracy sections and uses actual materials that patients might encounter in the healthcare setting, such as medication label instructions. The sum of the 2 sections yields the S-TOFHLA score, which ranges from 0 to 100. Scores on the S-TOFHLA are classified and interpreted as follows: inadequate health literacy (scores 0 to 53): individuals will often misread the simplest materials, including prescription bottles and appointment slips and the instructions for an upper gastrointestinal tract radiograph series; marginal health literacy (scores 54 to 66): individuals perform better on the simplest tasks but have difficulty comprehending the Medicaid rights and responsibilities passage; adequate health literacy (scores 67 to 100): individuals will successfully complete most of the tasks required to function in the healthcare setting, although many still have difficulty comprehending more difficult information (i.e., materials written above a 10th grade reading level). In this study patients with both inadequate and marginal health literacy are considered limited health literacy. The valid Persian version of the scale shows adequate internal reliability for numeracy (Cronbach's α =0.69) and for reading comprehension (Cronbach's α = 0.78) [27].

Participants of the study will undergo three measurements: on entry to the study (pretest) and 1 and 3 months after having gone through the intervention for following up. Selected patients will go through the pretest and a then one-month intervention, 1 and 3 months after intervention follow-up.

2.7. Randomization and Blinding. From all hypertensive patients who had medical records in the Haft-e-Tir comprehensive health services center and were eligible for the study, we will select for the invitation by simple random sampling. Then we will screen them for health literacy stage. After completing the inform consent form, limited health literacy patients will randomly allocate to either the control or the intervention group. Randomization of the participants will be done using permuted block randomization. Due to the nature of this intervention, blinding of the patients to the allocation will not be completely possible.

2.8. Outcome Measures. The outcome will be assessed at the baseline, one and 3-month after intervention [Figure 1]. Baseline measurement includes demographic (age, sex, marital status, education, job, income, smoking, and duration of the disease), HBM constructs questionnaire (perceived susceptibility, perceived severity, perceived barriers, perceived benefits, and self-efficacy), and self-care behaviors questionnaire.

2.9. Primary Outcome Measures

2.9.1. Self-Care Behavior. Self-care behaviors will be determined using the 31-item hypertension self-care activity level effects (H-scale) prepared by Findlow [28]. This scale aims to help physicians for a better guidance to hypertensive patients who are looking for attaining blood pressure control [29]. The H-scale surveys the level of self-care by questioning about the number of days per week on which an individual carries out a self-care behavior. The H-scale was previously validated in Persian patients with high blood pressure [28]. The Persian version consisted of 27 items that measure the hypertension self-care activities with the following domains: medication adherence (3 items), physical activity (2 items), low-salt diet (10 items), smoking (2 items), alcohol (1 item), and weight management (9 items). The Persian version of the scale shows adequate internal consistency. Cronbach alphas were as follows: medication adherence (Cronbach's α = 0.91), low-salt diet (Cronbach's α = 0.72), physical activity (Cronbach's α = 0.96), smoking (Cronbach's α = 0.91), and weight management (Cronbach's α = 0.85).

2.10. Secondary Outcome

2.10.1. Knowledge of Hypertension. Hypertension knowledge will be assess by using Hypertension Knowledge Level Scale (HK-LS); this 22-item scale is prepared by Erkoc et al. [30]. Hypertension Knowledge Level Scale (HK-LS) will assess respondents' knowledge in defining hypertension, lifestyle, medical treatment, drug compliance, diet, and complications of hypertension. Each item is a full sentence that is either correct or incorrect. And each item is prepared as part of a standard answer (correct, incorrect, or do not know). Motlagh et al. have validated this questionnaire in Iranian population [28]. In Persian version in the validation process, two items were excluded from the scale and the final version has 19 true/false items.

2.10.2. Health Belief Model Constructs. In order to assess the constructs of health belief model, a researcher made the questionnaire that will be used. Items developed for susceptibility, seriousness, benefits, barriers, and self-efficacy focused on self-care behaviors in hypertensive patients. 39 items with 5-point Likert answers will be used. Nine items for perceived benefits, 7 items for perceived barriers, 9 items for perceived susceptibility, 6 items for perceived severity, and 10 items for perceived self-efficacy were written. For determination of content validity, the list items were distributed to judges who were faculty members and PhD candidates and they were quite familiar with HBM constructs. In content validity, altering the format of questions and ignoring irrelevant questions were done. Then, mean Content Validity Index (CVI) and Content Validity Rate (CVR) of the questionnaire were calculated as 0.94 and 0.91, respectively.

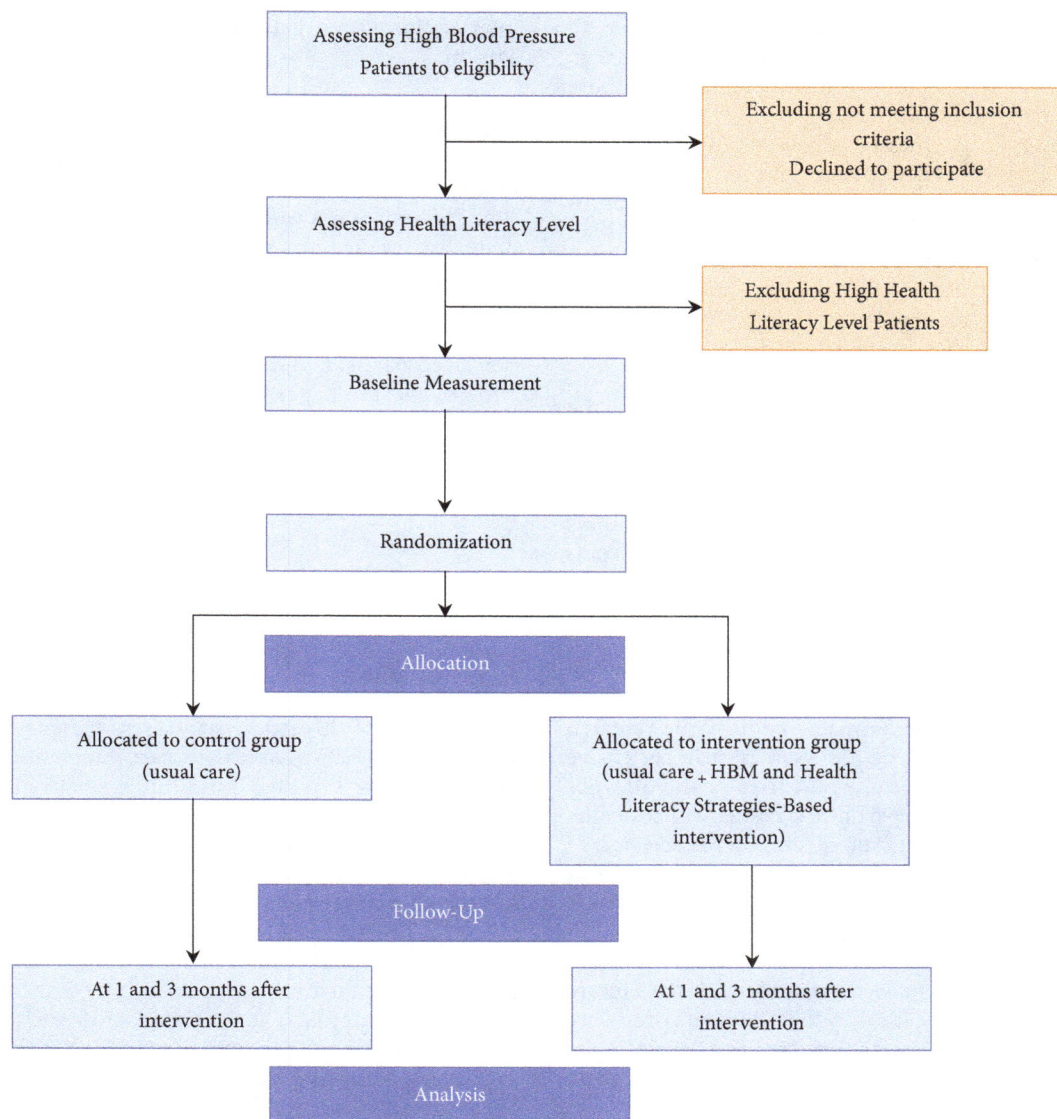

FIGURE 1: Study flow.

Reliability of the scale was calculated and the Cronbach's alpha values of knowledge questions were 0.71, 0.70, 0.70, 0.82, and 0.85 for perceived susceptibility, perceived severity, perceived barriers, perceived benefits, and perceived self-efficacy, respectively.

2.11. Intervention

2.11.1. Theoretical Framework. HBM constructs are the guidelines for the educational intervention design in this study. In the HBM model, perceived severity, perceived benefits, perceived barriers, and perceived self-efficacy are the determinant components. We will mainly establish the intervention model based on the principal HBM components. Patients randomized to the intervention group will receive four groups of educational sessions (lasting 50-60 min)

during four weeks. Topics of the first session are "what is high blood pressure?" and "what is self-care for hypertension?" This session will focus on the strategies to enhance perceived susceptibility and perceived severity of patients toward the disease. In this session, the patients will face the problem (risk of complications of hypertension problems) and they will be threatened (perceived susceptibility). Then, they will understand the depth of the risk and seriousness of complications (perceived severity).

In the second session, patients will learn and discuss healthy diet (such as low salt, low fat, fruit, and vegetable-rich diet). In the third session, patients will learn about physical activity and weight management. The fourth session will focus on medication adherence and avoidance of smoking and alcohol drinking. The importance of self-care behaviors, being physically active, adhering to medication, avoidance of smoking and alcohol drinking, and also possible barriers to a continuous healthy diet, will be discussed. In this session, brainstorming the possible and trained solutions for those barriers will cover the perceived barriers. By discussing the benefits and useful outcomes of adherence to the self-care behaviors, patients will believe the benefits and possibility of their behaviors (perceived benefits). Introducing an appropriate role model (strategy of vicarious experiences [Mrs. Karimi]) in video comics, providing solutions to address possible obstacles in removing the barriers, and giving verbal persuasions to positive expressions of the patients were used to enhance the self-efficacy of individuals for self-care behaviors.

Considering the limited health literacy level of the patients of the study, health literacy strategies will be used in educational material design for enhancing the quality of intervention. In order to cover these strategies, we will use four animated comics and fact sheets with a lot of illustrations and photos which are consistent with the HBM constructs and educational sessions' topics. Animated comics will be produced as media that will be shown to the intervention group patients at the beginning of each educational session to help them start discussing the topic and learn more about the self-care throughout the story of them.

In order to design these animated comics, the research team defines the characters of the story of a hypertensive patient (Mrs. Karimi), her family and friends and also her physician. The story of each part of the comic will cover the topic of the respective educational session. In the scenario of the animated comics we will make some recommendations for self-care behaviors to hypertensive patients. In the next step, the research team will design the storyboard of each part of the animated comic and then the characters and backgrounds will be illustrated compatible with the culture of the patients of the study using Adobe Illustrator software by a graphic designer. At last, the sounding and animating of each part of the storyboard will be done using Adobe After Effect software by an animation team.

The fact sheets that contain the most important recommendations and reminders of the educational topic will be designed based on existing standards and guidelines for designing simple and comprehensible educational media for limited health literacy patients, such as Simply-Put [31], which is provided by the Center for Disease Prevention and Control as a comprehensive guide for designing simple, understandable media. For optimal comprehension and compliance, it is suggested that patients' educational materials will be written at a sixth-grade or lower reading level, preferably including pictures and illustrations [32]. Therefore, Gunning Fog Index will be used to assess the readability of these written materials. This formula determines how difficult it is to read and understand a piece of writing. Readability will be calculated by the following formula: GFI = [(number of words/number of sentences) + number of "difficult words"] x 0.4 [33]. The number that results from the following calculation correlates with the grade level. All the sentences will design and modify in such a way that based on this indicator, scores less than 6 will be obtained for the readability level [32]. Each designed fact sheet will be given to the

intervention group patients at the end of each educational session.

2.12. Statistical Analysis. Survey data will be coded and analyzed using the Statistical Package for the Social Sciences (SPSS) version 22. In addition to providing descriptive statistics, Chi-square test will be used to compare the distribution of qualitative demographical characteristics between the two groups before intervention. T-test will be used to compare the mean scores of knowledge and health belief model constructs (perceived sensitivity, severity perceived benefits, perceived barriers, and perceived self-efficacy) between the two groups. The Repeated Measure ANOVA analysis will be used to examine and compare changes in the mean scores of knowledge and constructs during the study period in each group and the comparison between the two groups. The post hoc analysis will perform within per groups to compare the times. The Kolmogorov–Smirnov test will be used for checking the normality distribution of the data. The P value of <0.05 will be considered statistically significant.

3. Discussion

The purpose of this study is to assess the effectiveness of a theory-based (HBM-based) self-care intervention by the use of health literacy strategies in limited health literacy hypertensive patients. To our knowledge, there is no published study investigating the use of behavioral change theories and health literacy strategies simultaneously to design an intervention to improve self-care in patients with high blood pressure. This protocol has the potential to improve the standard care of patients with limited health literacy by a simple, accessible, and relatively inexpensive way that could improve signs and symptoms. It is hoped that such educational intervention will produce more favorable health outcomes.

In this study the intervention will be based on health belief model. Applying this model would decrease methodological errors of the study which, in turn, would allow us to apply the valid and reliable educational strategies. Consequently, we are likely to believe that designing this educational program based on HBM constructs would be the key to the possible success. If it is found that the intervention improves self-care behaviors, future experimental works will be required to identify the most important component of HBM-based intervention for hypertensive patients. The results of this study will provide useful insights into the role that health literacy strategies, and health literacy level can play a role in improving self-care and awareness of complications in hypertensive patients with limited health literacy. If successful, the intervention may be adopted in other patient populations and RCT study designs.

The proposed study has a number of potential limitations. First, there is only a limited time in which the participants can be recruited. Second, due to the nature of this intervention, blinding of the patients to the allocation is not completely possible in this study. Third, using self-report instruments for measuring self-care behaviors and adherence limits the ability to identify changes objectively. The fourth limitation is the use of questionnaires that their construct validity was not confirmed due to time limitation. However, appropriate content validity and reliability of the HBM questionnaires were properly met. Further studies should be done to measure long-term effects of the intervention as well as clinical outcomes.

References

[1] J.-E. Lee, H.-R. Han, H. Song et al., "Correlates of self-care behaviors for managing hypertension among Korean Americans: A questionnaire survey," *International Journal of Nursing Studies*, vol. 47, no. 4, pp. 411–417, 2010.

[2] A. A. Saeed, N. A. Al-Hamdan, A. A. Bahnassy, A. M. Abdalla, M. A. F. Abbas, and L. Z. Abuzaid, "Prevalence, awareness, treatment, and control of hypertension among Saudi adult population: a national survey," *International Journal of Hypertension*, vol. 2011, Article ID 174135, 8 pages, 2011.

[3] S. F. Zinat Motlagh, R. Chaman, S. R. Ghafari et al., "Knowledge, treatment, control, and risk factors for hypertension among adults in Southern Iran," *International Journal of Hypertension*, vol. 2015, Article ID 897070, 2015.

[4] M. Pereira, N. Lunet, A. Azevedo, and H. Barros, "Differences in prevalence, awareness, treatment and control of hypertension between developing and developed countries," *Journal of Hypertension*, vol. 27, no. 5, pp. 963–975, 2009.

[5] P. M. Kearney, M. Whelton, K. Reynolds, P. Muntner, P. K. Whelton, and J. He, "Global burden of hypertension: analysis of worldwide data," *The Lancet*, vol. 365, no. 9455, pp. 217–223, 2005.

[6] world health organization, *Silent killer, global public health crisis*, 2013, http://www.who.int/campaigns/world-health-day/2013/en/.

[7] E. M. Mutua, M. M. Gitonga, B. Mbuthia, N. Muiruri, J. J. Cheptum, and T. Maingi, "Level of blood pressure control among hypertensive patients on follow-up in a Regional Referral Hospital in Central Kenya," *Pan African Medical Journal*, vol. 18, article no. 278, p. 278, 2014.

[8] R. M. Peters and T. N. Templin, "Measuring blood pressure knowledge and self-care behaviors of African Americans," *Research in Nursing & Health*, vol. 31, no. 6, pp. 543–552, 2008.

[9] S. J. Flynn, J. M. Ameling, F. Hill-Briggs et al., "Facilitators and barriers to hypertension self-management in urban African Americans: perspectives of patients and family members," *Patient Preference and Adherence*, vol. 7, pp. 741–749, 2013.

[10] J. Chodosh, S. C. Morton, W. Mojica et al., "Meta-analysis: chronic disease self-management programs for older adults," *Annals of Internal Medicine*, vol. 143, no. 6, pp. 427–I32, 2005.

[11] J. Warren-Findlow, R. B. Seymour, and L. R. B. Huber, "The association between self-efficacy and hypertension self-care activities among African American adults," *Journal of Community Health*, vol. 37, no. 1, pp. 15–24, 2012.

[12] R. Shima, M. H. Farizah, and H. A. Majid, "A qualitative study on hypertensive care behavior in primary health care settings in Malaysia," *Patient Preference and Adherence*, vol. 8, pp. 1597–1609, 2014.

[13] R. S. Vasan, M. G. Larson, E. P. Leip, W. B. Kannel, and D. Levy, "Assessment of frequency of progression to hypertension in non-hypertensive participants in the Framingham Heart Study: a cohort study," *The Lancet*, vol. 358, no. 9294, pp. 1682–1686, 2001.

[14] A. Kamran, S. S. Ahari, M. Biria, A. Malpour, and H. Heydari, "Determinants of patient's adherence to hypertension medications: application of health belief model among rural patients," *Annals of Medical and Health Sciences Research*, vol. 4, no. 6, pp. 922–927, 2014.

[15] N. K. Janz and M. H. Becker, "The health belief model: a decade later," *Health Education Journal*, vol. 11, no. 1, pp. 1–47, 1984.

[16] R. Orji, J. Vassileva, and R. Mandryk, "Towards an effective health interventions design: an extension of the health belief model," *Online Journal of Public Health Informatics*, vol. 4, no. 3, 2012.

[17] M. Reisi, F. Mostafavi, H. Javadzade, B. Mahaki, and G. Sharifirad, "Assessment of some predicting factors of self-efficacy in patients with type 2 diabetes," *Iranian Journal of Endocrinology and Metabolism*, vol. 17, no. 1, pp. 44–52, 2015.

[18] A. Larki, R. Tahmasebi, and M. Reisi, "Factors Predicting Self-Care Behaviors among Low Health Literacy Hypertensive Patients Based on Health Belief Model in Bushehr District, South of Iran," *International Journal of Hypertension*, vol. 2018, pp. 1–7, 2018.

[19] R. J. Adams, "Improving health outcomes with better patient understanding and education," *Risk Management and Healthcare Policy*, vol. 3, pp. 61–72, 2010.

[20] A. Wallace, "Low health literacy: Overview, assessment, and steps toward providing high-quality diabetes care," *Diabetes Spectrum*, vol. 23, no. 4, pp. 220–227, 2010.

[21] S. A. Boren, "A review of health literacy and diabetes: opportunities for technology," *Journal of Diabetes Science and Technology*, vol. 3, no. 1, pp. 202–209, 2009.

[22] M. V. Williams, D. W. Baker, R. M. Parker, and J. R. Nurss, "Relationship of functional health literacy to patients' knowledge of their chronic disease: a study of patients with hypertension and diabetes," *JAMA Internal Medicine*, vol. 158, no. 2, pp. 166–172, 1998.

[23] Y. H. Tang, S. M. C. Pang, M. F. Chan, G. S. P. Yeung, and V. T. F. Yeung, "Health literacy, complication awareness, and diabetic control in patients with type 2 diabetes mellitus," *Journal of Advanced Nursing*, vol. 62, no. 1, pp. 74–83, 2008.

[24] F. L. Wilson, A. Mayeta-Peart, L. Parada-Webster, and C. Nordstrom, "Using the Teach-Back Method to Increase Maternal Immunization Literacy Among Low-Income Pregnant Women in Jamaica: A Pilot Study," *Journal of Pediatric Nursing*, vol. 27, no. 5, pp. 451–459, 2012.

[25] H. E. Ardebili, S. Fathi, H. Moradi, M. Mahmoudi, and A. B. Mahery, "Effect of educational intervention based on the health belief model in blood pressure control in hypertensive women," *Journal of Mazandaran University of Medical Sciences*, vol. 24, no. 119, pp. 62–71, 2014.

[26] D. W. Baker, M. V. Williams, R. M. Parker, J. A. Gazmararian, and J. Nurss, "Development of a brief test to measure functional health literacy," *Patient Education and Counseling*, vol. 38, no. 1, pp. 33–42, 1999.

[27] H. Javadzade, G. Sharifirad, M. Reisi, E. Tavassoli, and F. Rajati, "Health literacy among adults of Isfahan," *Health System Research*, vol. 9, no. 5, pp. 540–549, 2013.

[28] S. F. Zinat Motlagh, R. Chaman, E. Sadeghi, and A. Ali Eslami, "Self-care behaviors and related factors in hypertensive patients," *Iranian Red Crescent Medical Journal*, vol. 18, no. 6, Article ID e35805, 2016.

[29] J. Warren-Findlow, D. W. Basalik, M. Dulin, H. Tapp, and L. Kuhn, "Preliminary validation of the hypertension self-care activity level effects (H-SCALE) and clinical blood pressure among patients with hypertension," *The Journal of Clinical Hypertension*, vol. 15, no. 9, pp. 637–643, 2013.

6

A Systematic Review and Meta-Analysis on the Association between Hypertension and Tinnitus

Pan Yang,[1,2] Wenjun Ma,[2] Yiqing Zheng,[3] Haidi Yang,[3] and Hualiang Lin[2]

[1]School of Public Health, Sun Yat-sen University, Guangzhou, China
[2]Guangdong Provincial Institute of Public Health, Guangdong Provincial Center for Disease Control and Prevention, Guangzhou, China
[3]Department of Otolaryngology, Sun Yat-sen Memorial Hospital, Sun Yat-sen University, Guangzhou, China

Correspondence should be addressed to Hualiang Lin; linhualiang2002@163.com

Academic Editor: Claudio Borghi

Hypertension has been suggested to be one possible risk factor of tinnitus, but the association between hypertension and tinnitus remains uncertain. The authors performed a meta-analysis of the existing studies on the association between hypertension and tinnitus. We performed literature search of studies using SinoMed, CNKI, WanFang, PubMed, Scopus, Web of Science, and Google Scholar. Studies reported the odds ratio and 95% confidence interval (CI) (or provided sufficient information for calculation) of the association between hypertension and tinnitus were included. A total of 19 eligible studies with 20 effect estimates were used in this study. They included 63,154 participants with age ranging from 14 to 92. The pooled OR, which was pooled using a random effects model, was 1.37 (95% CI: 1.16 to 1.62). There was no evidence of publication bias ($p = 0.11$ for Begg's test, $p = 0.96$ for Egger's test). By meta-regression, we found that study design may be one possible factor of heterogeneity. Sensitivity analysis found that the result was stable. This study suggests that hypertension might be one risk factor of tinnitus, and hypertension prevention and control might be helpful in preventing tinnitus.

1. Introduction

Tinnitus is the perceived sensation of sound in the absence of a corresponding external acoustic stimulus [1]. It is a very bothersome symptom for many patients as it can affect the physical and mental health in different degree. The patients suffering from serious tinnitus may even commit suicide [2].

Hypertension has been suggested as one potential risk factor of tinnitus, but some other studies showed different results. Thirunavukkarasu and Geetha's retrospective study [3] showed that hypertension and giddiness were high risk factors for the occurrence of tinnitus. Nondahl et al.'s study [4] of ten-year incidence of tinnitus showed that hypertension was not associated with the incidence of tinnitus. Negrila-Mezei et al.'s case-control study [5] based on 471 ear-nose-throat department patients showed that hypertension was significantly associated with tinnitus, but de Moraes Marchiori's case-control study [6] did not find any significant association between hypertension and tinnitus.

Some cross-sectional surveys [7, 8] showed that hypertension was a risk of tinnitus, but some other cross-sectional surveys [9, 10] did not find any significant association. It is important to elucidate and quantify the association between hypertension and tinnitus. If the association holds, prevention and control of hypertension should then be included in the prevention measures of tinnitus.

In this study, we provided a meta-analysis of the tinnitus risk associated with hypertension. We also performed a meta-regression to examine possible sources of heterogeneity between the studies and examined the influence of single study on the overall meta-estimate.

2. Methods

2.1. Literature Search. Eligible studies were searched via databases. The databases included SinoMed, CNKI, WanFang, PubMed, Scopus, Web of Science, and Google Scholar.

Search strategies used subject headings and key words and did not have language and time restrictions. The presence of tinnitus was defined as answering "yes" to the question "In the past 12 months, have you ever heard a sound (buzzing, hissing, ringing, humming, roaring, machinery noise) originating in your ears?" or similar question in different phrase. Hypertension (high blood pressure) was defined as a systolic blood pressure (SBP) $\geq$ 140 mmHg or diastolic blood pressure (DBP) $\geq$ 90 mmHg or reported use of antihypertensive medication [11].

The studies were identified by combining the term "tinnitus" with several terms, such as hypertension, blood pressure, prevalence, risk factors, epidemiology, and characterization, which indicated that the study might provide the relevant information on the association between hypertension and tinnitus, such as OR (odds ratio) and 95% confidence intervals (95% CIs) or relevant information to calculate OR and 95% CIs. We also examined reference lists of the all identified studies and reviewed the cited literatures to identify any other relevant studies.

2.2. Inclusion and Exclusion Criteria. Studies were included in the current meta-analysis if they provided the information to examine the association between hypertension and tinnitus (OR and 95% CIs or relevant data to calculate OR and 95% CIs). Studies which reported one specific type of tinnitus (such as left ear tinnitus and pulsatile tinnitus) were excluded.

2.3. Meta-Analysis. To estimate the quantitative relationship between hypertension and tinnitus, we obtained estimates of the OR and 95% CIs from relevant studies. We used a random-effects model to combine estimates from the identified studies, which allowed between-study heterogeneity to contribute to the variance [12]. We assessed homogeneity of ORs with I^2 value which represented the estimated percent of total variance that could be explained by between-study heterogeneity [13]. Publication bias was assessed using Begg's test [14] and Egger's test [15]. Begg's funnel plot and Egger's publication bias plot were created to provide a visual investigation of possible publication bias. Meta-regression was used to explore whether the inconsistency in results across individual studies could be explained by variations in publication year, region (American and others), sample size, study design (case-control study and cross-sectional study), and confounder adjustment (the sets of potential confounders for which adjustment was made varied by study; we just assessed the difference between studies with adjusted ORs and studies with crude ORs) [16]. We performed both univariate and multivariate meta-regression analysis. Finally, we performed sensitivity analysis to examine the influence of individual studies, in which the meta-analysis estimates were derived by omitting one study at a time. The whole analyses were conducted using STATA software (v12.1).

3. Results

Of a total of 515 studies identified from the search strategy, 187 were epidemiological studies and 328 studies were literature reviews, experimental studies, clinical treatments, or others and were excluded from the analysis. We chose 20 studies reporting OR and 95% CIs of the association between hypertension and tinnitus or providing sufficient data for relevant calculation. Of the 20 studies, one study reported one specific type of tinnitus (left ear tinnitus, right ear tinnitus) and was excluded. Finally, we included a total of 19 studies which provided suitable information for the subsequent analysis (Figure 1).

We identified 3 case-control studies and 16 cross-sectional studies. Twenty population samples from 19 studies (Fujii et al.'s study [8] provided both men and women information) provided sufficient data for a meta-analysis. Details of the included studies were summarized in Table 1. Overall, this study included 63,154 participants from Italy, South Korea, China, Nigeria, USA, Brazil, Japan, Romania, Turkey, Australian, and Chile, the age of the subjects ranged from 14 to 92 years, sample size of the studies ranged between 120 and 14,178, and OR ranged between 0.73 (95% CI: 0.35 to 1.53) and 12.14 (95% CI: 5.04 to 29.23).

Figure 2 showed the forest plot of 20 effect estimates from 19 studies. Of them, eight studies showed a significant positive association between hypertension and tinnitus. The overall pooled OR was 1.37 (95% CI: 1.16 to 1.62).

Publication bias was not detected by Begg's test ($p = 0.11$) (Figure 3) and Egger's test ($p = 0.96$) (Figure 4). The heterogeneity test was significant ($Q = 155.06$, $p < 0.001$, $I^2 = 87.7\%$, and Tau-squared = 0.103). Meta-regression ($I^2 = 85.1\%$, Tau-squared = 0.090, and adjusted R-square = 73.6%) showed that, among various variables, study design was one significant contributor ($p = 0.002$) (Table 2).

The sensitivity analysis indicated that the omission of any of the studies led to changes in estimates between 1.29 (95% CI: 1.10 to 1.51) and 1.41 (95% CI: 1.19 to 1.68) (Figure 5).

4. Discussion

Tinnitus involves a large proportion of the general population and affects the quality of life and work efficiency. Most of tinnitus prevalence studies in Western Europe and USA have reported prevalence rates between 10% and 15% in the adult population [30]. For example, the largest study ($n = 48313$), which was undertaken as part of the National Study of Hearing in England, showed a prevalence of 10.1% among adults, with 2.8% of respondents describing it as moderately annoying, 1.6% as severely annoying, and 0.5% at a level severely affecting their normal life [31]. The mechanism of occurrence of tinnitus remains largely unknown; although several treatment strategies for tinnitus patients have been proposed, such as the tinnitus masking technique, pharmacological therapy, and surgery, no single effective cure exists for tinnitus [32]. It is necessary and important to study the risk factors of tinnitus, which will be helpful for formulating specific prevention measures for its prevention. This study provided a quantitative meta-analysis of the association between hypertension and tinnitus. The pooled OR was 1.37 (95% CI: 1.16 to 1.62), which supports that hypertension is significantly associated with tinnitus.

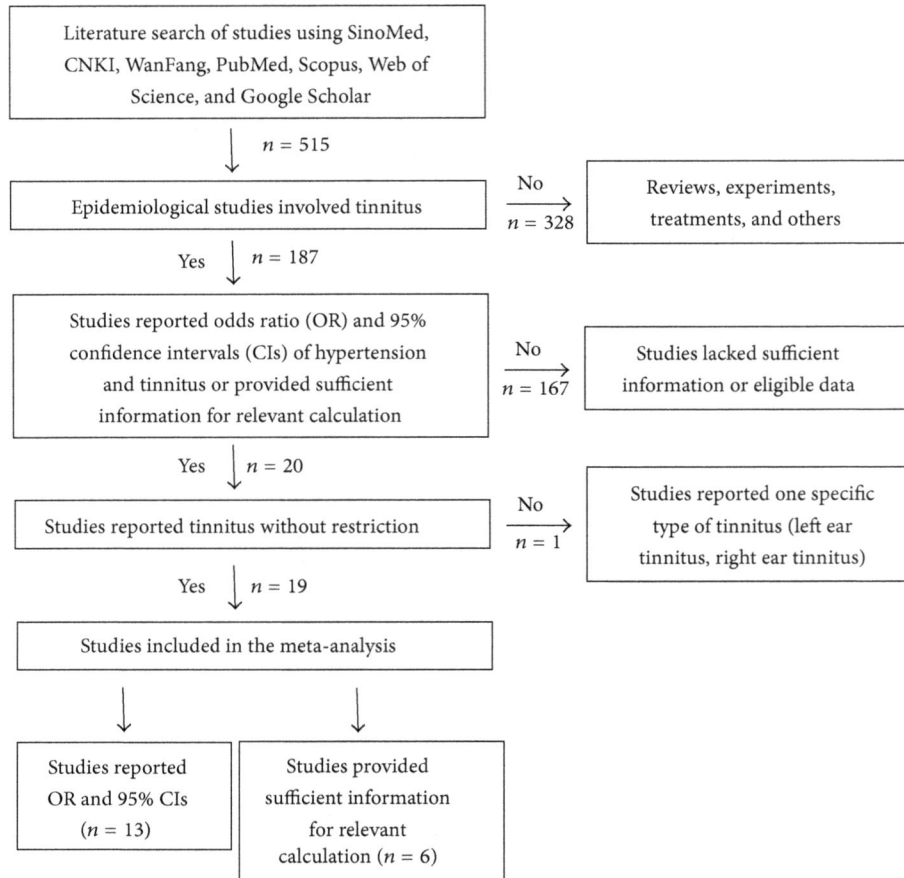

FIGURE 1: Flow diagram on the search process.

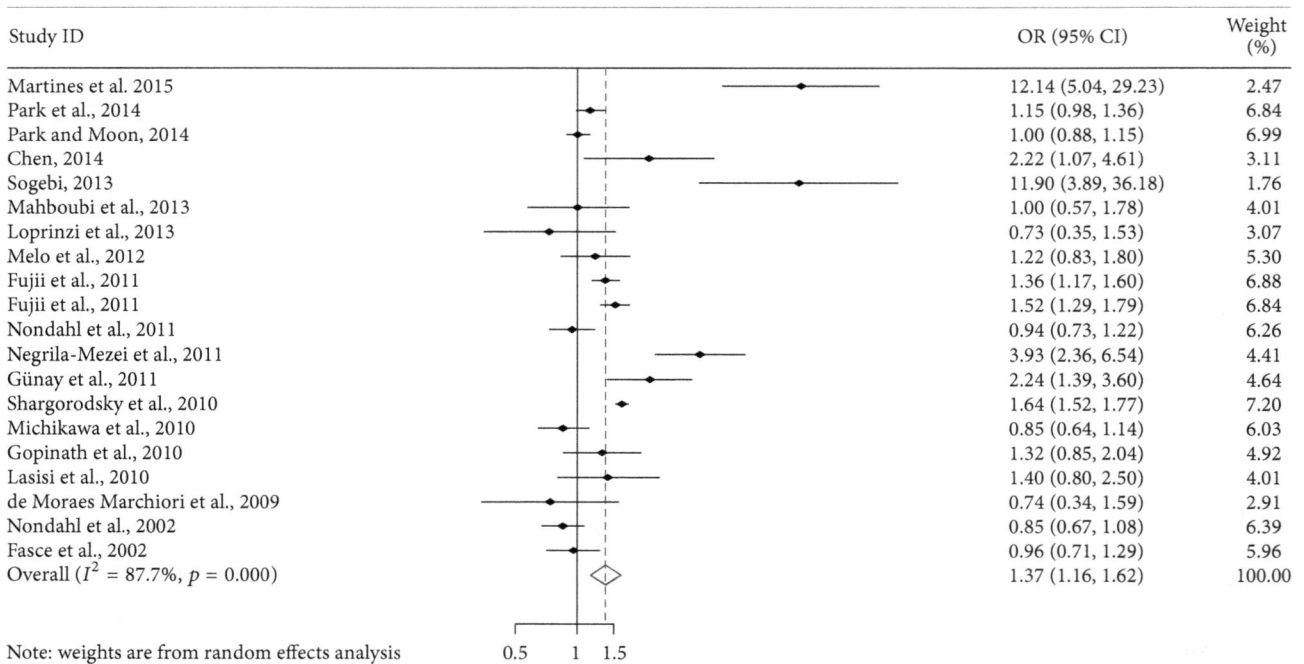

FIGURE 2: Forest plot of the associations between hypertension and tinnitus (OR and 95% CI indicate odds ratio and 95% confidence interval).

TABLE 1: Description of the study populations included in the meta-analysis ($n = 63154$).

First author	Year	Country	Study design	Sample size (n)	Age (years)
Martines [17]	2015	Italy	Case-control	120	14–85
Park [18]	2014	South Korea	Cross-sectional	5140	≥40
*Park [9]	2014	South Korea	Cross-sectional	10061	20–97
Chen [19]	2014	China	Case-control	204	NA
Sogebi [20]	2013	Nigeria	Cross-sectional	127	≥41
*Mahboubi [21]	2013	American	Cross-sectional	3520	12–19
*Loprinzi [22]	2013	American	Cross-sectional	473	70–85
*Melo [23]	2012	Brazil	Cross-sectional	498	≥60
*Fujii [8]	2011	Japan	Cross-sectional	6450 (men)	45–79
*Fujii [8]	2011	Japan	Cross-sectional	7973 (women)	45–79
*Nondahl [24]	2011	American	Cross-sectional	3267	21–84
Negrila-Mezei [5]	2011	Romania	Case-control	471	≥60
*Günay [7]	2011	Turkey	Cross-sectional	879	18–64
Shargorodsky [25]	2010	American	Cross-sectional	14178	NA
Michikawa [26]	2010	Japan	Cross-sectional	1286	≥65
Gopinath [27]	2010	Australian	Cross-sectional	1214	NA
*Lasisi [10]	2010	Nigeria	Cross-sectional	1302	≥65
de Moraes Marchiori [6]	2009	Brazil	Cross-sectional	154	45–64
Nondahl [28]	2002	American	Cross-sectional	3737	48–92
Fasce [29]	2002	Chile	Cross-sectional	2100	NA

*OR was adjusted; NA: not available.

TABLE 2: Parameter estimation of meta-regression.

Variable	Univariate		Multivariate	
	Coefficient	95% CI	Coefficient	95% CI
Publication year	0.07	$(-0.02, 0.16)$	0.04	$(-0.06, 0.13)$
Region	-0.49	$(-1.23, 0.25)$	-0.21	$(-0.86, 0.43)$
Sample size	$-3.46e-5$	$(-12.14e-5, 5.23e-5)$	$7.06e-6$	$(-6.71e-5, 8.12e-5)$
Study design	1.28	$(0.54, 2.02)$	1.10	$(0.07, 2.14)$
Confounder adjustment	0.34	$(-0.32, 1.01)$	0.10	$(-0.53, 0.73)$

95% CI indicates 95% confidence interval.

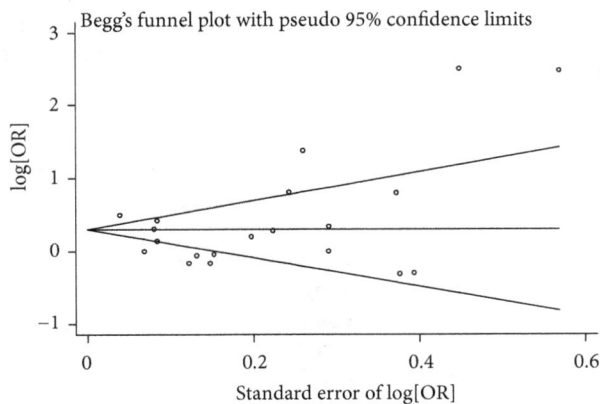

FIGURE 3: Begg's funnel plot for meta-analysis.

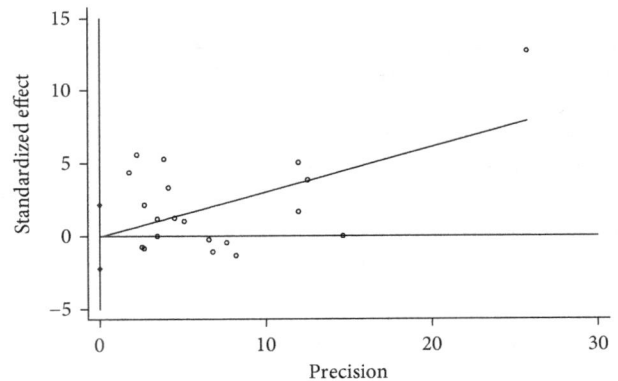

FIGURE 4: Egger's publication bias plot for meta-analysis.

Hypertension has been suggested as one potential risk factor of tinnitus in some studies. There are some studies about hypertension in patients with tinnitus; for example, Nowak et al.'s study [33] included 1200 patients getting treated in the Laryngological Rehabilitation Centre in Poznań due to

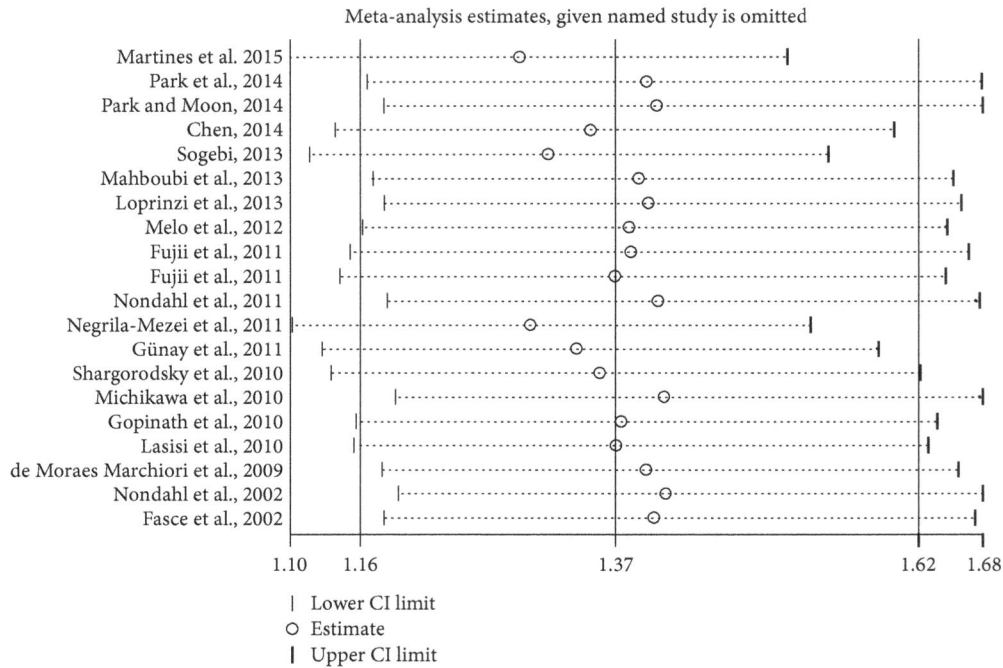

Meta-analysis estimates, given named study is omitted

	Lower CI limit
o	Estimate
	Upper CI limit

FIGURE 5: Sensitivity analysis.

tinnitus, in the examined group 34% suffered from systemic diseases, and among them the highest percentage (47%) suffered from hypertension; Sogebi's study [20] showed that, among 79 patients having complaints of tinnitus, 15.2% were suffering from hypertension. There are also some studies about tinnitus in patients with hypertension; for instance, Borghi et al.'s study [34] showed that 17.6% patients (aged 18 to 75 years, with uncontrolled hypertension) reported occasional or prolonged spontaneous tinnitus and suggested that systemic blood pressure might have played a prominent role in some tinnitus patients; Chávez-Delgado et al. conducted a cross-sectional study of 385 patients with hypertension, type 2 diabetes mellitus, and dyslipidemia with symptoms of hearing loss, vertigo, and tinnitus; the prevalence of tinnitus was 32% in patients with hypertension [35].

The pathophysiological mechanisms of tinnitus are still not clear. There are several possible mechanisms including increased spontaneous firing rate of neurons in the central auditory system, increased neural synchrony in the firing pattern across neurons in primary auditory cortex, and map reorganisation in the auditory modality [30]. The mechanisms underlying the relationship between hypertension and tinnitus are poorly understood. There are animal experiments [36, 37] indicating that hypertension may induce the occurrence of tinnitus or aggravate preexisting tinnitus through two principle mechanisms, high blood pressure might cause damage to the cochlear microcirculation, and diverse antihypertensive drugs might lead to ototoxicity. Tachibana et al. [37] suggested that the primary target of hypertensive damage in the rat cochlea is the stria vascularis, which feeds the organ of Corti. Przewoźny et al. [38] suggested that the subclinical damage to the stria vascularis includes the decrease in the

cochlear oxygen partial pressure and disturbance of the ionic K^+ recycling. Borghi et al. [34] suggested that the presence of tinnitus is the consequence of toxic damage of the labyrinth in most patients, which means that the onset of tinnitus might be an adverse event in patients treated with antihypertensive drugs. Another possibility pointed to the fact that when antihypertensive action exceeded the desired effects, subsequent abrupt hypotension would lead to cochlear hypoperfusion and circulatory impairment, which could disturb the sensorineural response, leading to the onset of tinnitus [34]. Clinical evidence also indicated an association between hypertension and tinnitus, which reinforces the hypothesis that alterations in the cochlear microcirculation, as causal or adjuvant factors in tinnitus pathophysiology, occur [39].

There is widespread recognition that consistency between research centers in the ways that patients with tinnitus are assessed and outcomes following interventions are measured would facilitate more effective cooperation and more meaningful evaluations and comparisons of outcomes [40]. But many studies still have methodological drawbacks, especially with production of an unambiguous definition of tinnitus and phrasing of appropriate epidemiological questions, which may be one of the main causes for the heterogeneity in the present study [30]. The other cause for heterogeneity of this research may include socioeconomic condition, ethnic differences, and public health service. Although the meta-analysis detected significant heterogeneity between studies, further sensitivity analyses and the exclusion of publication bias are in favor of a similar effect across the populations.

Hypertension is an important public health concern worldwide. Globally, the overall prevalence of hypertension in adults aged 18 years and over was around 22% in 2014 [41]. Kearney et al.'s study [42] estimated that 29% (about 1.56 billion) of the world's adult population would have hypertension by 2025. Since hypertension is one of the high incidence chronic diseases and has large numbers of patients, we must pay attention to the fact that tinnitus may be caused by hypertension and consider the ototoxicity of drugs for hypertension patients, which means that we may make a choice for hypertension medication to prevent tinnitus.

A few limitations should be noted. First, the included studies for this meta-analysis varied in the degree of controlling for potential confounders, such as age, gender, ethnicity, income, smoking, ear infecting, noise exposure, BMI, anemia, and hearing loss, only a few of the ORs were adjusted, and the adjusted ORs did not adjust for all the same factors. Second, the study design was either cross-sectional or case-control study; therefore it cannot determine temporal sequence and causality [43]. Third, our study did not investigate any causal mechanism of tinnitus and simply did quantitative analysis of the association between hypertension and tinnitus, this association may not be the direct causal role, and further studies are needed.

In conclusion, this meta-analysis suggests that hypertension might be a risk factor of tinnitus and should be considered in its prevention strategy.

Acknowledgment

This research was supported by Science and Technology Program of Guangzhou, China (no. 2014Y2-00511).

References

[1] B. Langguth, P. M. Kreuzer, T. Kleinjung, and D. De Ridder, "Tinnitus: causes and clinical management," *The Lancet Neurology*, vol. 12, no. 9, pp. 920–930, 2013.

[2] J. E. Lewis, S. D. G. Stephens, and L. McKenna, "Tinnitus and suicide," *Clinical Otolaryngology & Allied Sciences*, vol. 19, no. 1, pp. 50–54, 1994.

[3] K. Thirunavukkarasu and C. Geetha, "One-year prevalence and risk factors of tinnitus in older individuals with otological problems," *The International Tinnitus Journal*, vol. 18, no. 2, pp. 175–181, 2013.

[4] D. M. Nondahl, K. J. Cruickshanks, T. L. Wiley et al., "The ten-year incidence of tinnitus among older adults," *International Journal of Audiology*, vol. 49, no. 8, pp. 580–585, 2010.

[5] A. Negrila-Mezei, R. Enache, and C. Sarafoleanu, "Tinnitus in elderly population: clinic correlations and impact upon QoL," *Journal of Medicine and Life*, vol. 4, no. 4, pp. 412–416, 2011.

[6] L. L. de Moraes Marchiori, "Tinnitus complaint and blood hypertension in the aging process," *Revista Brasileira de Hipertensão*, vol. 16, no. 1, pp. 5–8, 2009.

[7] O. Günay, A. Borlu, D. Horoz, and I. Gün, "Tinnitus prevalence among the primary care patients in Kayseri, Turkiye," *Erciyes Tip Dergisi*, vol. 33, no. 1, pp. 39–46, 2011.

[8] K. Fujii, C. Nagata, K. Nakamura et al., "Prevalence of tinnitus in community-dwelling Japanese adults," *Journal of Epidemiology*, vol. 21, no. 4, pp. 299–304, 2011.

[9] R. J. Park and J. D. Moon, "Prevalence and risk factors of tinnitus: the Korean National Health and Nutrition Examination Survey 2010-2011, a cross-sectional study," *Clinical Otolaryngology*, vol. 39, no. 2, pp. 89–94, 2014.

[10] A. O. Lasisi, T. Abiona, and O. Gureje, "Tinnitus in the elderly: profile, correlates, and impact in the Nigerian study of ageing," *Otolaryngology: Head and Neck Surgery*, vol. 143, no. 4, pp. 510–515, 2010.

[11] F. Tesfaye, P. Byass, and S. Wall, "Population based prevalence of high blood pressure among adults in Addis Ababa: uncovering a silent epidemic," *BMC Cardiovascular Disorders*, vol. 9, no. 1, article 39, 2009.

[12] R. DerSimonian and N. Laird, "Meta-analysis in clinical trials," *Controlled Clinical Trials*, vol. 7, no. 3, pp. 177–188, 1986.

[13] J. P. T. Higgins, S. G. Thompson, J. J. Deeks, and D. G. Altman, "Measuring inconsistency in meta-analyses," *British Medical Journal*, vol. 327, no. 7414, pp. 557–560, 2003.

[14] C. B. Begg and M. Mazumdar, "Operating characteristics of a rank correlation test for publication bias," *Biometrics*, vol. 50, no. 4, pp. 1088–1101, 1994.

[15] J. L. Peters, A. J. Sutton, D. R. Jones, K. R. Abrams, and L. Rushton, "Comparison of two methods to detect publication bias in meta-analysis," *Journal of the American Medical Association*, vol. 295, no. 6, pp. 676–680, 2006.

[16] F. Song, T. A. Sheldon, A. J. Sutton, K. R. Abrams, and D. R. Jones, "Methods for exploring heterogeneity in meta-analysis," *Evaluation & the Health Professions*, vol. 24, no. 2, pp. 126–151, 2001.

[17] F. Martines, F. Sireci, E. Cannizzaro et al., "Clinical observations and risk factors for tinnitus in a Sicilian cohort," *European Archives of Oto-Rhino-Laryngology*, vol. 272, no. 10, pp. 2719–2729, 2015.

[18] K. H. O. Park, S. H. W. Lee, J.-W. Koo et al., "Prevalence and associated factors of tinnitus: data from the Korean national health and nutrition examination survey 2009–2011," *Journal of Epidemiology*, vol. 24, no. 5, pp. 417–426, 2014.

[19] Y. Chen, *Analysis on Risk Factors of Idiopathic Tinnitus*, Shanxi Medical University, 2014.

[20] O. A. Sogebi, "Characterization of tinnitus in Nigeria," *Auris Nasus Larynx*, vol. 40, no. 4, pp. 356–360, 2013.

[21] H. Mahboubi, S. Oliaei, S. Kiumehr, S. Dwabe, and H. R. Djalilian, "The prevalence and characteristics of tinnitus in the youth population of the United States," *The Laryngoscope*, vol. 123, no. 8, pp. 2001–2008, 2013.

[22] P. D. Loprinzi, H. Lee, B. Gilham, and B. J. Cardinal, "Association between accelerometer-assessed physical activity and tinnitus, NHANES 2005-2006," *Research Quarterly for Exercise and Sport*, vol. 84, no. 2, pp. 177–185, 2013.

[23] J. J. Melo, C. L. Meneses, and L. L. D. M. Marchiori, "Prevalence of tinnitus in elderly individuals with and without history of occupational noise exposure," *International Archives of Otorhinolaryngology*, vol. 16, no. 2, pp. 222–225, 2012.

[24] D. M. Nondahl, K. J. Cruickshanks, G.-H. Huang et al., "Tinnitus and its risk factors in the Beaver Dam Offspring study," *International Journal of Audiology*, vol. 50, no. 5, pp. 313–320, 2011.

[25] J. Shargorodsky, G. C. Curhan, and W. R. Farwell, "Prevalence and characteristics of tinnitus among US adults," *The American Journal of Medicine*, vol. 123, no. 8, pp. 711–718, 2010.

[26] T. Michikawa, Y. Nishiwaki, Y. Kikuchi et al., "Prevalence and factors associated with tinnitus: a community-based study of Japanese elders," *Journal of Epidemiology*, vol. 20, no. 4, pp. 271–276, 2010.

[27] B. Gopinath, C. M. McMahon, E. Rochtchina, M. J. Karpa, and P. Mitchell, "Risk factors and impacts of incident tinnitus in older adults," *Annals of Epidemiology*, vol. 20, no. 2, pp. 129–135, 2010.

[28] D. M. Nondahl, K. J. Cruickshanks, T. L. Wiley, R. Klein, B. E. K. Klein, and T. S. Tweed, "Prevalence and 5-year incidence of tinnitus among older adults: the epidemiology of hearing loss study," *Journal of the American Academy of Audiology*, vol. 13, no. 6, pp. 323–331, 2002.

[29] E. Fasce, M. Flores, and F. Fasce, "Prevalence of symptoms associated with blood pressure in normal and hypertensive population," *Revista Medica de Chile*, vol. 130, no. 2, pp. 160–166, 2002.

[30] D. Baguley, D. McFerran, and D. Hall, "Tinnitus," *The Lancet*, vol. 382, no. 9904, pp. 1600–1607, 2013.

[31] A. Davis and E. A. Rafaie, "Epidemiology of tinnitus," in *Tinnitus Handbook*, R. S. Tyler, Ed., pp. 1–23, Singular, San Diego, Calif, USA, 2000.

[32] N. Ahmad and M. Seidman, "Tinnitus in the older adult," *Drugs & Aging*, vol. 21, no. 5, pp. 297–305, 2004.

[33] K. Nowak, J. Banaszewski, P. Dabrowski, E. Szymiec, and W. Szyfter, "Tinnitus in systemic diseases," *Otolaryngologia Polska*, vol. 56, no. 2, pp. 213–216, 2002.

[34] C. Borghi, C. Brandolini, M. G. Prandin, A. Dormi, G. C. Modugno, and A. Pirodda, "Prevalence of tinnitus in patients withhypertension and the impact of different anti hypertensive drugs on the incidence of tinnitus: a prospective, single-blind, observational study," *Current Therapeutic Research*, vol. 66, no. 5, pp. 420–432, 2005.

[35] M. E. Chávez-Delgado, I. Vázquez-Granados, M. Rosales-Cortés, and V. Velasco-Rodríguez, "Cochleovestibular dysfunction in patients with diabetes mellitus, hypertension and dyslipidemia," *Acta Otorrinolaringologica Espanola*, vol. 63, no. 2, pp. 93–101, 2012.

[36] E. Borg and A. R. Moller, "Noise and blood pressure: effect of lifelong exposure in the rat," *Acta Physiologica Scandinavica*, vol. 103, no. 3, pp. 340–342, 1978.

[37] M. Tachibana, I. Yamamichi, S. Nakae, Y. Hirasugi, M. M. And, and O. Mizukoshi, "The site of involvement of hypertension within the cochlea: a comparative study of normotensive and spontaneously hypertensive rats," *Acta Oto-Laryngologica*, vol. 97, no. 3-4, pp. 257–265, 1984.

[38] T. Przewoźny, A. Gójska-Grymajło, M. Kwarciany, D. Gąsecki, and K. Narkiewicz, "Hypertension and cochlear hearing loss," *Blood Pressure*, vol. 24, no. 4, pp. 199–205, 2015.

[39] R. R. Figueiredo, A. A. de Azevedo, and N. de Oliveira Penido, "Tinnitus and arterial hypertension: a systematic review," *European Archives of Oto-Rhino-Laryngology*, vol. 272, no. 11, pp. 3089–3094, 2015.

[40] B. Langguth, R. Goodey, A. Azevedo et al., "Consensus for tinnitus patient assessment and treatment outcome measurement: tinnitus research initiative meeting, regensburg, July 2006," *Progress in Brain Research*, vol. 166, pp. 525–536, 2007.

[41] World Health Organization, *Global Status Report on Noncommunicable Diseases 2014*, World Health Organization, Geneva, Switzerland, 2014, http://apps.who.int/iris/bitstream/10665/148114/1/9789241564854_eng.pdf.

[42] P. M. Kearney, M. Whelton, K. Reynolds, P. Muntner, P. K. Whelton, and J. He, "Global burden of hypertension: analysis of worldwide data," *The Lancet*, vol. 365, no. 9455, pp. 217–223, 2005.

[43] F. P. Cappuccio, F. M. Taggart, N.-B. Kandala et al., "Meta-analysis of short sleep duration and obesity in children and adults," *Sleep*, vol. 31, no. 5, pp. 619–626, 2008.

7

Safety and Antihypertensive Effect of Selara (Eplerenone): Results from a Postmarketing Surveillance

Shoko Takahashi,[1] Megumi Hiramatsu,[2] Shinichi Hotta,[3] Yukie Watanabe,[3] Osamu Suga,[4] Yutaka Endo,[5] and Isamu Miyamori[6]

[1]Medical Affairs, Global Established Pharma Business, Pfizer Japan Inc., Shinjuku Bunka Quint Building, 3-22-7 Yoyogi, Shibuya-ku, Tokyo 151-8589, Japan
[2]PMS Planning & Operation, Pfizer Japan Inc., Shinjuku Bunka Quint Building, 3-22-7 Yoyogi, Shibuya-ku, Tokyo 151-8589, Japan
[3]Clinical Informatics and Innovation, Pfizer Japan Inc., Shinjuku Bunka Quint Building, 3-22-7 Yoyogi, Shibuya-ku, Tokyo 151-8589, Japan
[4]Medical Writing and Document Management, Pfizer Japan Inc., Shinjuku Bunka Quint Building, 3-22-7 Yoyogi, Shibuya-ku, Tokyo 151-8589, Japan
[5]Clinical Statistics, Pfizer Japan Inc., Shinjuku Bunka Quint Building, 3-22-7 Yoyogi, Shibuya-ku, Tokyo 151-8589, Japan
[6]University of Fukui, 23-3 Matsuokashimoaizuki, Eiheiji-cho, Yoshida-gun, Fukui Prefecture 910-1193, Japan

Correspondence should be addressed to Shoko Takahashi; shoko.takahashi@pfizer.com

Academic Editor: Kazuomi Kario

Prospective postmarketing surveillance of Selara (eplerenone), a selective mineralocorticoid receptor antagonist, was performed to confirm its safety and efficacy for hypertension treatment in Japan. The change in blood pressure after initiation of eplerenone treatment was also examined. Patients with essential hypertension who were eplerenone-naïve were recruited regardless of the use of other antihypertensive drugs. For examination of changes in blood pressure, patients were excluded if eplerenone was contraindicated or used off-label. Patients received 50–100 mg of eplerenone once daily and were observed for 12 weeks. No treatments including antihypertensive drugs were restricted during the surveillance period. Across Japan, 3,166 patients were included for safety analysis. The incidence of adverse drug reactions was 2.4%. The major adverse drug reactions observed were hyperkalemia (0.6%), dizziness, renal impairment, and increased serum potassium (0.2% each). The mean systolic blood pressure decreased from 152.1 ± 19.0 mmHg to 134.8 ± 15.2 mmHg at week 12, and the mean diastolic blood pressure decreased from 85.8 ± 13.7 mmHg to 77.7 ± 11.4 mmHg. There were no significant new findings regarding the type or incidence of adverse reactions, and eplerenone had a clinically significant antihypertensive effect, leading to favorable blood pressure control.

1. Introduction

Hypertension is a major public health issue in many countries. In Japan, 53% of individuals aged 40–74 years and 79% of those aged 75 years and older were diagnosed with hypertension based on systolic blood pressure (SBP) ≥ 140 mmHg, diastolic blood pressure (DBP) ≥ 90 mmHg, and/or treatment with an antihypertensive drug, according to the 2013 National Health and Nutrition Survey published by the Ministry of Health, Labor, and Welfare [1]. The risk for cardiovascular events has been shown to be high among patients with hypertensive conditions, particularly among those who have comorbidities such as diabetes, chronic kidney disease (CKD), metabolic syndrome, cerebrovascular disorders, or organ dysfunction including heart disease. Therefore, it is important to provide guidance for lifestyle modifications and to administer strict treatment with antihypertensive drugs according to the target blood pressure (BP) levels, depending on the comorbidities [2]. The Eighth Joint National Committee [3], American Heart Association/American College of Cardiology/Centers for Disease Control and Prevention [4], and 2014 Guidelines for the Management of Hypertension by the Japanese Society of Hypertension (JSH 2014) [2] have recommended diuretics, calcium channel blockers (CCBs), angiotensin II receptor blockers (ARBs), and angiotensin-converting enzyme (ACE) inhibitors as first-line antihypertensive drugs [5]. In addition, combination therapy consisting of drugs with different mechanisms of action has been recommended to further lower BP without causing adverse drug reactions (ADRs) [2].

Mineralocorticoid receptor antagonists (MRAs) have been shown to exert antihypertensive effects by binding to mineralocorticoid receptors (MRs) and blocking MR-dependent signal transduction. Hyperkalemia is a known major ADR for the MRAs eplerenone and spironolactone [6], as MRAs enhance sodium excretion and potassium reabsorption upon binding to MRs in the renal tubules. Hyperkalemia occurs more frequently after combined treatment with an ARB/ACE inhibitor and an MRA; thus, MRAs should be used carefully, especially when used in combination.

As of March 2016, eplerenone has been approved in over 70 countries (the brand name of eplerenone is Selara in Japan and Inspra® in other countries) for heart failure after acute myocardial infarction and/or heart failure with mild symptoms. However, it has been approved for the treatment of hypertension in only 11 countries including Japan, the United States, Canada, and Singapore. This postmarketing surveillance (PMS) was conducted to identify unknown ADRs that are not stated in the package insert of Selara tablets [7], estimate the incidence of ADRs including hyperkalemia in general practice, and elucidate the factors that affect the safety of the drug when it is used in Japanese hypertensive patients. Additionally, the antihypertensive effects of eplerenone were evaluated.

2. Methods

2.1. Data Collection and Analysis.
Between May 2008 and April 2012, we conducted a PMS that targeted hypertensive patients in Japan who had not previously been treated with eplerenone. The surveillance was conducted in accordance with Articles 14-4 and 14-6 of the Pharmaceutical Affairs Law and in accordance with a protocol approved by the Ministry of Health, Labor, and Welfare (MHLW) of Japan. A written agreement was obtained from participating institutions. The study was also in accordance with the standard of Good Postmarketing Study Practice (GPSP). GPSP is the authorized standard for PMS studies of approved drugs in clinical practice, and no formal ethics committee approval or informed consent was necessary to conduct surveillance under this ordinance.

Because a PMS does not restrict the administration of the study drug or concomitant treatments, the outcomes observed in the PMS reflect the overall consequences of administration of the study drug and concomitant treatments in real-world settings. We aimed to collect 3,000 cases using a centralized registration method to be able to detect unknown ADRs at a frequency of 0.1% with a reliability of 95%.

2.2. Patients.
Patients were eplerenone-naïve and had essential hypertension diagnosed by physicians in charge. There were no exclusion criteria for patient registration. The physicians in charge were encouraged to consult the Guidelines for the Management of Hypertension 2004 to determine the severity of hypertension in a comprehensive manner. For hepatic function abnormality and renal impairment, categories determined by the physician in charge were adopted. Although precise definitions of severity were not provided, the physicians in charge were asked to judge the severity in a comprehensive manner, considering the disease duration, complications, concomitant medications, and other relevant factors.

2.3. Dosage and Administration.
In principle, patients received 50–100 mg of eplerenone once a day orally, and the dose was adjusted as necessary. Administration of any concomitant treatment including other antihypertensive drugs was not restricted. The observation period was 12 weeks and began upon initiation of treatment.

2.4. Assessment of Safety.
Adverse events (AEs) were assessed as a safety endpoint. All unfavorable or unintended signs, symptoms, and diseases that occurred in patients who received eplerenone, regardless of whether there was a clear causal relationship with eplerenone, were considered AEs. If there was a clear causal relationship between eplerenone and an AE, it was considered an ADR. Events were categorized as ADRs when either the physician in charge or the sponsoring company (Pfizer Japan Inc.), or both, determined that the categorization was appropriate. "Hyperkalemia" and "increased serum potassium levels" were categorized as different ADRs based on the terms reported by the physician in charge, because increased serum potassium levels are not necessarily equivalent to hyperkalemia.

A severe ADR was defined as (1) death, (2) a life-threatening event, (3) hospitalization or extension of the hospitalization period, (4) a permanent or remarkable disorder/dysfunction, (5) a congenital abnormality/defect, (6) another medically significant event, or (7) an event that could lead to disability.

Of the patients that were surveyed, it was confirmed that those included in the safety analysis had taken eplerenone at least once during the observation period. However, patients that did not meet the requirements for determining safety according to the selection criteria (i.e., cases involving a breach of contract/imperfect contract and/or registration violations, cases in which target drug use was unable to be confirmed, and cases in which information regarding the presence of AEs was unknown) were excluded from the safety analysis.

2.5. Assessments of Effectiveness.
The effectiveness of blood pressure reduction was assessed 12 ± 2 weeks after initiation of eplerenone treatment. The population for the effectiveness analysis excluded patients from the safety analysis with contraindicated/off-label use of eplerenone. The exclusion criteria included the following: (1) eplerenone at a dosage of <25 mg or >100 mg per day during the PMS; (2) hyperkalemia (diagnosed by a physician in charge) or high serum potassium levels (>5.0 mEq/L) at baseline; (3) diabetes with

microalbuminuria or proteinuria; (4) moderate or severe renal impairment (creatinine clearance rate <50 mL/min); (5) severe hepatic function disorder; and (6) treatment with potassium supplements, potassium-sparing diuretics, itraconazole, ritonavir, or nelfinavir. Creatinine clearance was calculated using the Cockcroft-Gault formula.

2.6. Statistics. The use of the terminology for AEs and the classification of events into System Organ Classes were conducted in accordance with the International Conference in Harmonization of Technical Requirements for Registration of Pharmaceuticals for Human Use Medical Dictionary for Regulatory Activities, version 17.1. The number and incidence ((%): (the number of ADR events)/(the number of surveyed cases)) of ADRs were determined by using the System Organ Classes and terminology for AEs. If the severity, treatment, or outcome of an AE was missing, it was considered "unknown."

In the analysis of the binary data, the frequencies and incidence of AEs were calculated. The 95% two-sided confidence intervals for the incidence were calculated. Fisher's exact test was used to test relationships with nominal data, whereas the Cochran-Armitage test (exact method) was used to test relationships with ordinal data. The data from the analyses were presented (unless otherwise noted) as the mean ± standard deviation or as the percentage of total patients (%). Data processing and analysis were performed using SAS Version 9 (SAS Institute, Cary, NC).

3. Results

In the current PMS, 3,374 patients were registered from 400 of 557 contracted institutions. Filled case report forms for 3,318 of these patients were collected from 386 institutions. The participating institutions mainly included private practices and clinics (60.6%). The other institutions included national, public, and private university hospitals. Of the 3,318 cases in which the PMS had been completed, 152 were excluded because of a breach of contract or imperfect contract ($N = 96$), lack of information regarding AEs (no revisit, $N = 39$), violation of registration ($N = 14$), or a lack of information regarding eplerenone treatment ($N = 3$). In total, 3,166 patients were therefore included in the safety analysis. The effect of eplerenone on BP was analyzed in 1,024 patients who met the criteria stated in the method section.

3.1. Subject Characteristics. Among the 3,166 patients included in the safety analysis, 51.8% were male, and the mean age was 67.6 ± 12.8 years. Elderly individuals 65 years of age or older accounted for 62.0% of the patients (Table 1). The mean body mass index was 24.4 ± 4.1 kg/m². The severity of hypertension was mild in 29.1%, moderate in 48.9%, and severe in 12.5% of the patients. The mean serum potassium levels were 4.1 ± 0.5 mEq/L at baseline. Concomitant diabetes was observed in 20.0% of the patients, whereas concomitant heart failure was observed in 16.2%. Concomitant renal impairment was observed in 13.5% of the patients, and the mean creatinine clearance rate was 77.6 ± 33.9 mL/min. Patients who received 50 mg of eplerenone at baseline accounted for 74.5% of the total patients, and the

TABLE 1: Patient characteristics.

Factors	Categories	Analysis populations Safety analysis population, $N = 3,166$ (%)
Sex	Male	1,640 (51.8)
Age (years)	Mean ± SD	67.6 ± 12.8
	<35	21 (0.7)
	35 to <45	149 (4.7)
	45 to <55	343 (10.8)
	55 to <65	689 (21.8)
	65 to <75	897 (28.3)
	75 to <85	845 (26.7)
	≥85	222 (7.0)
BMI (kg/m²)	Mean ± SD	24.4 ± 4.1
	<25	1,411 (44.6)
	≥25	875 (27.6)
	Unknown	880 (27.8)
Targeted disease	Hypertension	2,919 (92.2)
	Other reasons	247 (7.8)
Severity of hypertension	Mild	922 (29.1)
	Moderate	1,548 (48.9)
	Severe	395 (12.5)
	Unknown	54 (1.7)
Inpatients/outpatients	Inpatients	191 (6.0)
	Outpatients	2,975 (94.6)
Fasting glucose (mg/dL)	Mean ± SD	110.0 ± 36.8
	<110	1,271 (40.1)
	110 to <126	255 (8.1)
	≥126	294 (9.3)
	Not examined	1,346 (42.5)
HbA1c (%)	Mean ± SD	5.7 ± 1.0
	<5.8	1,106 (34.9)
	5.8 to <6.5	289 (9.1)
	≥6.5	247 (7.8)
	Not examined	1,524 (48.1)
Hepatic function disorder	No	2,647 (83.6)
	Yes	472 (14.9)
	Mild	405 (12.8)
	Moderate	47 (1.5)
	Severe	6 (0.2)
	Unknown	14 (0.4)
	Unknown	47 (1.5)
Renal impairment	No	2,697 (85.2)
	Yes	426 (13.5)
	Mild	323 (10.2)
	Moderate	88 (2.8)
	Severe	11 (0.3)
	Unknown	4 (0.1)
	Unknown	43 (1.4)
Heart failure	No	2,631 (83.1)
	Yes	513 (16.2)
	Unknown	22 (0.7)

TABLE 1: Continued.

Factors	Categories	Analysis populations Safety analysis population, N = 3,166 (%)
NYHA functional class	I	197 (6.2)
	II	199 (6.3)
	III	56 (1.8)
	IV	13 (0.4)
	Unknown	70 (2.2)
Diabetes	No	2,490 (78.6)
	Yes	634 (20.0)
	Unknown	42 (1.3)
Primary aldosteronism	No	3,121 (98.6)
	Yes	45 (1.4)
Initial dose of eplerenone (mg/day)	Mean ± SD	45.5 ± 13.7
	25	718 (22.7)
	50	2,358 (74.5)
	75	6 (0.2)
	100	78 (2.5)
	Other reasons	6 (0.2)
Serum potassium concentrations (mEq/L)	Mean ± SD	4.1 ± 0.5
	≤3.5	239 (7.5)
	>3.5 to ≤5.0	1,991 (62.9)
	>5.0	59 (1.9)
	Unknown	877 (27.7)
Creatinine clearance (mL/min)	Mean ± SD	77.6 ± 33.9
	>80	851 (26.9)
	≥50 to ≤80	753 (23.8)
	≥30 to <50	345 (10.9)
	<30	87 (2.7)
	Unknown	1,130 (35.7)

SD: standard deviation; BMI: body mass index; HbA1c: glycated hemoglobin A1c; NYHA: New York Heart Association; CrCl: creatinine clearance.

mean daily dosage was 45.5 ± 13.7 mg. The mean duration of eplerenone treatment was 128.0 ± 93.5 days, and the median was 106.0 days. At the time eplerenone treatment was initiated, 74.3% of the patients had been treated with other antihypertensive drugs (e.g., CCB, ARB, ACE inhibitor, direct renin inhibitor, thiazide diuretic, loop diuretic, alpha-blocker, or beta-blocker). CCB (49.0%) was the drug most frequently administered concomitantly with eplerenone, followed by ARB (46.6%). Among the patients included in the safety analysis, eplerenone treatment was discontinued in 10.0% of the patients. The reasons for discontinuation were AEs (19.2%), loss to follow-up (18.2%), insufficient clinical effectiveness (16.7%), cure (effective) (15.1%), abnormal clinical laboratory test results (3.8%), death of the patient (3.8%), or other reasons (23.3%). All the deaths were judged as not attributable to eplerenone.

3.2. Safety

3.2.1. Adverse Drug Reactions.
Among the patients included in the safety analysis, ADRs were observed in 75, and the incidence was 2.4%. The most common ADRs were hyperkalemia (0.6%), dizziness (0.2%), renal impairment (0.2%), and increased serum potassium (0.2%). ADRs that were unpredictabl efrom the pa ck age insert of Selara tabl ts were observed in 11 patients and included renal impairment (N = 3), shingles (N = 1), acute myeloid leukemia (N = 1), lymphadenitis (N = 1), loss of appetite (N = 1), spasm (N = 1), ear fullness (N = 1), gastric ulcer (N = 1), fecal incontinence (N = 1), and photosensitivity reaction (N = 1). No clinically significant change in the mean pulse rate was observed.

3.2.2. Serious Adverse Drug Reactions.
Among the patients included in the safety analysis, serious ADRs were observed in 0.5% (Table 3). These included hyperkalemia (0.3%), renal impairment (0.1%), increased serum potassium (0.1%), acute myeloid leukemia (0.03%), decreased appetite (0.03%), hepatic function abnormal (0.03%), and drug interactions (0.03%). The outcomes of these ADRs were "unrecovered" for a patient with acute myeloid leukemia and a patient with hepatic function abnormal and "unknown" for a patient with hyperkalemia, whereas the ADRs "disappeared/recovered" or "became less severe" for all the other patients.

3.2.3. Changes in Serum Potassium Levels.
There have been concerns regarding a possible increase in serum potassium levels caused by the pharmacological actions of eplerenone. Hyperkalemia or increased serum potassium was observed in 20 and 6 patients, respectively (Table 2). Among these patients, 88.5% were at least 65 years old and 26.9% were at least 80 years old, and concomitant heart failure and diabetes were observed in 34.6% and 26.9% of these patients, respectively. The ADRs were judged serious in 11 of 26 patients (Table 3). Of these patients, 3 had moderate or mild hepatic function disorder, 8 had moderate or mild renal impairment, and 3 had functional class II heart failure according to the New York Heart Association (NYHA) classification system. The ADRs in all of these patients "disappeared/recovered" or "became less severe," except for 1 patient with an "unknown" outcome. Among the patients whose outcomes were known, 9 halted or withdrew from eplerenone treatment, and 1 did not change the dose.

The incidence of adverse events was 4.7% in patients with renal impairment, which was 2.4-fold higher than that in patients without renal impairment. Of these adverse events, hyperkalemia accounted for 45%.

Serum potassium levels during the surveillance period slightly increased in patients who had serum potassium levels ≤ 4.5 mEq/L (Table 4) at baseline. The incidence of potassium increase in the patients with baseline serum potassium levels ≤ 3.5 mEq/L was 21.6%, which was higher than that of patients with serum potassium levels over 3.5 mEq/L to 4.5 mEq/L at baseline (6.4%). Very little change in the serum potassium level was observed in patients with serum potassium levels of over 4.5 to 5.0 mEq/L at baseline, whereas the levels slightly decreased in those with serum potassium levels over 5.0 mEq/L at baseline. In contrast, the percentage of patients

TABLE 2: Incidence of adverse drug reactions in safety analysis population.

Adverse drug reactions: SOC	N (%)	Major types: PT (occurrence ≥ 0.1%) (N (%))
Number of patients in safety analysis population	3,166 (100)	
Patients with adverse drug reactions	75 (2.37)	
Total number of adverse drug reactions	82	
Infections and infestations	1 (0.03)	
Neoplasms (benign, malignant, and unspecified, including cysts and polyps)	1 (0.03)	
Blood and lymphatic system disorders	1 (0.03)	
Metabolism and nutrition disorders	25 (0.79)	Hyperkalemia: 20 (0.63)
Nervous system disorders	10 (0.32)	Dizziness: 7 (0.22)
Ear and labyrinth disorders	1 (0.03)	
Cardiac disorders	1 (0.03)	
Vascular disorders	3 (0.09)	
Respiratory, thoracic, and mediastinal disorders	1 (0.03)	
Gastrointestinal disorders	6 (0.19)	
Hepatobiliary disorders	2 (0.06)	
Skin and subcutaneous tissue disorders	5 (0.16)	
Renal and urinary disorders	10 (0.32)	Renal impairment: 7 (0.22)
General disorders and administration site conditions	4 (0.13)	
Investigations	11 (0.35)	Increased serum potassium: 6 (0.19)

Calculated with MedDRA/J17.1 System Organ Class and preferred terms.

TABLE 3: Incidence of serious adverse drug reactions.

Serious adverse drug reactions	N (%)
Safety analysis population	3,166
Patients with adverse drug reactions	16 (0.51)
Neoplasms (benign, malignant, and unspecified, including cysts and polyps)	*1 (0.03)*
Acute myeloid leukemia	1 (0.03)
Metabolism and nutrition disorders	*10 (0.32)*
Hyperkalemia	9 (0.28)
Decreased appetite	1 (0.03)
Hepatobiliary disorders	*1 (0.03)*
Hepatic function abnormal	1 (0.03)
Renal and urinary disorders	*3 (0.09)*
Renal impairment	3 (0.09)
General disorders and administration site conditions	*1 (0.03)*
Drug interaction	1 (0.03)
Investigations	*2 (0.06)*
Blood potassium increased	2 (0.06)

Calculated with MedDRA/J17.1 System Organ Class and preferred terms.

with serum potassium values over 5.5 mEq/L increased as the baseline serum potassium levels increased. One case of hyperkalemia was observed among the 158 patients who received 100 mg of eplerenone, which was the maximum approved dosage per day, on at least 1 day during the surveillance period. The hyperkalemia disappeared/recovered without changing of the dose in the patient. Importantly, eplerenone is contraindicated in patients with serum potassium levels > 5.5 mEq/L according to the package insert of Selara tablets [7].

3.2.4. Adverse Drug Reactions in Patients with Lower Creatinine Clearance. There were 6 cases that had ADRs with CCr < 30 mL/min at baseline, and the incidence of any ADR was 6.9%. The major ADRs of these patients were hyperkalemia (3.4%) and renal impairment (2.3%). The incidence of ADRs in patients with baseline CCr from greater than or equal to 30 mL/min to less than 50 mL/min was 4.1%, and their major ADRs were also hyperkalemia (1.2%) and increased serum potassium (0.9%). In contrast, the incidence of ADRs in patients with baseline CCr from greater than or equal to 50 mL/min up to 80 mL/min was 2.5%, and major ADRs were also hyperkalemia and increased serum potassium (both 0.4%). It is important to note that eplerenone is contraindicated in patients with CCr < 50 mL/min according to the package insert of Selara tablets.

3.2.5. Adverse Drug Reactions in Patients Prescribed Other Antihypertensive Drugs. Among the 2,355 patients who were prescribed antihypertensive medications other than eplerenone at the time of initiation of eplerenone treatment, 2 cases developed hypotension. Both were prescribed more than 2 antihypertensive drugs in addition to eplerenone. The incidence of hyperkalemia among patients prescribed ACE inhibitors or ARBs concomitantly with eplerenone was 1.1%

TABLE 4: Serum potassium levels during eplerenone treatment relative to baseline levels.

Baseline level (mEq/L)	N	Maximal value (mEq/L)	Changes from baseline (mEq/L)	% changes from baseline (%)	Patients with ≥5.5 mEq/L (N (% [95% CI]))
Serum potassium ≤ 3.5	195	3.9 ± 0.4	0.69 ± 0.45	21.6 ± 15.5	0 (0.0 [0.0–1.9])
3.5 < serum potassium ≤ 4.5	1315	4.3 ± 0.4	0.25 ± 0.42	6.4 ± 10.6	19 (1.4 [0.9–2.2])
4.5 < serum potassium ≤ 5.0	263	4.7 ± 0.5	−0.02 ± 0.51	−0.27 ± 10.7	14 (5.3 [2.9–8.8])
Serum potassium > 5.0	51	5.0 ± 0.6	−0.41 ± 0.80	−7.1 ± 13.7	10 (19.6 [9.8–33.1])

Mean ± standard deviation. CI: confidence interval. The cases who had serum potassium data at baseline and additional timings during the PMS were included in this table. The number of the cases was 1,824 out of the safety analysis population (N = 3,166).

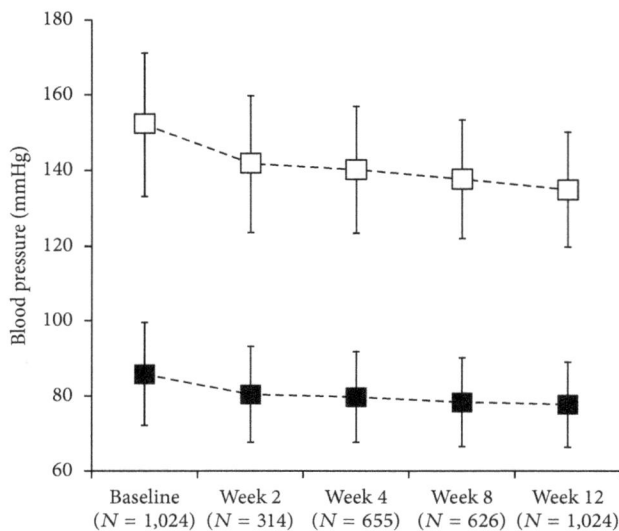

FIGURE 1: Changes in systolic (open square) and diastolic (closed square) blood pressure at each observation time point from baseline to week 12 (mean ± standard deviation) during the 12-week treatment period in the effectiveness analysis population.

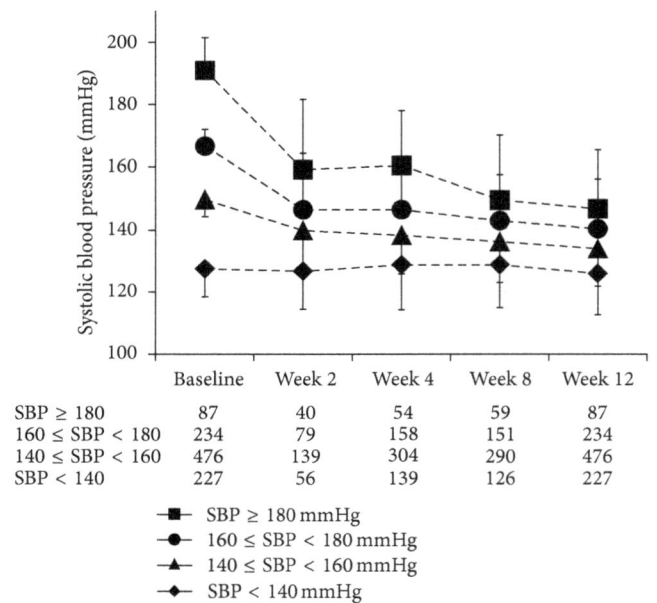

FIGURE 2: Changes in systolic blood pressure (mean ± standard deviation) from baseline to each observation time point during the 12-week treatment period in the effectiveness analysis population. The number of patients at each time point is indicated by the SBP levels under the chart.

and 0.8%, respectively, and that of patients without concomitant use of ACE inhibitors or ARBs was 0.6% and 0.5%, respectively. The incidence of hyperkalemia among patients prescribed thiazide diuretics or loop diuretics together with eplerenone was 0% and 0.9%, respectively, and the incidence in patients treated without these drugs was 0.7% and 0.6%, respectively. The incidence of adverse drug reactions classified according to the concomitant antihypertensive medication is presented in the Supplementary Material (Table S2 to S9). Serious adverse events were seen in 15 among 2,355 patients who were taking concomitant antihypertensive medications at the time of initiation of eplerenone. The most frequent serious adverse events were hyperkalemia (8 cases) followed by renal impairment (3 cases).

3.3. Effectiveness

3.3.1. Blood Pressure Control. Of the 1,024 patients for whom the effect of eplerenone on BP was analyzed, the mean SBP and the mean DBP at baseline were 152.1 ± 19.0 mmHg and 85.8 ± 13.7 mmHg, respectively (Figure 1). The changes in

mean SBP and DBP from baseline to week 12 were −17.3 ± 18.4 mmHg (percent change from baseline: −10.6 ± 11.4%) and −8.1 ± 11.8 mmHg (−8.3 ± 13.4%), respectively. The changes in mean SBP and DBP from baseline to week 2 were −13.5 ± 18.1 and −6.7 ± 11.1 mmHg, respectively. The changes in SBP from baseline to week 12 in < 140 mmHg, 140 mmHg to < 160 mmHg, 160 mmHg to < 180 mmHg, and ≥ 180 mmHg groups were the following: −1.5 ± 14.7 mmHg, −15.6 ± 12.0 mmHg, −26.3 ± 15.5 mmHg, and −44.1 ± 19.6 mmHg (Figure 2). The BP changes from baseline were larger in the groups with higher baseline BP, and there was little change in the group with the lowest BP level at baseline.

4. Discussion

4.1. Subjects Included in the Analysis. Among the patients registered in this PMS, patients over 55 years of age accounted for approximately 80%, which is similar to the fraction of elderly hypertensive patients in Japan [2]. In this surveillance, more than 70% of the patients had been prescribed at least one antihypertensive drug at the time that eplerenone treatment was initiated. MRAs are not the first-line drugs recommended by the JSH 2009 or JSH 2014 guidelines [8], but they are recommended for treatment of resistant hypertension. This PMS showed that CCBs and ARBs, which are recommended as first-line drugs by the guidelines, were the most frequent drugs to be prescribed concomitantly with eplerenone.

4.2. Safety Analysis. In the current PMS, the most common ADRs were hyperkalemia (0.6%), dizziness (0.2%), renal impairment (0.2%), and increased serum potassium (0.2%). The ADRs most frequently observed in the clinical trials cited in the new-drug application of eplerenone in Japan included headache (6.1%), dizziness (2.6%), nausea (1.9%), hyperkalemia (1.7%), fatigue (1.6%), increased alanine aminotransferase (1.4%), increased gamma-glutamyl transferase (1.3%), indigestion (1.2%), increased aspartate aminotransferase (1.2%), muscle spasms (1.0%), and hyperuricemia (1.0%). The types of ADRs observed in this PMS were similar to those observed in the clinical trials, and no notable new ADRs were observed. The difference in the frequency of ADRs between the PMS and the clinical trials is attributable to differences in study design, as a PMS is an observational study and the clinical trials were interventional studies.

According to a survey by the Japanese Society of Nephrology [9], the frequency of CKD increases with age among Japanese men and women. In particular, most patients had stage 3 CKD (glomerular filtration rate: 30–59 mL/min/1.73 m^2): 15.6% of men in their 60s and 43.1% of men over 80 years of age. In this PMS, patients who were reported to have hyperkalemia or increased serum potassium accounted for 88.5% of patients aged 65 years or over, and 26.9% of patients aged 80 years or over. Retention of serum potassium is known to occur more frequently in patients with renal impairment. In this PMS, the occurrence of adverse events was more frequent in patients with renal impairment, and many of the events were hyperkalemia. Therefore, the results of this surveillance also suggest that patients with renal impairment are more prone to hyperkalemia and that serum potassium levels should be properly monitored according to the package insert. Regarding the change in serum potassium levels during the treatment period, it is possible that the physicians adjusted the eplerenone dosage or withdrew other potassium-retaining drugs that had been administered concomitantly in patients with high baseline serum potassium levels.

In this PMS, some patients were prescribed eplerenone even though they met the contraindication criteria for Selara tablets. Patients with a serum potassium value over 5.0 mEq/L comprised 1.9% of the safety analysis population. There were 14.8% patients whose CCr was less than 50 mL/min calculated from their sex, age, and weight by Pfizer Japan Inc. or judged by the physicians as having as moderate or severe renal impairment. In addition, patients with severe hepatic function comprised 0.2% of the safety analysis population. Clinicians should pay careful attention to the contraindications listed on the package insert when prescribing drugs and conducting regular monitoring of serum potassium levels.

The incidence of hypotension among patients prescribed antihypertensive drugs in addition to eplerenone was considered as not high and the symptoms were improved. Although the incidence of hyperkalemia tended to be higher among patients prescribed ACE inhibitors or ARBs concomitantly with eplerenone, it was considered within the scope of the package insert of Selara tablets. There was no tendency for the incidence of hyperkalemia to increase when eplerenone was used with either thiazide diuretics or loop diuretics. Therefore, we concluded that it is not necessary to call for special attention or implement new measures to ensure safety for concomitant use of eplerenone and other antihypertensive drugs.

4.3. Antihypertensive Effects. In an analysis of the antihypertensive effects of eplerenone based on the BP at baseline, the degree of BP reduction appeared to vary depending on the BP value at the time of initiation of eplerenone. Because we aimed to investigate the effects of the drugs in real-world settings and because the dosage of all of the antihypertensive drugs including eplerenone could have been modified, the results do not necessarily reflect the effects of eplerenone treatment alone.

However, considering that, on average, clinically significant effectiveness against hypertension was observed during the observation period, the effectiveness of eplerenone as an antihypertensive drug was shown under the conditions in which it is currently used.

Because a relatively large antihypertensive effect was observed immediately after initiation of eplerenone treatment followed by a gradual decrease in BP, a decrease of several mmHg after week 12 was expected. The finding that eplerenone gradually reduced BP over 2-3 months is consistent with a previous report [9]. The reason for the gradual decrease in BP and the antihypertensive effects of eplerenone may involve the complex mechanism of action of the drug. Aldosterone, a ligand for MRs, is a hormone involved in the reabsorption of sodium by the kidneys. However, recent studies have demonstrated that MRs are expressed in various organs including vascular endothelial and smooth muscle cells found in all cardiovascular tissues [10–14]. Therefore, various factors might contribute to BP reduction through MR blockade.

4.4. Organ Damage with Aldosterone. Recent studies have revealed that organ damage occurs in the cardiovascular system and kidneys when aldosterone coexists with high sodium. This organ damage includes ventricular remodeling [15, 16], renal impairment [17–19], and vascular endothelial dysfunction [20]. Furthermore, aldosterone, which exerts its activity in adipocytes, is involved in abnormal production/secretion of adipocytokines by adipocytes [21] and contributes to increases in oxidative stress [22] and decreases insulin sensitivity in adipose tissue [23, 24]. Eplerenone is thought to suppress the adverse effects of aldosterone in in various organs including the endothelium by inhibiting aldosterone activity through binding to MRs [25]; thus, eplerenone is a pharmacologically promising drug to prevent end organ damage induced by aldosterone.

4.5. Study Limitations. This surveillance has several limitations. First, PMSs including this study are not required to monitor the data consistency between the medical record and the data reported to the pharmaceutical company, although the data consistency within the case report forms is systematically confirmed. Second, as stated above, because the PMS does not restrict the administration of eplerenone or other antihypertensive drugs, the outcomes observed in this surveillance would reflect the overall consequences of antihypertensive treatments in real-world settings; thus, the treatment could have been changed based on observed AEs or change in blood pressure during the surveillance. Third, because there were no exclusion criteria in this study, patients with severe conditions such as active malignancy were not excluded, which might have affected the safety and efficacy parameters. Fourth, this PMS was conducted as a noninterventional study under real-world settings and the results should be interpreted within this context. For example, potassium concentration data were unavailable (unknown) in 877 subjects, which comprised 27.7% of the safety analysis population (Table 1), because the clinical data could only be collected when the lab tests were conducted in the usual care settings. Fifth, because the method for measuring BP was not standardized, that is, the measuring device and method varied at each institution, it is possible that the assessment of antihypertensive effects varied. However, even if this potential variability is taken into account, our results still showed a decrease in the mean SBP/DBP (17.3/8.1 mmHg); thus, the conclusion of a significant clinical difference would not be affected. Sixth, although this PMS was conducted in patients with essential hypertension, patients with secondary hypertension such as primary aldosteronism (PA) may have also been included without a definite diagnosis. Because PA responds well to MRAs, inclusion of such patients might have contributed to a reduction in the mean BP to some extent. However, as the prevalence of PA is only approximately 10% among patients with essential hypertension [26], the influence on the mean BP would not be substantial. Despite these limitations, this PMS has provided important information regarding the effect of eplerenone in patients with essential hypertension in real-world settings.

5. Conclusions

In this PMS, patients treated with eplerenone showed a marked blood pressure reduction over 12 weeks after initiation of treatment. There was no significant difference in the type or incidence of ADRs in this surveillance compared to results reported prior to approval of the drug. With respect to hyperkalemia, the current PMS confirmed that it is important to adhere to the contraindications stated on the package insert. Eplerenone is contraindicated in patients with CCr < 50 mL/min; administration should be very carefully conducted in the elderly. Because recent studies have revealed that aldosterone can contribute to organ damage (e.g., damage to the heart and kidneys), the use of a selective MRA such as eplerenone can provide benefit for patients who need antihypertensive treatment.

Competing Interests

Shoko Takahashi, Megumi Hiramatsu, Shinichi Hotta, Yukie Watanabe, Osamu Suga, and Yutaka Endo are employed by Pfizer Japan Inc. Isamu Miyamori has received honoraria for lectures from Pfizer Japan Inc.

Acknowledgments

This PMS was sponsored by Pfizer Japan Inc. Planning, data collection, and data analyses of the PMS were performed by Pfizer Japan Inc. The authors would like to thank all of the physicians who participated in this surveillance and provided valuable information. They also thank Cactus Communications for their editorial support. This study was funded by Pfizer Japan Inc., Tokyo, Japan.

References

[1] "Office of Nutrition Cancer Measures and Health Promotion Division Health Service, Ministry of Health, Labour and Welfare, Japan," 2013, http://www.mhlw.go.jp/bunya/kenkou/eiyou/dl/h25-houkokus.pdf.

[2] K. Shimamoto, K. Ando, T. Fujita et al., "The Japanese Society of Hypertension guidelines for the management of hypertension (JSH 2014)," *Hypertension Research*, vol. 37, no. 4, pp. 253–390, 2014.

[3] P. A. James, S. Oparil, B. L. Carter et al., "2014 evidence-based guideline for the management of high blood pressure in adults: report from the panel members appointed to the Eighth Joint National Committee (JNC 8)," *Journal of the American Medical Association*, vol. 311, no. 5, pp. 507–520, 2014.

[4] A. S. Go, M. A. Bauman, S. M. Coleman King et al., "An effective approach to high blood pressure control: a science advisory from the American Heart Association, the American College Of Cardiology, and the Centers for Disease Control and Prevention," *Hypertension*, vol. 63, no. 4, pp. 878–885, 2014.

[5] G. Mancia, R. Fagard, K. Narkiewicz et al., "2013 ESH/ESC guidelines for the management of arterial hypertension: the Task Force for the management of arterial hypertension of the European Society of Hypertension (ESH) and of the European Society of Cardiology (ESC)," *Journal of Hypertension*, vol. 34, no. 28, pp. 2159–2219, 2013.

[6] M. Lainscak, F. Pelliccia, G. Rosano et al., "Safety profile of mineralocorticoid receptor antagonists: spironolactone and eplerenone," *International Journal of Cardiology*, vol. 200, pp. 25–29, 2015.

[7] Selara, *Selara® Tablets 25 mg, Selara® Tablets 50 mg, Selara® Tablets 100 mg*, Pfizer Japan, Tokyo, Japan, 2011 (Japanese).

[8] T. Ogihara, K. Kikuchi, H. Matsuoka et al., "The Japanese Society of Hypertension guidelines for the management of hypertension (JSH 2009)," *Hypertension Research*, vol. 32, no. 1, pp. 3–107, 2009.

[9] Japan Nephrology Society, "Special issue: clinical practice guidebook for diagnosis and treatment of chronic kidney disease 2012," *Nihon Jinzo Gakkai Shi*, vol. 54, no. 8, pp. 1034–1191, 2012 (Japanese).

[10] W. J. Meyer III and N. R. Nichols, "Mineralocorticoid binding in cultured smooth muscle cells and fibroblasts from rat aorta," *Journal of Steroid Biochemistry*, vol. 14, no. 11, pp. 1157–1168, 1981.

[11] J. W. Funder, P. T. Pearce, R. Smith, and J. Campbell, "Vascular type I aldosterone binding sites are physiological mineralocorticoid receptors," *Endocrinology*, vol. 125, no. 4, pp. 2224–2226, 1989.

[12] M. Lombes, M.-E. Oblin, J.-M. Gasc, E. E. Baulieu, N. Farman, and J.-P. Bonvalet, "Immunohistochemical and biochemical evidence for a cardiovascular mineralocorticoid receptor," *Circulation Research*, vol. 71, no. 3, pp. 503–510, 1992.

[13] M. Lombès, N. Alfaidy, E. Eugene, A. Lessana, N. Farman, and J.-P. Bonvalet, "Prerequisite for cardiac aldosterone action: mineralocorticoid receptor and 11β-hydroxysteroid dehydrogenase in the human heart," *Circulation*, vol. 92, no. 2, pp. 175–182, 1995.

[14] M. Lombès, N. Farman, J. P. Bonvalet, and M.-C. Zennaro, "Identification and role of aldosterone receptors in the cardiovascular system," *Annales d'Endocrinologie*, vol. 61, no. 1, pp. 41–46, 2000.

[15] M. Yamamuro, M. Yoshimura, M. Nakayama et al., "Direct effects of aldosterone on cardiomyocytes in the presence of normal and elevated extracellular sodium," *Endocrinology*, vol. 147, no. 3, pp. 1314–1321, 2006.

[16] A. Urabe, T. Izumi, Y. Abe, I. Taniguchi, and S. Mochizuki, "Effects of eplerenone and salt intake on left ventricular remodeling after myocardial infarction in rats," *Hypertension Research*, vol. 29, no. 8, pp. 627–634, 2006.

[17] E. R. Blasi, R. Rocha, A. E. Rudolph, E. A. G. Blomme, M. L. Polly, and E. G. McMahon, "Aldosterone/salt induces renal inflammation and fibrosis in hypertensive rats," *Kidney International*, vol. 63, no. 5, pp. 1791–1800, 2003.

[18] A. Nishiyama, L. Yao, Y. Nagai et al., "Possible contributions of reactive oxygen species and mitogen-activated protein kinase to renal injury in aldosterone/salt-induced hypertensive rats," *Hypertension*, vol. 43, no. 4, pp. 841–848, 2004.

[19] W. Kawarazaki, M. Nagase, S. Yoshida et al., "Angiotensin II- and salt-induced kidney injury through Rac1-mediated mineralocorticoid receptor activation," *Journal of the American Society of Nephrology*, vol. 23, no. 6, pp. 997–1007, 2012.

[20] N. de las Heras, M. Ruiz-Ortega, M. Miana et al., "Interactions between aldosterone and connective tissue growth factor in vascular and renal damage in spontaneously hypertensive rats," *Journal of Hypertension*, vol. 25, no. 3, pp. 629–638, 2007.

[21] D. Kraus, J. Jäger, B. Meier, M. Fasshauer, and J. Klein, "Aldosterone inhibits uncoupling protein-1, induces insulin resistance, and stimulates proinflammatory adipokines in adipocytes," *Hormone and Metabolic Research*, vol. 37, no. 7, pp. 455–459, 2005.

[22] A. Hirata, N. Maeda, A. Hiuge et al., "Blockade of mineralocorticoid receptor reverses adipocyte dysfunction and insulin resistance in obese mice," *Cardiovascular Research*, vol. 84, no. 1, pp. 164–172, 2009.

[23] R. Garg, S. Hurwitz, G. H. Williams, P. N. Hopkins, and G. K. Adler, "Aldosterone production and insulin resistance in healthy adults," *Journal of Clinical Endocrinology and Metabolism*, vol. 95, no. 4, pp. 1986–1990, 2010.

[24] C. Catena, R. Lapenna, S. Baroselli et al., "Insulin sensitivity in patients with primary aldosteronism: A Follow-Up Study," *Journal of Clinical Endocrinology and Metabolism*, vol. 91, no. 9, pp. 3457–3463, 2006.

[25] K. Eguchi, T. Kabutoya, S. Hoshide, S. Ishikawa, and K. Kario, "Add-on use of eplerenone is effective for lowering home and ambulatory blood pressure in drug-resistant hypertension," *The Journal of Clinical Hypertension*, 2016.

[26] J. W. Funder, "Primary aldosteronism and salt," *Pflugers Archiv*, vol. 467, no. 3, pp. 587–594, 2015.

8

Value of Assessing Autonomic Nervous Function by Heart Rate Variability and Heart Rate Turbulence in Hypertensive Patients

Yijun Yu, Yanling Xu, Mingjing Zhang, Yuting Wang, Wusong Zou, and Ye Gu ⓘ

Department of Cardiology, Wuhan Fourth Hospital, Puai Hospital Affiliated to Tongji Medical College, Huazhong University of Science and Technology, Wuhan 430030, China

Correspondence should be addressed to Ye Gu; yegu2003cn@163.com

Guest Editor: Chengxing Shen

Purpose. To explore the relationship between blood pressure control and autonomic nervous function assessing by heart rate variability (HRV) and heart rate turbulence (HRT) in hypertensive patients. *Methods.* A total of 120 consecutive hypertensive patients and 80 nonhypertensive patients (N-HP group) were enrolled in this study. The hypertensive patients were divided into controlled blood pressure and uncontrolled blood pressure groups according to their blood pressure on admission. All subjects underwent 24-hour Holter monitoring. This study compared HRV and HRT in nonhypertensive and hypertensive patients and hypertensive patients with controlled and uncontrolled blood pressure. HRV parameters include square root of mean of the sum of squares of successive NN interval differences (rMSSD), number of successive NN intervals differing by > 50ms divided by the total number of successive NN intervals (pNN50), very low frequency (VLF) at frequency between 0.0033 and 0.04 Hz, low frequency (LF) at frequency between 0.04 and 0.15 Hz, and high frequency (HF) at frequency between 0.15 and 0.4 Hz. Turbulence slope (TS) belongs to HRT parameters. *Results.* TS, rMSSD, pNN50, VLF, LF, and HF values were significantly lower in the HP group than in the N-HP group. Multiple logistic regression analysis showed that reduced TS, rMSSD, pNN50, LF, and HF values were risk factors of hypertension. TS, rMSSD, pNN50, VLF, LF, and HF values were significantly lower in hypertensive patients with uncontrolled blood pressure than in hypertensive patients with controlled blood pressure. Multiple logistic regression analysis showed that reduced TS, rMSSD, pNN50, VLF, LF, and HF values were risk factors for uncontrolled blood pressure. *Conclusions.* This study indicates impaired autonomic nervous function in hypertensive patients, especially in hypertensive patients with uncontrolled blood pressure despite guideline recommended antihypertensive medications.

1. Introduction

Hypertension is a major disease that damages people's health. Long-term hypertension could impair major organs such as heart, brain, kidneys, and blood vessels, which is related to considerable mortality [1]. Sympathetic overactivation and autonomous imbalance play important roles in the pathogenesis of hypertension. Heart rate variability (HRV) and heart rate turbulence (HRT) reflect the autonomic regulation of cardiac function. HRV is the response of autonomic nervous system to external environmental stimuli, and HRT is the response to autonomic nervous function triggered by endogenous ventricular premature beat. Abnormal HRV and HRT reflected autonomous imbalance and were related to worse cardiovascular outcome [2–5]. Abnormal HRV or

HRT was demonstrated in hypertensive patients in previous studies [6–8]. However, there was scantly research on the relationship between HRV, HRT, and blood pressure control with hypertensive patients. The present study analyzed the HRV and HRT between nonhypertensive (N-HP) patients and hypertensive patients and between hypertensive patients with uncontrolled blood pressure and controlled blood pressure after hypertensive medication.

2. Materials and Methods

2.1. Study Population. A total of 120 consecutive hospitalized hypertensive patients and 80 N-HP patients were included in this retrospective study from June 2016 to June 2018. The hypertensive patients were divided into controlled blood pressure (n=66) and uncontrolled blood pressure (n=54) groups according to their blood pressure on admission.

Patients with Diabetes Mellitus (DM), Acute Coronary Syndrome (ACS), valvular heart disease and known non-ischemic cardiomyopathy, atrial fibrillation, atrial flutter, 2nd- or 3rd-degree atrioventricular block, and pacemaker implantation and patients without premature ventricular contraction (PVC) of 24-hour Holter monitoring were excluded. All hypertensive patients received antihypertensive medication. All patients gave informed consent for participation in this study, and the study protocol was approved by the ethical committees of Wuhan Fourth Hospital, Puai Hospital affiliated to Tongji Medical College, Huazhong University of Science and Technology, Wuhan, China.

2.2. HRV Analysis. All participants underwent 24-hour Holter monitoring (GE MARS Software and Seer Light recording box). Quantitative HRV analysis was performed according to the guidelines of the European Society of Cardiology and the North American Society of Pacing and Electrophysiology [9]. HRV parameters were derived from Holter monitoring including time domain and frequency domain. The following four time domain and four frequency domain indexes were analyzed: standard deviation of NN intervals (SDNN), standard deviation of all 5-minute average NN intervals (SDANN), square root of mean of the sum of squares of successive NN interval differences (rMSSD), number of successive NN intervals differing by > 50ms divided by the total number of successive NN intervals (pNN50), very low frequency (VLF) at frequency between 0.0033 and 0.04 Hz, low frequency (LF) at frequency between 0.04 and 0.15 Hz, high frequency (HF) at frequency between 0.15 and 0.4 Hz, and low frequency/high frequency ratio (LF/HF).

2.3. HRT Analysis. HRT parameters were also derived from Holter monitoring including turbulence onset (TO) and turbulence slope (TS). TO was the amount of sinus acceleration following a PVC. TO was expressed as a percentage and was calculated with the following formula: TO (%) = 100 × [(RR1 + RR2) − (RR−1 +RR−2)]/(RR−1 + RR−2), where RR1 and RR2 were the first and second sinus RR intervals after the PVC, and RR−1 and RR−2 were the first and second sinus intervals preceding the PVC. TO value < 0% indicated early sinus acceleration and was considered normal. TO ≥ 0% indicated that normal sinus heart rate acceleration phenomenon after PVC disappeared and was described as abnormal [5]. TS was late deceleration phenomenon of sinus rhythm after PVC following the sinus acceleration. TS was defined as the maximum regression slope measured on any 5- consecutive sinus beats within the first 15-sinus intervals after a PVC. TS could not be calculated when there were fewer than 15-sinus beats after the PVC. TS value > 2.5 ms/RR interval indicated the normal expected late deceleration. TS ≤ 2.5 ms/RR interval is described as abnormal [5]. TO and TS were computed as an average of the responses to all PVC on Holter record.

2.4. Statistical Analysis. Continuous data were presented as mean ± standard deviation (SD). Normal distribution of continuous variables was performed by Kolmogorov-Smirnov test. Continuous variables with normal distribution were assessed by Student's *t*-test. Nonnormal distribution data were tested by two-tailed Mann–Whitney *U* test. The chi-square test was used to compare categorical variables as percentages. The risk factors for hypertension were determined by multivariate logistic regression model after adjusting for age, gender, and beta-blockers use. Spearman correlation analysis of the hypertensive patients was performed between HRV and HRT. *P* values less than 0.05 were considered statistically significant. Statistical analyses were performed using IBM SPSS (version 22.0) for Windows (SPSS).

3. Results

3.1. Clinical Features of Patients in N-HP and HP Groups. BMI, triglyceride level, interventricular septum (IVS) thickness, and incidence of stable CAD were significantly higher in the HP group compared to the N-HP group. Blood pressure on admission was significantly higher in the HP group compared to the N-HP group. The proportions of beta-blockers and diuretics uses were higher in the HP group than in the N-HP group (Table 1). TS, rMSSD, pNN50, VLF, LF, and HF values were significantly lower in the HP group than in the N-HP group (Figure 1). Multiple regression analysis showed that history of stable CAD, higher BMI, and reduced TS, rMSSD, pNN50, LF, and HF values were risk factors of hypertension after adjusting for gender, age, and beta-blockers use (Table 2).

3.2. Clinical Features of Hypertensive Patients with Controlled and Uncontrolled Blood Pressure. The percentage of hypertensive patients receiving combined antihypertensive drug therapy was significantly higher and percentage of patients treating with monotherapy was significantly lower in hypertensive patients with uncontrolled blood pressure compared to hypertensive patients with controlled blood pressure (Table 3). TS, rMSSD, pNN50, VLF, LF, and HF values were significantly lower in hypertensive patients with uncontrolled blood pressure compared to hypertensive patients with controlled blood pressure (Figure 2). Multiple logistic regression analysis showed that reduced TS, rMSSD, pNN50, VLF, LF, and HF values were risk factors for blood pressure control after adjusting for age, gender, and beta-blockers use (Table 4).

3.3. Spearman Correlation of HRV and HRT for Hypertensive Patients. Spearman correlation analysis of the hypertensive patients showed that LF and LF/HF were negatively correlated with TO, while SDNN, SDANN, rMSSD, PNN50, VLF, LF, and HF were positively correlated with TS (Table 5).

4. Discussion

The present study found that TS, rMSSD, pNN50, VLF, LF, and HF values were significantly lower in hypertensive patients compared to N-HP patients, and TS, rMSSD,

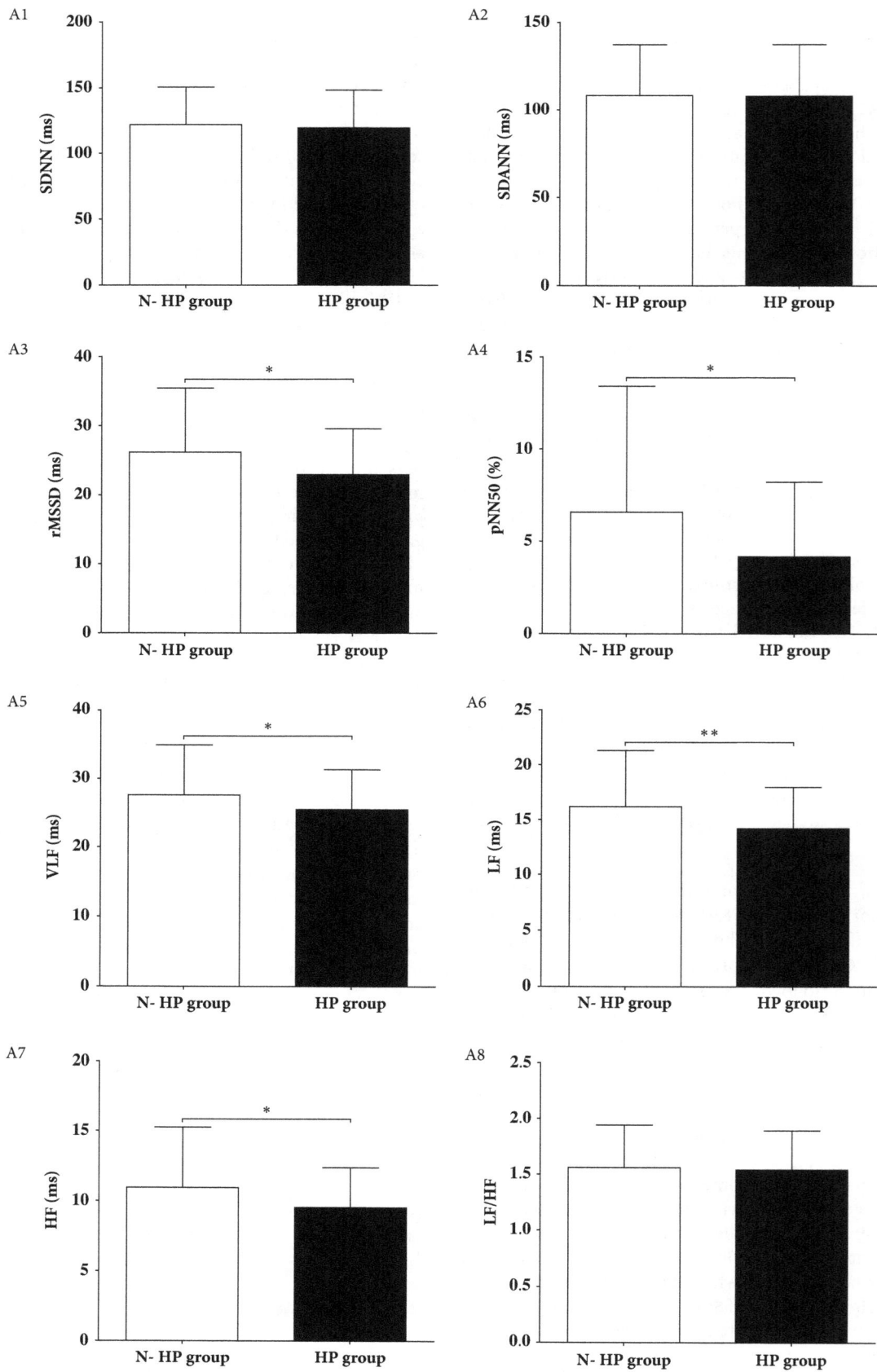

FIGURE 1: Continued.

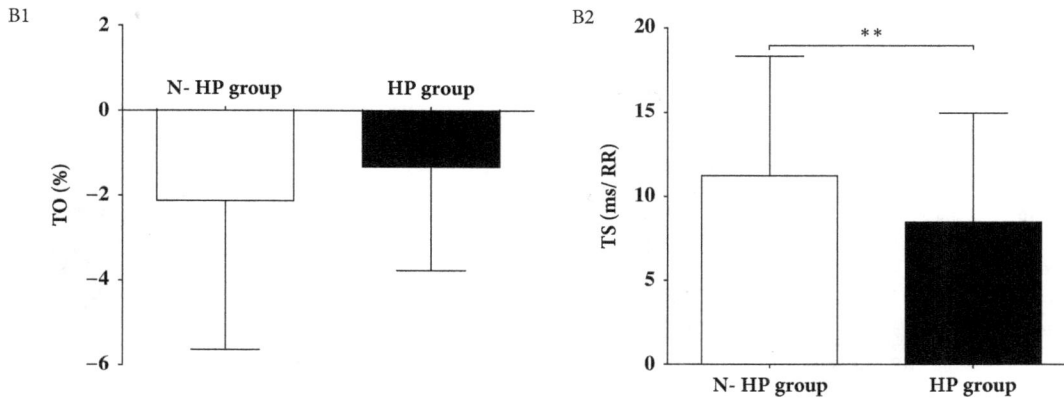

FIGURE 1: HRV and HRT analysis of N-HP and HP groups; *P<0.05; **P<0.01. HRV, heart rate variability; HRT, heart rate turbulence; N-HP, nonhypertensive; HP, hypertensive; SDNN, standard deviation of NN intervals; SDANN, standard deviation of all 5-minute average NN intervals; rMSSD, square root of mean of the sum of squares of successive NN interval differences; pNN50, number of successive NN intervals differing by >50ms divided by the total number of successive NN intervals; VLF, very low frequency; LF, low frequency; HF, high frequency; TO, turbulence onset; TS, turbulence slope.

TABLE 1: Clinical characteristic of N-HP group and HP group.

	N-HP group (n=80)	HP group (n=120)	P value
Age (yr)	56.66±6.62	58.05±7.55	0.183
Male gender (n, %)	39/80 (48.5%)	54/120 (45.0%)	0.602
BMI (kg/m^2)	23.60±2.78	25.20±3.29	<0.0001
Smoker (n, %)	21/80 (26.3%)	40/120 (33.3%)	0.286
Stable CAD (n, %)	12/80 (15.0%)	37/120 (30.8%)	0.011
Dyslipidemia (n, %)	64/80 (80.0%)	105/120 (87.5%)	0.151
Systolic blood pressure (mmHg)	118.50±11.75	134.98±14.95	<0.0001
Diastolic blood pressure (mmHg)	76.10±7.48	81.98±10.15	<0.0001
Heart rate (bpm)	74.18±6.62	73.11±8.16	0.307
Creatinine (μM)	67.44±16.33	67.34±14.63	0.839
CHOL (mM)	4.67±0.91	4.83±1.00	0.228
TG (mM)	1.59±0.98	2.13±2.10	0.002
LDL-c (mM)	2.96±0.83	2.92±0.82	0.742
HDL-c (mM)	1.09±0.25	1.10±0.27	0.848
Ejection fraction (%)	61.61±4.95	61.91±5.17	0.657
LVEDd (cm)	4.39±0.39	4.40±0.44	0.843
IVS (cm)	0.93±0.12	0.99±0.19	0.010
Medication			
Bata-blockers use (n, %)	23/80 (28.8%)	60/120 (50.0%)	0.003
Diuretics use (n, %)	0/80 (0.0%)	12/120 (10.0%)	0.009

N-HP, nonhypertensive; HP, hypertensive; BMI, body mass index; CAD, coronary artery disease; CHOL, cholesterol; TG, triglyceride; LDL-c, low-density lipoprotein cholesterol; HDL-c, high-density lipoprotein cholesterol; LVEDd, left ventricular end diastolic diameter; IVS, interventricular septum.

pNN50, VLF, LF, and HF values were significantly lower in hypertensive patients with uncontrolled blood pressure compared to hypertensive patients with controlled blood pressure. Our study results thus indicate impaired autonomic nervous function in hypertensive patients, especially in hypertensive patients with uncontrolled blood pressure despite guideline recommended antihypertensive medications. To the best of our knowledge, this is the first study describing the association between autonomic nervous function, evaluated by HRV and HRT changes, and blood pressure control in hypertensive patients.

4.1. Reduced HRV and HRT in Hypertensive Patients. HRV and HRT changes could reflect sympathetic and vagal function in hypertensive patients. HRV reflects the fluctuation of heart rate as time changes in response to external environmental stimulation; HRV changes were related to various cardiovascular diseases [3]. HRT reflects the start

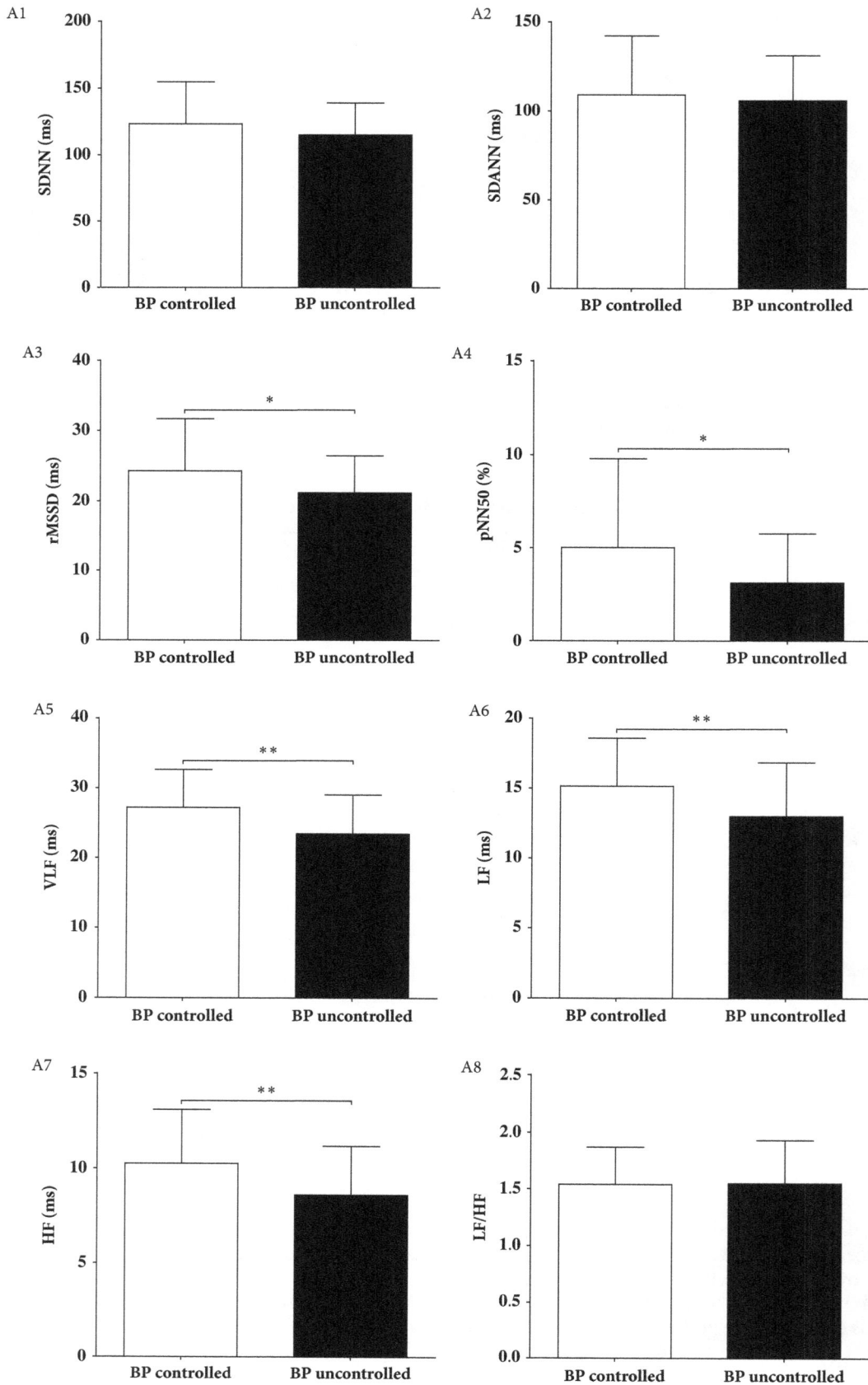

FIGURE 2: Continued.

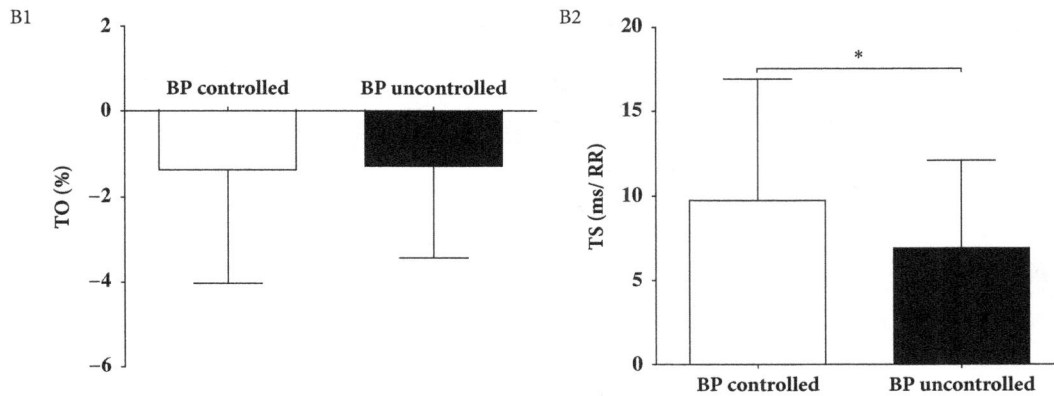

FIGURE 2: HRV and HRT analysis of BP controlled and BP uncontrolled groups, $*P<0.05$; $**P<0.01$. HRV, heart rate variability; HRT, heart rate turbulence; BP, blood pressure; SDNN, standard deviation of NN intervals; SDANN, standard deviation of all 5-minute average NN intervals; rMSSD, square root of mean of the sum of squares of successive NN interval differences; pNN50, number of successive NN intervals differing by >50ms divided by the total number of successive NN intervals; VLF, very low frequency; LF, low frequency; HF, high frequency; TO, turbulence onset; TS, turbulence slope.

TABLE 2: Multivariate logistic regression results for risk of hypertension.

	B	S.E	Wald	P value	Exp	95% CI lower limit	95% CI upper limit
BMI	0.196	0.053	13.788	0.000	1.217	1.097	1.350
Stable CAD	0.832	0.395	4.431	0.035	2.297	1.059	4.982
TG	0.413	0.163	6.387	0.011	1.511	1.097	2.082
rMSSD (ms)	0.044	0.020	4.804	0.028	1.045	1.005	1.086
pNN50 (%)	0.070	0.031	5.249	0.022	1.073	1.010	1.139
VLF (ms)	0.039	0.024	2.716	0.099	1.041	0.993	1.091
LF (ms)	0.100	0.037	7.187	0.007	1.105	1.027	1.189
HF (ms)	0.096	0.046	4.356	0.037	1.100	1.006	1.203
TS (ms/ RR)	0.055	0.023	5.684	0.017	1.057	1.010	1.106

BMI, body mass index; CAD, coronary artery disease; TG, triglyceride; rMSSD, square root of mean of the sum of squares of successive NN interval differences; pNN50, number of successive NN intervals differing by >50ms divided by the total number of successive NN intervals; VLF, very low frequency; LF, low frequency; HF, high frequency; TS, turbulence slope.

acceleration and the late deceleration of the heart rate after ventricular premature contraction and refers the endogenous stimulus triggered pressure reflex regulation and could also be used to evaluate the balance and coordination of the cardiac autonomic nervous system [5]. Combined analysis with HRV and HRT parameters makes it possible to comprehensively evaluate the autonomic nervous system regulation and response status to internal and external stimuli in hypertensive patients. Pal and colleagues [7] demonstrated enhanced sympathetic nerve activity and inhibited vagal activity in prehypertensive patients and found that the vagal inhibition was more prominent than sympathetic overactivity in hypertensive patients. Erdem [10] explored the relationship between autonomic nervous regulation and blood pressure in prehypertensive patients and found that TO was significantly higher and TS was significantly lower in nondipper blood pressure group than in dipper blood pressure group, hinting at impaired autonomous balance in prehypertensive patients with nondipper blood pressure. Another study [11] reported that heart rate was increased and HRV was decreased in patients with refractory hypertension, suggesting that overactivation of the sympathetic nervous system might play an important role in patients with refractory hypertension. In a previous study [12], we demonstrated significant differences on autonomous balance in hypertensive patients with controlled and uncontrolled blood pressure. The present study showed that TS (reflecting vagus function triggered by endogenous ventricular premature beat [13]), rMSSD (reflecting vagus function by external environmental stimuli [14]), pNN50 (reflecting vagus function by external environmental stimuli [14]), VLF (reflecting sympathetic activity by external environmental stimuli [15]), LF (reflecting balance of sympathetic and vagal activity [14]), and HF (reflecting vagus function by external environmental stimuli [14]) values were significantly lower in hypertensive patients compared to N-HP patients, and TS, rMSSD, pNN50, VLF, LF, and HF values were also significantly lower in hypertensive patients with uncontrolled blood pressure compared to hypertensive patients with controlled blood pressure. This novel finding demonstrated that autonomic nervous function was impaired

TABLE 3: Clinical characteristics of hypertensive patients with controlled blood pressure group and uncontrolled blood pressure group.

	BP controlled group (n=66)	BP uncontrolled group (n=54)	P value
Age (yr)	57.03±6.81	59.30±8.26	0.109
Male gender (n, %)	27/66 (40.9%)	27/54 (50.0%)	0.319
BMI (kg/m^2)	25.19±3.34	25.22±3.25	0.954
Smoker (n, %)	20/66 (30.3%)	20/54 (37.0%)	0.436
Stable CAD (n, %)	18/66 (27.3%)	19/54 (35.1%)	0.350
Dyslipidemia (n, %)	58/66 (87.9%)	47/54 (87.0%)	0.890
SBP (mmHg)	124.97±9.72	147.20±10.45	<0.0001
DBP (mmHg)	78.02±7.43	86.82±10.97	0.000
Heart rate (bpm)	72.35±8.27	74.03±8.00	0.364
Creatinine (μM)	67.14±14.87	67.59±14.46	0.867
CHOL (mM)	4.83±0.93	4.84±1.08	0.945
TG (mM)	2.00±1.49	2.29±2.68	0.663
LDL-c (mM)	2.97±0.81	2.86±0.84	0.472
HDL-c (mM)	1.11±0.25	1.09±0.30	0.436
Ejection fraction (%)	62.33±4.78	61.39±5.60	0.321
LVEDd (cm)	4.40±0.48	4.41±0.39	0.907
IVS (cm)	1.00±0.15	1.00±0.22	0.891
Medication			
Bata-blockers (n, %)	32/66 (48.5%)	28/54 (51.9%)	0.714
ACEI (n, %)	14/66 (21.2%)	12/54 (22.2%)	0.894
ARBs (n, %)	19/66 (28.8%)	23/54 (42.6%)	0.115
CCB (n, %)	37/66 (56.1%)	39/54 (72.2%)	0.068
Diuretics (n, %)	6/66 (9.1%)	6/54 (11.1%)	0.714
Categories of drugs			0.021
Monotherapy (n,%)	32/66 (48.5%)	15/54 (27.7%)	
≥Two-drug therapy (n, %)	34/66 (51.5%)	39/54 (72.2%)	

BP, blood pressure; BMI, body mass index; CAD, coronary artery disease; SBP, systolic blood pressure; DBP, diastolic blood pressure; CHOL, cholesterol; TG, triglyceride; LDL-c, low-density lipoprotein cholesterol; HDL-c, high-density lipoprotein cholesterol; LVEDd, left ventricular end diastolic diameter; IVS, interventricular septum; ACEI, angiotensin-converting enzyme inhibitor; ARBs, angiotensin receptor blocker; CCB, calcium channel blocker.

TABLE 4: Multivariate logistic regression results for risk of uncontrolled blood pressure.

	B	S.E	Wald	P value	Exp	95% CI lower limit	95% CI upper limit
rMSSD (ms)	0.073	0.032	5.363	0.021	1.075	1.011	1.144
pNN50 (%)	0.131	0.058	5.130	0.024	1.140	1.017	1.277
VLF (ms)	0.128	0.038	11.358	0.001	1.136	1.055	1.225
LF (ms)	0.166	0.058	8.245	0.004	1.181	1.054	1.321
HF (ms)	0.213	0.076	7.957	0.005	1.238	1.067	1.435
TS (ms/ RR)	0.071	0.034	4.453	0.035	1.073	1.005	1.147

rMSSD, square root of mean of the sum of squares of successive NN interval differences; pNN50, number of successive NN intervals differing by >50ms divided by the total number of successive NN intervals; VLF, very low frequency; LF, low frequency; HF, high frequency; TS, turbulence slope.

in hypertensive patients compared to N-HP patients. Moreover, autonomic nervous function damage was more severe in hypertensive patients with uncontrolled blood pressure than in hypertensive patients with controlled blood pressure, as expressed by sympathetic overactivity and vagal withdrawal triggered by external environmental stimuli and vagal withdrawal triggered by endogenous ventricular premature beat. In our study, the percentage of hypertensive patients receiving combined antihypertensive drug therapy was significantly higher and percentage of patients treated with monotherapy was significantly lower in hypertensive patients with uncontrolled blood pressure compared to hypertensive patients with controlled blood pressure, indicating that the uncontrolled blood pressure observed in our patient cohort is probably not due to the insufficient hypertensive medication; future studies are warranted to explore the role of the

TABLE 5: Spearman correlation analysis of HRV and HRT in HP patients.

	TO		TS	
	r value	P value	r value	P value
SDNN	-0.008	0.930	0.298	0.001
SDANN	0.023	0.800	0.260	0.004
rMSSD	0.006	0.945	0.292	0.001
pNN50	-0.012	0.895	0.228	0.012
VLF	-0.143	0.120	0.438	<0.0001
LF	-0.237	0.009	0.441	<0.0001
HF	-0.027	0.767	0.343	<0.0001
LF/HF	-0.241	0.008	0.095	0.301

HRV, heart rate variability; HRT, heart rate turbulence; HP, hypertensive; SDNN, standard deviation of NN intervals; SDANN, standard deviation of all 5-minute average NN intervals; rMSSD, square root of mean of the sum of squares of successive NN interval differences; pNN50, number of successive NN intervals differing by >50ms divided by the total number of successive NN intervals; VLF, very low frequency; LF, low frequency; HF, high frequency; TO, turbulence onset; TS, turbulence slope.

more severe autonomous function impairment in hypertensive patients with uncontrolled blood pressure despite the treatment of guideline recommended antihypertensive medications and to see if options targeting the autonomic nervous function might help the blood pressure control on top of combined antihypertensive therapy [16].

Previous studies found that DM and beta-blockers use might affect the HRV [15, 17]. Patients with DM were thus excluded in our study. Results of logistic regression analysis showed that reduced TS, rMSSD, pNN50, VLF, LF, and HF values were risk factors for uncontrolled blood pressure after adjusting for age, gender, and beta-blockers use. Therefore, the difference in HRV and HRT values between the uncontrolled and controlled blood pressure groups was unlikely induced by beta-blockers use.

HRV mainly reflected the interaction between neural modulatory and sinus node function, while HRT could be considered as parameter reflecting the physiological response to endogenous stimulus. Spearman correlation analysis between HRV and HRT showed that LF and LF/HF were negatively correlated with TO, and SDNN, SDANN, rMSSD, PNN50, VLF, LF, and HF were positively correlated with TS, which suggested the close correlation between HRV and TS, and HRV and HRT could be considered as complementary parameters reflecting autonomic nervous function change.

4.2. Clinical Implications. Impaired autonomic function played an important role in the pathogenesis of hypertension. Long-term sympathetic excitation might lead to left ventricular remodeling and atherosclerosis. Poreba et al. [8] found that TO was significantly higher and TS was significantly lower in hypertensive patients with left ventricular hypertrophy than in hypertensive patients without left ventricular hypertrophy. Therefore, the detection of autonomic nervous function in hypertensive patients might be useful in predicting the target organ damage in hypertensive patients. Abnormal HRV and HRT in hypertensive patients might suggest the presence of autonomic nervous system dysfunction. The present results found abnormal HRV and HRT in hypertensive patients, especially in hypertensive patients with uncontrolled blood pressure. It is thus clinically

important to monitor HRV and HRT during antihypertensive therapy, aiming to improve the autonomic nervous system function in hypertensive patients, which might reduce the incidence of target organ damage and improve the prognosis of hypertensive patients.

4.3. Study Limitations. There were some limitations in this study. First, this was a retrospective single-center clinical study with a small number of patients. Our results need to be confirmed by a multicenter prospective clinical study with larger patient cohort to explore the impact of autonomic nervous dysfunction on prognosis of hypertensive patients. Second, HRV and HRT evaluation was not suitable to hypertensive patients with nonsinus rhythm such as atrial fibrillation, atrial flutter or pacemaker implantation, or 2nd- or 3rd-degree atrioventricular block and without PVC on Holter monitoring. Third, we did not quantify cardiac remodeling parameters including left ventricular posterior wall thickness and diastolic function parameters as E/A and E/e' in this patient cohort. Finally, this study did not analyze potential impact of the disease stage as well as the duration of antihypertensive medication on HRV and HRT because many elderly patients in this patient cohort could not provide us with the inquired data. Above study limitations should be considered when interpreting results demonstrated in this study.

5. Conclusions

The present study shows that autonomic nervous dysfunction, as expressed by reduced HRV and HRT, exists in hypertensive patients, especially in hypertensive patients with uncontrolled blood pressure. Monitoring HRV and HRT parameters, which jointly reflect autonomic nervous system's regulation and response to internal and external stimuli, might be helpful to evaluate the autonomic nervous function status of the patients and supply useful information to optimize therapeutic efficacy aiming to improve autonomic nervous function balance for hypertensive patients. Future studies are warranted to explore if targeting the autonomic nervous function on top of antihypertensive medication might obtain better clinical efficacy on blood pressure control for patients with refractory hypertension.

Acknowledgments

This work was supported by the Natural Science Foundation of Hubei Province, China (Grant no. 2018CFB761).

References

[1] A. V. Chobanian, "Time to reassess blood-pressure goals," *The New England Journal of Medicine*, vol. 373, no. 22, pp. 2093–2095, 2015.

[2] H. V. Huikuri and P. K. Stein, "Heart rate variability in risk stratification of cardiac patients," *Progress in Cardiovascular Diseases*, vol. 56, no. 2, pp. 153–159, 2013.

[3] F. Lombardi and P. K. Stein, "Origin of heart rate variability a ap nd turbulence: an praisal of autonomic modulation of cardiovascular function," *Frontiers in Physiology*, vol. 2, p. 95, 2011.

[4] P. K. Stein, J. I. Barzilay, P. H. M. Chaves, P. P. Domitrovich, and J. S. Gottdiener, "Heart rate variability and its changes over 5 years in older adults," *Age and Ageing*, vol. 38, no. 2, pp. 212–218, 2009.

[5] G. Schmidt, M. Malik, P. Barthel et al., "Heart-rate turbulence after ventricular premature beats as a predictor of mortality after acute myocardial infarction," *The Lancet*, vol. 353, no. 9162, pp. 1390–1396, 1999.

[6] A. De La Sierra, D. A. Calhoun, E. Vinyoles et al., "Heart rate and heart rate variability in resistant versus controlled hypertension and in true versus white-coat resistance," *Journal of Human Hypertension*, vol. 28, no. 7, pp. 416–420, 2014.

[7] G. K. Pal, C. Adithan, D. Amudharaj et al., "Assessment of sympathovagal imbalance by spectral analysis of heart rate variability in prehypertensive and hypertensive patients in indian population," *Clinical and Experimental Hypertension*, vol. 33, no. 7, pp. 478–483, 2011.

[8] R. Poreba, A. Derkacz, and M. Silber, "Assessment of cardiac arrhythmias in patients suffering from essential hypertension," *Polskie Archiwum Medycyny Wewnętrznej*, vol. 111, no. 2, pp. 183–189, 2004.

[9] "Heart rate variability: standards of measurement, physiological interpretation and clinical use. Task Force of the European Society of Cardiology and the North American Society of Pacing and Electrophysiology," *Circulation*, vol. 93, no. 5, pp. 1043–1065, 1996.

[10] A. Erdem, M. Uenishi, Z. Küçükdurmaz et al., "Cardiac autonomic function measured by heart rate variability and turbulence in pre-hypertensive subjects," *Clinical and Experimental Hypertension*, vol. 35, no. 2, pp. 102–107, 2013.

[11] G. F. Salles, F. M. Ribeiro, G. M. Guimarães, E. S. Muxfeldt, and C. R. L. Cardoso, "A reduced heart rate variability is independently associated with a blunted nocturnal blood pressure fall in patients with resistant hypertension," *Journal of Hypertension*, vol. 32, no. 3, pp. 644–651, 2014.

[12] Y. Yu, T. Liu, J. Wu et al., "Heart rate recovery in hypertensive patients: Relationship with blood pressure control," *Journal of Human Hypertension*, vol. 31, no. 5, pp. 354–360, 2017.

[13] S. G. Priori, E. Aliot, C. Blomstrom-Lundqvist et al., "Task Force on sudden cardiac death of the European Society of Cardiology," *European Heart Journal*, vol. 22, no. 16, pp. 1374–1450, 2001.

[14] F. S. Routledge, T. S. Campbell, J. A. McFetridge-Durdle, and S. L. Bacon, "Improvements in heart rate variability with exercise therapy," *Canadian Journal of Cardiology*, vol. 26, no. 6, pp. 303–312, 2010.

[15] A. I. Vinik and D. Ziegler, "Diabetic cardiovascular autonomic neuropathy," *Circulation*, vol. 115, no. 3, pp. 387–397, 2007.

[16] H. Jaques, "NICE Guideline on hypertension," *European Heart Journal*, vol. 34, no. 6, pp. 406–408, 2013.

[17] V. Jokinen, J. M. Tapanainen, T. Seppänen, and H. V. Huikuri, "Temporal changes and prognostic significance of measures of heart rate dynamics after acute myocardial infarction in the beta-blocking era," *American Journal of Cardiology*, vol. 92, no. 8, pp. 907–912, 2003.

9

Prevalence of Hypertension and its Associated Risk Factors among 34,111 HAART Naïve HIV-Infected Adults

Marina Njelekela,[1] Alfa Muhihi,[2,3] Akum Aveika,[2] Donna Spiegelman,[4,5] Claudia Hawkins,[6] Catharina Armstrong,[7] Enju Liu,[8,9] James Okuma,[8] Guerino Chalamila,[2] Sylvia Kaaya,[10] Ferdinand Mugusi,[11] and Wafaie Fawzi[4,8,9]

[1] Department of Physiology, Muhimbili University of Health and Allied Sciences, Dar es Salaam, Tanzania
[2] Management and Development for Health, HIV/AIDS Care and Treatment Program, Dar es Salaam, Tanzania
[3] Africa Academy for Public Health, P.O. Box 79810, Dar es Salaam, Tanzania
[4] Department of Epidemiology, Harvard TH Chan School of Public Health, Boston, MA, USA
[5] Department of Biostatistics, Harvard TH Chan School of Public Health, Boston, MA, USA
[6] Feinberg School of Medicine, Northwestern University, Chicago, IL, USA
[7] Tufts University School of Medicine, Boston, MA, USA
[8] Department of Nutrition, Harvard TH Chan School of Public Health, Boston, MA, USA
[9] Department of Global Health and Population, Harvard TH Chan School of Public Health, Boston, MA, USA
[10] Department of Psychiatry and Mental Health, Muhimbili University of Health and Allied Sciences, Dar es Salaam, Tanzania
[11] Department of Internal Medicine, Muhimbili University of Health and Allied Sciences, Dar es Salaam, Tanzania

Correspondence should be addressed to Marina Njelekela; madaula@yahoo.com

Academic Editor: Tomohiro Katsuya

Background. Elevated blood pressure has been reported among treatment naïve HIV-infected patients. We investigated prevalence of hypertension and its associated risk factors in a HAART naïve HIV-infected population in Dar es Salaam, Tanzania. *Methods.* A cross-sectional analysis was conducted among HAART naïve HIV-infected patients. Hypertension was defined as systolic blood pressure (SBP) $\geq$ 140 mmHg and/or diastolic blood pressure (DBP) $\geq$ 90 mmHg. Overweight and obesity were defined as body mass index (BMI) between $25.0–29.9 \, kg/m^2$ and $\geq 30 \, kg/m^2$, respectively. We used relative risks to examine factors associated with hypertension. *Results.* Prevalence of hypertension was found to be 12.5%. After adjusting for possible confounders, risk of hypertension was 10% more in male than female patients. Patients aged ≥ 50 years had more than 2-fold increased risk for hypertension compared to 30–39-years-old patients. Overweight and obesity were associated with 51% and 94% increased risk for hypertension compared to normal weight patients. Low CD4+ T-cell count, advanced WHO clinical disease stage, and history of TB were associated with 10%, 42%, and 14% decreased risk for hypertension. *Conclusions.* Older age, male gender, and overweight/obesity were associated with hypertension. Immune suppression and history of TB were associated with lower risk for hypertension. HIV treatment programs should screen and manage hypertension even in HAART naïve individuals.

1. Introduction

The introduction of Highly Active Antiretroviral Therapy (HAART) marked a milestone in the prognosis, course of infection, and quality of life for people living with human immunodeficiency virus (HIV) in both developed and developing countries [1, 2]. Cardiovascular diseases (CVDs) are increasingly observed in HIV-infected people especially in developed countries where people with HIV/AIDS are living much longer [3]. In addition to increased patient longevity, data indicate that increased incidence of CVDs is also attributable to HIV infection itself and use of HAART [4, 5].

Generally, the impact of HIV and HAART on hypertension remains controversial. A recent systematic review with meta-analysis of over 44,000 HIV-infected patients has shown the mean systolic blood pressure and risk of hypertension to be significantly higher among HAART exposed compared to HAART naïve individuals [6]. Studies conducted in Europe and US found higher rates of hypertension among HIV-infected adults on HAART than uninfected adults [7] with others indicating no difference [8, 9]. However, results from a multicenter AIDS cohort study of men with blood pressure measurements between 1984 and 2003 indicated a significant association between prolonged use of HAART with systolic hypertension [10].

A systematic review and meta-analysis from sub-Saharan Africa found lower blood pressure levels among HIV-infected than uninfected adults [11]. Another large, population-based study from South Africa indicated hypertension to be less common among HIV-infected adults [12]. However, both studies from Africa lacked data on long-term HAART use. Hypertension may develop as a result of long-term HAART use due to weight gain, drug toxicity, and some immune-related phenomenon. A study conducted in Nigeria reported no association between HIV infection and HAART status with hypertension [13]. However, this study had a relatively small sample size and was of short duration of HAART in the treated group. Reports from other studies indicate a slightly higher prevalence of CVD risk factors among HIV-infected individuals, especially those on HAART [14, 15].

Data from resource-limited settings among non-HIV-infected people has indicated increasing rates of traditional risk factors associated with CVD such as hypertension, diabetes mellitus, and dyslipidemia, primarily as a result of obesity and urbanization [16–18]. These risk factors contribute to a significant proportion of overall disease burden in Africa [19, 20]. The prevalences of metabolic syndrome and hypertension are reported to be increasing in Africa [18, 21]. Metabolic syndrome is defined as a cluster of several cardiometabolic risk factors, including abdominal obesity, hyperglycemia, dyslipidemia, and elevated blood pressure [22].

In view of existing gap of knowledge and scarcity of data on the prevalence and correlates of CVD risk factors especially among HIV-infected population in resource-limited settings, we conducted this analysis to assess the prevalence of hypertension and its associated risk factors in a cohort of HIV-infected, HAART naïve in Dar es Salaam, Tanzania.

2. Methods

2.1. Study Design, Site, and Population. Data for this cross-sectional analysis were collected at 12 HIV Care and Treatment Clinics (CTCs) affiliated to Management and Development for Health (MDH) and supported by President's Emergency Plan for AIDS Relief (PEPFAR) in Dar es Salaam, Tanzania. The MDH-PEPFAR program was established in 2004 and provided infrastructure, laboratory, and technical support to HIV CTCs, Prevention of Mother to Child

Transmission (PMTCT) clinics, and Tuberculosis facilities in Dar es Salaam region. Dar es Salaam has a population of more than four million people with an HIV prevalence of 6.9% [23]. This analysis is comprised of patients who had blood pressure (BP) measurement taken, were ≥15 years of age, and were nonpregnant at the time of enrolment.

2.2. Blood Pressure Measurement. Blood pressure measurements were taken on arrival to the clinic using a standardized digital blood pressure measuring machine (AD Medical Inc.). Three blood pressure readings were taken on the left upper arm with the participant in a seated position following at least 5 to 10 minutes of rest. The average of the three readings was used in this analysis.

2.3. Anthropometric Measurement. Body weight and height were taken following standard procedures. Body weight (to the nearest 0.5 kg) was taken with the participant in light clothing using a SECA scale. Height (to the nearest 0.5 cm) was measured using a stadiometer with participants wearing no shoes. Body mass index (BMI) was then calculated as weight in kilograms divided by square of height in meters (kg/m^2). Overweight was defined as BMI between 25.0 and 29.9 kg/m^2 and obesity as BMI ≥ 30 kg/m^2.

2.4. Clinical and Laboratory Procedures. Clinical care of all HIV-infected patients at MDH-supported CTCs follows the Tanzanian National guidelines for management of HIV patients [24]. Following HIV diagnosis, patients were enrolled in the CTC clinic and had WHO clinical stage, CD4+ T-cell count, and HAART eligibility status determined. Eligible patients were subsequently initiated on HAART after adherence counseling and were followed up by physicians and nurses at two weeks after HAART initiation for assessment and management of any toxicity. They were then assessed at monthly clinic visits. Patients not yet meeting HAART initiation criteria were followed up at 6 monthly HIV care and monitoring visits.

Blood samples were collected and separated within 6 to 8 hours of specimen collection and stored at −80-degree centigrade for four weeks. Batch testing of samples was performed by a senior technician at Muhimbili University of Health and Allied Sciences (MUHAS). Daily calibration of instruments was done following standardized procedures. The MUHAS laboratory participates in the College of American Pathologists proficiency testing programs where three general chemistry panels including lipids and two calibration verification panels are taken annually. Immunologic assessment with CD4+ T-cell count was performed using the FACS Calibur System (Becton Dickinson, San Jose, California, USA).

TB screening was performed to all patients at baseline using a TB screener form containing five questions:

(i) History of cough for ≥2 weeks

(ii) History of hemoptysis

(iii) History of fever for ≥2 weeks

(iv) Noticeable weight loss for new patients or weight loss ≥ 3.0 kg in a month

(v) Excessive night sweats for ≥2 weeks.

All patients who were screened positive for TB (had at least one of the abovementioned symptoms) had a chest radiograph and sputum analysis conducted for diagnosis of TB.

2.5. Data Collection and Management. Physicians and nurses completed standard forms capturing demographic, clinical, laboratory, and therapeutic information at baseline and follow-up visits. Data reviewers were stationed at each clinic to ensure completeness of data recording by physicians and nurses. Data collected was then entered into a secure computerized database using unique patient identifiers. The database was updated daily by dedicated data entry clerks trained to use a prospective data collection instrument.

Weekly quality assurance checks were performed by the data management team to ensure data accuracy. Data collected for this analysis included baseline demographics, age, weight, height, blood pressure, midupper arm circumference (MUAC), body mass index (BMI), WHO clinical disease stage, and history of prior or current TB.

2.6. Outcomes and Definitions. The primary outcome of interest was hypertension, which was defined according to the guidelines for management of hypertension in HIV. The Joint National Committee VII (JNC VII) report released in 2003 categorizes blood pressure as follows: normal blood pressure (systolic (SBP)/diastolic (DBP) < 120/80 mmHg); prehypertension (SBP 120–139 mmHg or DBP 80–89 mmHg); stage 1 hypertension (SBP 140–159 mmHg or DBP 90–99 mmHg); and stage 2 hypertension (SBP ≥ 160 mmHg or DBP ≥ 100 mmHg) [25].

2.7. Ethical Approval. The study was approved by institutional review boards for human research at Harvard TH Chan School of Public Health and the Research Ethics Review Committee of the Muhimbili University of Health and Allied Sciences. Patients were recruited for participation and enrolled in the MDH-supported CTCs following written informed consent.

2.8. Statistical Analysis. Sociodemographic and cardiometabolic characteristics of the study population were described using mean (SD) or percentage. To examine the factors associated with hypertension, prevalence ratios (relative risks) were estimated using Generalized Estimating Equations (GEE) with the log link function and the binomial variance [26, 27]. All multivariate analyses were adjusted for age (<30, 30–39, 40–49, and ≥50 years); gender (male/female); district (Ilala, Kinondoni, and Temeke); calendar year and season of enrolment; BMI (underweight, normal weight, overweight, and obesity); CD4+ T-cell count (<350, 350–<500, and ≥500); WHO clinical disease stage (I, II, III, and IV); history of TB; and current TB/HIV coinfected. The median score test was used to assess the significance of any trends observed and a Wald test was used for binary variables. The missing indicator method was used in the multivariate models [28]. Statistical analyses were performed with the statistical software package SAS (release 9.2). All tests were two-sided, and a $p < 0.05$ was considered statistically significant.

Table 1: Sociodemographic and clinical characteristics of the participants.

Characteristic	Mean ± SD or N (%)
Age (years)	36.6 ± 9.5
Age categories	
<30	7760 (22.9)
30–39	14877 (43.9)
40–49	7964 (23.4)
≥50	3317 (9.8)
Gender	
Male	11199 (32.8)
Female	22912 (67.2)
BMI (kg/m^2)	21.4 ± 4.8
BMI-defined categories	
Underweight (BMI < 18.5 kg/m^2)	9235 (27.6)
Normal (BMI 18.5–24.9 kg/m^2)	18160 (54.4)
Overweight (BMI 25.0–29.9 kg/m^2)	4322 (12.9)
Obesity (BMI ≥ 30 kg/m^2)	1693 (5.1)
CD4+ cell count (cells/μL)	
<350	23050 (75.5)
350–<500	3748 (12.3)
≥500	3720 (12.2)
WHO clinical disease stage	
Stage I	4910 (14.9)
Stage II	6228 (18.9)
Stage III	15128 (45.9)
Stage IV	6686 (20.3)
History of TB infection	
Yes	7739 (23.3)
No	25539 (76.7)
Current TB/HIV coinfection	
Yes	3245 (9.7)
No	30246 (90.3)

BMI: body mass index; BP: blood pressure; CD4+: cluster of differentiation 4; HIV: human immunodeficiency virus; TB: tuberculosis; WHO: World Health Organization.

3. Results

3.1. Sociodemographic and Clinical Characteristics of the Study Population. A total of 34,111 nonpregnant, HAART naïve patients who had blood pressure measurement taken were included in the analysis. The baseline demographic and clinical characteristics of the study patients are summarized in Table 1. The mean age and BMI of the patients were 36.6 ± 9.5 years and 21.4 ± 4.8 kg/m^2, respectively, and women constituted two-thirds of the study participants. Three-quarters (75.5%) of the participants had CD4+ T-cell count of less than 350 cells/μL and two-thirds (66.2%) had a WHO clinical disease stage III or stage IV. Nearly quarter of the participants (23.3%) had a positive history of TB and about one-tenth (9.7%) were currently TB/HIV coinfected receiving anti-TB treatment.

TABLE 2: Mean systolic and diastolic blood pressures and prevalence of hypertension.

Variable	Mean ± SD or N (%)
Systolic blood pressure, SBP (mmHg)	114.1 ± 18.1
Diastolic blood pressure, DBP (mmHg)	73.1 ± 12.9
Blood pressure categories	
Normal BP	19859 (58.2)
Prehypertension	9967 (29.2)
Stage 1 hypertension	2668 (7.8)
Stage 2 hypertension	1617 (4.7)
Hypertension	
Yes	4285 (12.5)
No	29826 (87.4)

BP: blood pressure; SD: standard deviation.

3.2. Blood Pressure and Prevalence of Hypertension. Results on blood pressure measurements are summarized in Table 2. The mean systolic and diastolic blood pressures were 114.1 ± 18.1 mmHg and 73.1 ± 12.9 mmHg, respectively. More than half (58.2%) of the patients had their blood pressure measurement within the normal range and more than quarter (29.2%) had their blood pressure in the prehypertension range. The prevalence of hypertension (combined stages 1 and 2 hypertension) found in this study population was 12.5%.

3.3. Sociodemographic and Clinical Characteristics Associated with Hypertension. The various sociodemographic and clinical factors associated with hypertension among study patients are summarized in Table 3. Older age (≥50 years), male gender, overweight and obesity, CD4+ T-cell count (≥500 cells/μL), and WHO clinical disease stage I were all significantly associated with higher prevalence of hypertension. WHO clinical disease stage IV, history of TB, and being TB/HIV coinfected were significantly associated with a lower prevalence of hypertension.

3.4. Relationship between Age, Gender, and Body Mass Index with Prevalence of Hypertension. Results for univariate and multivariate analyses for risk factors associated with hypertension are summarized in Table 4. After adjusting for district (Ilala, Kinondoni, and Temeke), calendar year and season of enrolment, age (<30, 30–39, 40–49, and ≥50 years), gender (male/female), BMI (underweight, normal weight, overweight, and obesity), CD4+ T-cell count (<350, 350–<500, and ≥500), WHO clinical disease stage (I, II, III, and IV), history of TB, and current TB/HIV coinfected, patients aged 40–49 years and those aged ≥50 years had a 43% [ARR 1.43 (95% CI 1.33, 1.53)] and 2-fold [ARR 2.52 (95% CI 1.92, 3.30)] increased risk for hypertension compared to patients aged 30–39 years. Male patients had 10% [ARR 1.10 (95% CI 1.04, 1.17)] increased risk of hypertension compared to female patients. Overweight and obesity were associated with 51% [ARR 1.51 (95% CI 1.40, 1.62)] and 94% [ARR 1.94 (95% CI 1.78, 2.12)], respectively, increased risk for hypertension compared to normal weight patients.

Prevalence of hypertension was significantly lower in patients with immune suppression at baseline. Hypertension was 10% (ARR 0.90; 95% CI 0.83, 0.98) lower in patients with CD4+ T-cell count < 350 cells/μL compared to those with CD4+ T-cell count ≥ 500 cells/μL. Similarly, patients with advanced WHO clinical disease stage had significantly lower risk of hypertension. Patients with WHO clinical disease stages II and III had 12% and 28% decreased risk for hypertension compared to patients with stage I disease. WHO clinical disease stage IV was associated with 42% decreased risk for hypertension compared to stage I disease.

History of TB was observed to be protective against hypertension. Patients with history of TB had statistically significant 14% decreased risk for hypertension compared to patients with no history of TB. On the contrary, patients who were current TB/HIV coinfected had a nonsignificant 5% increased risk for hypertension.

4. Discussion

We report an appreciable prevalence of hypertension in a cohort of HAART naïve HIV-infected adults in Tanzania. We found significant associations between older age, male gender, and overweight/obesity with higher prevalence of hypertension. Furthermore, the prevalence of hypertension was inversely associated with level of immune suppression. This study is one among few published studies examining the prevalence of hypertension as one of the key risk factors associated with CVD in HIV-infected population from resource-limited settings.

Arterial hypertension is a major CVD risk factor. However, there are few studies that have analyzed the relationship between blood pressure and HIV infection [7, 8]. In our study, we observed a prevalence of hypertension (combined stages 1 and 2) of 12.5%. The prevalence of hypertension observed in this study is lower than that reported by studies conducted elsewhere in Africa [13, 29–31]. Although we did not compare the prevalence of hypertension to patients on HAART, several studies have reported higher prevalence of hypertension among HIV-infected patients on HAART [29, 30, 32, 33], supporting that HAART is associated with hypertension. Other studies have found no association between HAART use and hypertension [9, 34]. Ogunmola et al. reported no significant difference in the prevalence of hypertension, mean SBP, and mean DBP between HIV-negative, HIV-positive on HAART, and HIV-positive HAART naïve patients [13].

The variability in the prevalence of hypertension observed in our study to that reported by other studies may be explained by several factors, one of them being the cut-off for defining hypertension. For example, in most of these studies, their cut-off point was 160/95 mmHg compared to the definition we used (SBP ≥ 140 mmHg and/or DBP ≥ 90 mmHg). Other factors such as differences in age, ethnicity, and levels of obesity may also explain the variations in the observed prevalence of hypertension. In our study, inclusion of HAART naïve patients only may partly explain the observed low prevalence of hypertension. Further analysis comparing with patients on HAART is warranted.

Several mechanisms have been proposed to explain the link between HIV and CVD [31, 35]. HIV infection, chronic inflammation, hypercoagulability, and platelet activation

TABLE 3: Sociodemographic and clinical characteristics associated with hypertension.

Parameter	All $N = 34{,}111$	Normotensive N (%)	Hypertensive N (%)	p value
Age (years)				**<0.001**
<30	7760	7131 (91.9%)	629 (8.1%)	
30–39	14877	3289 (89.3%)	1588 (10.7%)	
40–49	7964	6756 (84.8%)	1208 (15.2%)	
≥50	3317	2505 (75.5%)	813 (24.5%)	
Gender				**<0.001**
Male	11199	8423 (75.2%)	2776 (24.8%)	
Female	22912	21409 (93.4%)	1503 (6.6%)	
BMI-defined obesity				**<0.001**
Underweight (BMI < 18.5 kg/m^2)	9235	8643 (93.6%)	592 (6.4%)	
Normal (BMI 18.5–24.9 kg/m^2)	18160	15884 (87.5%)	2276 (12.5%)	
Overweight (BMI 25.0–29.9 kg/m^2)	4322	3440 (79.6%)	882 (20.4%)	
Obesity (BMI ≥ 30 kg/m^2)	1693	1228 (72.5%)	465 (27.5%)	
CD4+ cell count (cells/μL)				**<0.001**
<350	23050	20414 (88.6%)	2636 (11.4%)	
350–<500	3748	3177 (84.8%)	571 (15.2%)	
≥500	3720	3120 (83.9%)	600 (16.1%)	
WHO clinical disease stage				**<0.001**
Stage I	4910	3982 (81.1%)	928 (18.9%)	
Stage II	6228	5234 (84.0%)	994 (16.0%)	
Stage III	15128	13392 (88.5%)	1736 (11.5%)	
Stage IV	6686	6139 (91.8%)	547 (8.2%)	
History of TB				**<0.001**
Yes	7739	6993 (90.4%)	746 (9.6%)	
No	25539	22097 (86.5%)	3442 (13.5%)	
Current TB/HIV coinfection				**<0.001**
Yes	3245	2940 (90.6%)	305 (9.4%)	
No	30246	26345 (87.1%)	3901 (12.9%)	

BMI: body mass index; CD4+: cluster of differentiation 4; HIV: human immunodeficiency virus; TB: tuberculosis; WHO: World Health Organization.

mediated by HIV infection itself contribute to endothelial dysfunction and subsequent increased CVD risk [15, 36]. It has been proposed that HIV influences endothelial function via activated monocytes and resultant cytokine secretion and via a direct effect of the secreted HIV proteins tat and gp120 [37]. Another mechanism involves free radical physiology, where excess nitric oxide reacts with oxygen radicals to produce peroxynitrite, which then causes oxidative damage to the vascular endothelium, and decreased flow mediated dilation [38]. Use of HAART in patients infected with HIV-1 has been shown to reduce markers of endothelial function and coagulation [15, 31, 35].

We observed a significant association between older age, male gender, and overweight/obesity and increased risk for hypertension. These findings are in agreement with other studies conducted among HIV-infected individuals. In addition to HAART exposure, these studies found male gender, advancing age, high body mass index, greater waist circumference, HIV-hepatitis C coinfection, and ethnicity to be associated with increased risk of developing hypertension and coronary heart disease (CHD) in HIV-infected patients [7, 33]. We have also demonstrated increased mortality among male patients with HIV in one of our publications [39].

We observed an inverse association between advanced HIV disease (defined as low CD4+ T-cell count and advanced WHO clinical disease stage) and risk for hypertension. Participants with low CD4+ T-cell count < 350 cells/μL and those with WHO clinical disease stage IV had lower risk for hypertension. This finding is contrary to results from other studies which show that low CD4+ T-cell count is a risk for CVD [40–43]. The proposed mechanism for association between low immunity and risk of CVD is that chronic inflammation that accompanies uncontrolled

TABLE 4: Univariate and multivariate adjusted demographic, body mass index, and clinical and immunological factors associated with prevalence of hypertension.

	Unadjusted RR (95% CI)	p value	Adjusted RR (95% CI)	p value
Age group (years)		**0.002**		**<0.001**
15–29	0.76 (0.70–0.83)		0.74 (0.67–0.81)	
30–39	Reference		Reference	
40–49	1.42 (1.32–1.52)		1.43 (1.33–1.53)	
50	2.30 (2.14–2.49)		2.52 (1.92–3.30)	
Gender		**<0.001**		**0.002**
Female	Reference		Reference	
Male	1.11 (1.05–1.18)		1.10 (1.04–1.17)	
BMI-defined obesity		**0.003**		**<0.001**
Underweight (BMI < 18.5 kg/m^2)	0.51 (0.47–0.56)		0.57 (0.52–0.62)	
Normal (BMI 18.5–24.9 kg/m^2)	Reference		Reference	
Overweight (BMI 25.0–29.9 kg/m^2)	1.63 (1.52–1.74)		1.51 (1.40–1.62)	
Obesity (BMI ≥ 30 kg/m^2)	2.19 (2.00–2.38)		1.94 (1.78–2.12)	
CD4+ cell count (cells/μL)		**<0.001**		**0.003**
<350	0.49 (0.44–0.54)			
350–<500	0.77 (0.72–0.82)			
>500	Reference		Reference	
WHO Clinical disease stage		**<0.001**		**<0.001**
Stage I	Reference		Reference	
Stage II	0.83 (0.77–0.90)		0.88 (0.81–0.96)	
Stage III	0.58 (0.54–0.63)		0.72 (0.66–0.78)	
Stage IV	0.42 (0.38–0.47)		0.58 (0.52–0.64)	
History of TB		**<0.001**		**<0.001**
Yes	0.72 (0.66–0.77)		0.86 (0.78–0.94)	
No	Reference		Reference	
Current TB/HIV coinfection		**0.410**		**0.420**
Yes	1.08 (0.89–1.18)		1.05 (0.92–1.20)	
No	Reference		Reference	

BMI: body mass index; CI: confidence interval; HIV: human immune deficiency virus; RR: risk ratio; TB: tuberculosis; WHO: World Health Organization. The final model for multivariate analyses included district (Ilala, Kinondoni, and Temeke), calendar year and season of enrolment, age (<30, 30–39, 40–49, and ≥50 years), gender (male/female), BMI (underweight, normal weight, overweight, and obesity), CD4+ cell count (<350, 350–<500, and ≥500), WHO clinical disease stage (I, II, III, and IV), history of TB, and current TB/HIV coinfected. The median score test was used to assess the significance of any trends observed and a Wald test was used for binary variables.

or more advanced HIV disease is associated with elevated levels of serum markers of inflammation and increased levels of activated CD4+ T-cells and proinflammatory cytokines that destabilize atherosclerotic plaques leading to CVD event [42, 44].

Participants with history of TB had a 10% decreased risk for hypertension, but this protective effect was not observed among those who were currently TB/HIV coinfected. Few studies have explored the association between TB and CVD risk and have reported contradicting conclusions. An age and sex matched study conducted by Giral et al. [45] showed that past TB was not associated with a higher prevalence of atherosclerotic lesions in patients with hypercholesterolemia patients, while Wu et al. [46] reported that non-CNS TB does not increase the risk of subsequent ischemic stroke. In

contrary, Sheu et al. [47] found patients with a diagnosis of TB to be at an increased risk for ischemic stroke. Our finding of history of TB conferring protective effect against hypertension further increases the need for further research to investigate the relationship between TB and CVD and its risk factors.

While the major strength of this analysis is its large sample size, it has several limitations worth mentioning. First, the cross-sectional design of the study does not provide proof of causal association between HIV, immune suppression, and the development of hypertension. Secondly, the analysis was limited to hypertension and obesity. We did not evaluate the contribution of other conversional risk factors such as diabetes, lipid profile, smoking, alcohol drinking, physical activity, dietary, and other lifestyle related factors. Third, inclusion of HAART naïve only in the analysis made it impossible to make comparisons with counterpart HIV-infected patients on HAART or HIV-negative as in other studies [13, 30]. Fourth, selection bias might have been introduced by inclusion of patients who attended MDH-supported CTCs only, thus affecting generalizability of the findings. However, MDH-supported CTCs are publicly accessible and patients attending these clinics may be similar to those attending other public health facilities CTCs in Dar es Salaam. Despite the abovementioned limitations, this study remains an important analysis of blood pressure and its associated risk factors in a large cohort of HIV-infected HAART naïve patients from resource-limited settings.

In conclusion, we observed that older age, male gender, and BMI-defined overweight/obesity were significantly associated with higher prevalence of hypertension even after adjusting for potential confounders. Furthermore, immune suppression (defined by low CD4+ T-cell count and advanced WHO clinical diseased stage) and history of TB were associated with decreased risk for hypertension. Screening and regular monitoring for complications associated with use of HAART among HIV-infected people have been a routine clinical practice. HIV treatment programs are recommended to conduct routine screening and monitoring for hypertension and other CVD risk factors even prior to initiation of HAART especially among healthy-looking individuals. Traditional hypertension control measures such as physical exercise, weight control, and healthy diet should be recommended to HIV-infected individuals. Further research is warranted to investigate the association between TB, immune suppression, and CVD risk observed in this study.

Competing Interests

The authors declare that they have no competing interests.

Authors' Contributions

Wafaie Fawzi, Donna Spiegelman, Guerino Chalamila, Sylvia Kaaya, and Ferdinand Mugusi conceived and designed the experiment. Wafaie Fawzi, Donna Spiegelman, Guerino Chalamila, Sylvia Kaaya, and Ferdinand Mugusi performed the experiment. Marina Njelekela, Akum Aveika, Enju Liu, and Alfa Muhihi analyzed the data. Wafaie Fawzi, Donna Spiegelman, Catharina Armstrong, and James Okuma contributed reagents/materials/analysis tools. Wafaie Fawzi, Donna Spiegelman, Guerino Chalamila, Sylvia Kaaya, Ferdinand Mugusi, Marina Njelekela, Alfa Muhihi, Claudia Hawkins, Enju Liu, Catharina Armstrong, and James Okuma wrote the paper. All authors read and approved the final version.

Acknowledgments

The PEPFAR funded National HIV Care and Treatment in Dar es Salaam program was implemented by Management and Development for Health (MDH) in collaboration with Dar es Salaam City Council, Harvard TH Chan School of Public Health (HSPH), Muhimbili University of Health and Allied Sciences (MUHAS) and the Ministry of Health, Community Development, Gender, Elderly and Children in Tanzania. The authors thank the Fogarty International Fellowship Grant through MUHAS-Harvard Collaboration for supporting Dr. Marina Njelekela during data analysis and manuscript writing. The authors also extend their gratitude to all the study participants as well as staff of the MDH-supported care and treatment sites who contributed tirelessly to making these findings known.

References

[1] O. O. Oguntibeju, "Quality of life of people living with HIV and AIDS and antiretroviral therapy," *HIV/AIDS—Research and Palliative Care*, vol. 4, pp. 117–124, 2012.

[2] J. Beard, F. Feeley, and S. Rosen, "Economic and quality of life outcomes of antiretroviral therapy for HIV/AIDS in developing countries: a systematic literature review," *AIDS Care*, vol. 21, no. 11, pp. 1343–1356, 2009.

[3] J. E. Sackoff, D. B. Hanna, M. R. Pfeiffer, and L. V. Torian, "Causes of death among persons with aids in the era of highly active antiretroviral therapy: New York City," *Annals of Internal Medicine*, vol. 145, no. 6, pp. 397–406, 2006.

[4] A. d'Arminio, C. A. Sabin, A. N. Phillips et al., "Cardio- and cerebrovascular events in HIV-infected persons," *AIDS*, vol. 18, no. 13, pp. 1811–1817, 2004.

[5] G. Guaraldi, "Cardiovascular complications in HIV-infected individuals," *Current Opinion in HIV and AIDS*, vol. 1, no. 6, pp. 507–513, 2006.

[6] C. U. Nduka, S. Stranges, A. M. Sarki, P. K. Kimani, and O. A. Uthman, "Evidence of increased blood pressure and hypertension risk among people living with HIV on antiretroviral therapy: a systematic review with meta-analysis," *Journal of Human Hypertension*, vol. 30, no. 6, pp. 355–362, 2016.

[7] C. Gazzaruso, R. Bruno, A. Garzaniti et al., "Hypertension among HIV patients: prevalence and relationships to insulin resistance and metabolic syndrome," *Journal of Hypertension*, vol. 21, no. 7, pp. 1377–1382, 2003.

[8] C. Jericó, H. Knobel, M. Montero et al., "Hypertension in HIV-infected patients: prevalence and related factors," *American Journal of Hypertension*, vol. 18, no. 11, pp. 1396–1401, 2005.

[9] B. M. Bergersen, L. Sandvik, O. Dunlop, K. Birkeland, and J. N. Bruun, "Prevalence of Hypertension in HIV-Positive Patients on Highly Active Retroviral Therapy (HAART) compared with HAART-Naïve and HIV-Negative Controls: results from a Norwegian Study of 721 patients," *European Journal of Clinical Microbiology and Infectious Diseases*, vol. 22, no. 12, pp. 731–736, 2003.

[10] E. C. Seaberg, A. Muñoz, M. Lu et al., "Association between highly active antiretroviral therapy and hypertension in a large cohort of men followed from 1984 to 2003," *AIDS*, vol. 19, no. 9, pp. 953–960, 2005.

[11] D. G. Dillon, D. Gurdasani, J. Riha et al., "Association of HIV and ART with cardiometabolic traits in sub-Saharan Africa: a systematic review and meta-analysis," *International Journal of Epidemiology*, vol. 42, no. 6, pp. 1754–1771, 2013.

[12] A. Malaza, J. Mossong, T. Bärnighausen, and M.-L. Newell, "Hypertension and obesity in adults living in a high HIV prevalence rural area in South Africa," *PLoS ONE*, vol. 7, no. 10, article e47761, 2012.

[13] O. J. Ogunmola, O. Y. Oladosu, and A. M. Olamoyegun, "Association of hypertension and obesity with HIV and antiretroviral

therapy in a rural tertiary health center in Nigeria: a cross-sectional cohort study," *Vascular Health and Risk Management*, vol. 10, pp. 129–137, 2014.

[14] A. G. Pacheco, S. H. Tuboi, J. C. Faulhaber, L. H. Harrison, and M. Schechter, "Increase in non-AIDS related conditions as causes of death among HIV-infected individuals in the HAART era in Brazil," *PLoS ONE*, vol. 3, no. 1, Article ID e1531, 2008.

[15] A. Calmy, A. Gayet-Ageron, F. Montecucco et al., "HIV increases markers of cardiovascular risk: results from a randomized, treatment interruption trial," *AIDS*, vol. 23, no. 8, pp. 929–939, 2009.

[16] A. A. Motala, M. A. K. Omar, and F. J. Pirie, "Diabetes in Africa. Epidemiology of type 1 and type 2 diabetes in Africa," *Journal of Cardiovascular Risk*, vol. 10, no. 2, pp. 77–83, 2003.

[17] M. Njelekela, H. Negishi, Y. Nara et al., "Cardiovascular risk factors in Tanzania: a revisit," *Acta Tropica*, vol. 79, no. 3, pp. 231–239, 2001.

[18] R. Fuentes, N. Ilmaniemi, E. Laurikainen, J. Tuomilehto, and A. Nissinen, "Hypertension in developing economies: a review of population-based studies carried out from 1980 to 1998," *Journal of Hypertension*, vol. 18, no. 5, pp. 521–529, 2000.

[19] E. Mutimura, N. J. Crowther, A. Stewart, and W. T. Cade, "The human immunodeficiency virus and the cardiometabolic syndrome in the developing world: an African perspective," *Journal of the Cardiometabolic Syndrome*, vol. 3, no. 2, pp. 106–110, 2008.

[20] S. Wild, G. Roglic, A. Green, R. Sicree, and H. King, "Global prevalence of diabetes: estimates for the year 2000 and projections for 2030," *Diabetes Care*, vol. 27, no. 10, pp. 2568–2569, 2004.

[21] A. R. Hosseinpoor, N. Bergen, S. Mendis et al., "Socioeconomic inequality in the prevalence of noncommunicable diseases in low- and middle-income countries: results from the World Health Survey," *BMC Public Health*, vol. 12, no. 1, article 474, 2012.

[22] S. M. Grundy, J. I. Cleeman, S. R. Daniels et al., "Diagnosis and management of the metabolic syndrome: an American Heart Association/National Heart, Lung, and Blood Institute scientific statement," *Circulation*, vol. 112, no. 17, pp. 2735–2752, 2005.

[23] TACAIDS, *Tanzania HIV/AIDS and Malaria Indicator Survey, 2011/2012*, Dar es Salaam, 2012.

[24] NACP. The United Republic of Tanzania-Ministry of Health and Social Welfare, *National Guidelines for the Management of HIV and AIDS*, Ministry of Health and Social Welfare, Dar es Salaam, Tanzania, 5th edition, 2015.

[25] A. V. Chobanian, G. L. Bakris, H. R. Black et al., "Seventh report of the joint national committee on prevention, detection, evaluation, and treatment of high blood pressure," *Hypertension*, vol. 42, no. 6, pp. 1206–1252, 2003.

[26] L. Alfredsson and A. Ahlbom, "Binomial regression in GLIM: estimating risk ratios and risk differences," *American Journal of Epidemiology*, vol. 125, no. 1, pp. 174–184, 1987.

[27] S. Wacholder, "Binomial regression in GLIM: estimating risk ratios and risk differences," *American Journal of Epidemiology*, vol. 123, no. 1, pp. 174–184, 1986.

[28] O. Miettinen, *Theoretical Epidemiology*, Wiley-Blackwell, New York, NY, USA, 1985.

[29] S. Muhammad, M. U. Sani, and B. N. Okeahialam, "Cardiovascular disease risk factors among HIV-infected Nigerians receiving highly active antiretroviral therapy," *Nigerian Medical Journal*, vol. 54, no. 3, pp. 185–190, 2013.

[30] C. A. Dimala, J. Atashili, J. C. Mbuagbaw, A. Wilfred, and G. L. Monekosso, "Prevalence of hypertension in HIV/AIDS patients on highly active antiretroviral therapy (HAART) compared with HAART-naïve patients at the limbe regional hospital, Cameroon," *PLoS ONE*, vol. 11, no. 2, Article ID e0148100, 2016.

[31] K. Wolf, D. A. Tsakiris, R. Weber, P. Erb, and M. Battegay, "Antiretroviral therapy reduces markers of endothelial and coagulation activation in patients infected with human immunodeficiency virus type 1," *Journal of Infectious Diseases*, vol. 185, no. 4, pp. 456–462, 2002.

[32] L. G. Ekali, L. K. Johnstone, J. B. Echouffo-Tcheugui et al., "Fasting blood glucose and insulin sensitivity are unaffected by HAART duration in Cameroonians receiving first-line antiretroviral treatment," *Diabetes and Metabolism*, vol. 39, no. 1, pp. 71–77, 2013.

[33] J. I. Bernardino de la Serna, F. X. Zamora, M. L. Montes, J. García-Puig, and J. R. Arribas, "Hypertension, HIV infection, and highly active antiretroviric therapy," *Enfermedades Infecciosas y Microbiologia Clinica*, vol. 28, no. 1, pp. 32–37, 2010.

[34] O. Jung, M. Bickel, T. Ditting et al., "Hypertension in HIV-1-infected patients and its impact on renal and cardiovascular integrity," *Nephrology Dialysis Transplantation*, vol. 19, no. 9, pp. 2250–2258, 2004.

[35] E. Jong, S. Louw, E. C. M. Van Gorp, J. C. M. Meijers, H. Ten Cate, and B. F. Jacobson, "The effect of initiating combined antiretroviral therapy on endothelial cell activation and coagulation markers in South African HIV-infected individuals," *Thrombosis and Haemostasis*, vol. 104, no. 6, pp. 1228–1234, 2010.

[36] C. Fourie, J. Van Rooyen, M. Pieters, K. Conradie, T. Hoekstra, and A. Schutte, "Is HIV-1 infection associated with endothelial dysfunction in a population of African ancestry in South Africa?" *Cardiovascular Journal of Africa*, vol. 22, no. 3, pp. 134–140, 2011.

[37] E. R. Kline and R. L. Sutliff, "The roles of HIV-1 proteins and antiretroviral drug therapy in HIV-1-associated endothelial dysfunction," *Journal of Investigative Medicine*, vol. 56, no. 5, pp. 752–769, 2008.

[38] D. Torre, "Nitric oxide and endothelial dysfunction in HIV type 1 infection," *Clinical Infectious Diseases*, vol. 43, no. 8, pp. 1086–1087, 2006.

[39] C. Hawkins, G. Chalamilla, J. Okuma et al., "Sex differences in antiretroviral treatment outcomes among HIV-infected adults in an urban Tanzanian setting," *AIDS*, vol. 25, no. 9, pp. 1189–1197, 2011.

[40] K. A. Lichtenstein, C. Armon, K. Buchacz et al., "Low CD4+ T cell count is a risk factor for cardiovascular disease events in the HIV Outpatient Study," *Clinical Infectious Diseases*, vol. 51, no. 4, pp. 435–447, 2010.

[41] I. W. Manner, M. Trøseid, O. Oektedalen, M. Baekken, and I. Os, "Low nadir CD4 cell count predicts sustained hypertension in HIV-infected individuals," *Journal of Clinical Hypertension*, vol. 15, no. 2, pp. 101–106, 2013.

[42] R. C. Kaplan, L. A. Kingsley, S. J. Gange et al., "Low CD4+ T-cell count as a major atherosclerosis risk factor in HIV-infected women and men," *AIDS*, vol. 22, no. 13, pp. 1615–1624, 2008.

[43] V. A. Triant, S. Regan, H. Lee, P. E. Sax, J. B. Meigs, and S. K. Grinspoon, "Association of immunologic and virologic factors with myocardial infarction rates in a US healthcare system," *Journal of Acquired Immune Deficiency Syndromes*, vol. 55, no. 5, pp. 615–619, 2010.

[44] P. Y. Hsue, S. G. Deeks, and P. W. Hunt, "Immunologic basis of cardiovascular disease in HIV-infected adults," *Journal of Infectious Diseases*, vol. 205, no. 3, pp. S375–S382, 2012.

[45] P. Giral, J.-F. Kahn, J.-M. André et al., "Carotid atherosclerosis is not related to past tuberculosis in hypercholesterolemic patients," *Atherosclerosis*, vol. 190, no. 1, pp. 150–155, 2007.

[46] C.-H. Wu, L.-S. Chen, M.-F. Yen et al., "Does non-central nervous system tuberculosis increase the risk of ischemic stroke? A population-based propensity score-matched follow-up study," *PLoS ONE*, vol. 9, no. 7, article e98158, 2014.

[47] J.-J. Sheu, H.-Y. Chiou, J.-H. Kang, Y.-H. Chen, and H.-C. Lin, "Tuberculosis and the risk of ischemic stroke: a 3-year follow-up study," *Stroke*, vol. 41, no. 2, pp. 244–249, 2010.

10

Prevalence and Associated Factors of Hypertension: A Community-Based Cross-Sectional Study in Municipalities

Raja Ram Dhungana,[1] Achyut Raj Pandey,[2] Bihungum Bista,[2]
Suira Joshi,[3] and Surya Devkota[4]

[1]Nepal Family Development Foundation, Kathmandu, Nepal
[2]Nepal Health Research Council, Kathmandu, Nepal
[3]Ministry of Health and Population, Kathmandu, Nepal
[4]Manmohan Cardiothoracic, Vascular and Transplant Centre, Institute of Medicine, Tribhuvan University, Kathmandu, Nepal

Correspondence should be addressed to Raja Ram Dhungana; raja.dhungana@gmail.com

Academic Editor: Roberto Pontremoli

Objective. This study aimed to assess the prevalence and associated factors of hypertension in newly declared municipalities of Kathmandu, Nepal. *Design, Settings, and Participants*. This was a community-based cross-sectional study conducted in the municipalities of Kathmandu District, Nepal, between January and July 2015. Study participants were aged 18 to 70 years, residing permanently in the study sites. Municipalities, Wards, households, and respondents were selected randomly. *Results*. Of the 587 participants, 58.8% were females, mean (SD) age was 42.3 (13.5) years, 29.3% had no formal education, 35.1% were Brahmins, and 41.2% were homemakers. Prevalence of hypertension was 32.5% (95% CI: 28.7–36.3). Age, gender, education, ethnicity, occupation, smoking, alcohol consumption, physical activity, diabetes, menopausal history, and family history of cardiovascular disease (CVD) and hypertension were significantly associated with hypertension. In multivariable analysis, smoking, alcohol consumption, physical activity, body mass index, and diabetes were identified as significant explanatory variables for hypertension. *Conclusion*. This study demonstrated that the people living in newly established municipalities of Kathmandu, Nepal, have a high burden of hypertension as well as its associated factors. Therefore, community-based preventive approaches like lifestyle modification and early detection and treatment of hypertension might bring a substantial change in tackling the burden effectively.

1. Background

Worldwide levels of hypertension represent the global public health crisis. Hypertension affects around 22% of people aged 18 years and over and is responsible for an estimated 9.4 million deaths per year globally [1, 2]. Raised blood pressure mostly remains asymptomatic while increasing the risk of heart disease, stroke, and renal failure [3]. It contributes to at least 45% of deaths due to heart disease and 51% of deaths as a result of stroke [1]. Additionally, around 10% of healthcare expenditure is directly related to hypertension and its complications [3].

The increasing prevalence of hypertension in developing countries is a major concern. According to recent estimates from the World Health Organization, two-thirds of hypertensive people live in developing countries [4]. Africa has the highest prevalence of hypertension (29.6%) followed by the Eastern Mediterranean (26.9%), South East Asia (24.7%), Europe (23.3%), the Western Pacific (18.7%), and America (18.2%) [2]. Among South Asian countries, Nepal reported the second highest proportion of hypertensive people (27.3%) after Afghanistan (29%) [2].

There are a range of factors that increase the risk of developing hypertension [5]. Tobacco use increases the incidence of cardiovascular diseases including hypertension [6]. Alcohol consumption is related to 5% to 30% of hypertension cases in the general population [7, 8]. Similarly, about 30% of cases are attributed to increased salt consumption and 20% to physical inactivity [9]. Hypertension has also well-established relationship with obesity and diabetes [10, 11]. Recent reports have provided evidence that increasing rates of noncommunicable diseases, including hypertension, are associated with other determinants like increases in rapid unplanned urbanization, globalization, and sociodemographic and nutritional transition [12, 13].

The surroundings of Kathmandu metropolitan city have many of the characteristics that can lead to an increase in noncommunicable diseases or conditions like hypertension. These factors include high internal migration from other regions of Nepal, increasing sedentary lifestyles, inadequate development and planning, high levels of air pollution, and changes in the dietary habits of residents [14]. However, there is little evidence on the prevalence and risk factors of hypertension in the periurban areas of Kathmandu District. Therefore, this study was conducted to estimate the prevalence of hypertension and to quantify health and social determinants related to hypertension in periurban areas of Kathmandu.

2. Methods

2.1. Study Design, Settings, and Participants. This was a community-based, cross-sectional study conducted in the newly established (established in December 2014) municipalities of Kathmandu District, Nepal, between January and July 2015. The ten municipalities are located on the outskirts of Kathmandu metropolitan city and are areas with rapid, unplanned urbanization and with high immigration of people from other areas of Nepal [14]. These municipalities contain a total population of more than 300,000 people [15].

Study participants were aged between 18 and 70 years, holding permanent resident status in the study areas at the time of study. Individuals diagnosed with any mental disorder or pregnant women were excluded from the study.

Of the ten municipalities in Kathmandu, two municipalities were randomly selected, one each from the eastern (Kageshwari-Manohara) and western (Nagarjun) clusters. These municipalities consist of around 130,000 people living in 27 Wards. From the total Wards, four Wards, two from each municipality, were randomly selected. The sample was proportionately allocated to each Ward based on the number of households in the Ward. A systematic random sampling method was then applied to choose 600 households from around 5600 households. The study area was mapped and each household was assigned a number, beginning from clockwise direction from first lane of eastern corner of the sites. One household was randomly selected from the first 10 houses using random number table, and then every 10th household from that initial household was approached systematically until the sample size was completed. Among adult members of each household, one individual from that household was enrolled in the study by KISH method [16].

2.2. Data Collection. Data were collected by face-to-face interview, anthropometric measurements, and clinical examinations. Fifteen medical professionals were recruited and trained in data collection methods.

2.2.1. Interview. The survey questionnaire (WHO STEPwise questionnaires) covered the demographics and health behaviors of respondents [17]. Demographic information included age, sex, ethnicity, marital status, years at school, and primary occupation. The health behaviors included tobacco use, alcohol consumption, fruit and vegetable consumption, and physical activity.

Tobacco Use. Questions were asked to identify current users, daily users, and past users.

Alcohol Consumption. Questions were asked to determine the current users of alcohol. Detailed information, such as the number of standard drinks consumed in the last 30 days, was obtained from current users. Pictorial cards showing different kinds of glasses and bowls most commonly used in Nepal were used to help the participants recall the amount of alcohol consumed. The amount, as identified by the respondent, was then used to estimate the number of standard drinks of alcohol consumed (one standard drink being defined as 10 grams of ethanol).

Diet. Seventy-two hours dietary recall was used to estimate fruit and vegetable consumption. Determination of the amount of fruit and vegetables consumed was aided by pictorial show cards and standard measuring cups.

Physical Activity. Seven-day history of physical activity was recorded. The physical activities related to work, transport, and recreational activities were categorized into vigorous, moderate, and low levels of activity in accordance with published guidelines [18, 19]. Vigorous physical activity was defined as any activity that had more than six Metabolic Equivalent of Task (MET) values. Moderate physical activity was defined as any activity that had MET values between three and six [18]. Physical activity having less than three METs, like spending time sitting at a desk or travelling in a car, bus, or train, was considered low or sedentary physical activity.

Diabetes. Participants were requested to provide information on status of diabetes or diabetic medication history.

2.2.2. Anthropometric Measurement. Height and weight were measured using the digital weighing machines and the portable standard stature scales, respectively, from which body mass index (BMI) was calculated. Waist and hip circumferences were also measured by Johnson's nonstretchable measuring tape in order to determine the waist-hip ratio.

2.2.3. Clinical Examination. Trained data collectors measured blood pressure using an aneroid sphygmomanometer. Before taking the measurements, respondents were requested to sit quietly and rest for 15 minutes with legs uncrossed. Three readings of the systolic and diastolic blood pressure were taken with three-minute rest between each reading and the mean of second and third reading was used for analysis.

2.2.4. Operational Definitions.

Standard operational definitions were adopted for key variables to maintain consistency and uniformity of the information.

Poor. Poor was defined as those having income less than 40,933 Nepalese Rupees per annum [20].

Current Smoker. Current smokers were defined as those who reported smoking any tobacco product within last 30 days. Respondents who reported smoking at least 100 cigarettes in their lifetime and who, at the time of the survey, did not smoke were defined as past smoker [21].

Current Alcohol Drinkers. Those who consumed alcohol within last 30 days were considered current alcohol drinkers [21].

Sufficient Fruit and Vegetables Intake. Intake of at least 400 gm of fruit and vegetables in a day was regarded as sufficient [22].

Sufficient Physical Activity. Sufficient physical activity was defined as ≥600 METs of moderate and vigorous activity in a week [18].

Hypertension. The diagnostic criterion for hypertension was set as a systolic blood pressure ≥ 140 mmHg and/or a diastolic blood pressure ≥ 90 mmHg as recommended by Joint National Committee-VII. Those research participants who were using antihypertensive medicine were also considered as hypertensive [23].

Diabetes. Self-reported status or the use of any antidiabetic medication was the diagnostic criteria for diabetes.

2.3. Sample Size.

Sample size was calculated for a single sample of the estimated population using the specified absolute precision formula ($N = z2pq/d2$) [24]. For estimation of sample size, prevalence of hypertension was taken as 25.7% [25] with 5% of allowable error. The sample size was adjusted with design effect (multiplied by 2) and nonresponse rate (2%). The total calculated sample size was 600.

2.4. Data Management and Analysis.

Data were compiled, edited, and checked to maintain consistency. Duplications and omissions of data were corrected before coding and entering them in Epidata V.2.1. Data were then exported to SPSS V.16.0 for analysis.

Frequencies and percentages were calculated to identify the distribution of sociodemographic characteristics. Chi-square and independent *t*-tests were conducted for comparing proportions of categorical and mean of continuous variables. Nonnormally distributed data were analyzed by Mann-Whitney U test. For multivariable analysis, hypertension was considered as a dichotomous dependent variable. Study variables having significant association with hypertension in bivariate analysis were entered in logistic model using Stepwise Forward Conditional method. The result was validated using Backward Conditional method. Variables having collinearity and confounding effects (waist circumference and hip circumference with BMI; age with diabetes) were excluded from the analysis. All tests were two-tailed and $p < 0.05$ was considered statistically significant.

3. Results

3.1. Sociodemographic Characteristics.

The total number of study participants was 587, excluding 13 who did not respond well. Of these, 58.8% were females. The mean (SD) age of participants was 42.3 (13.5) years. Nearly one-third (29.3%) of participants had no formal education. Of total participants, Brahmins comprised the largest proportion (35.1%), followed by Chetris (29.1%) and Newars (20.3%). Nearly half of the respondents were homemakers (41.2%) and were living below the poverty line (49%).

The difference in male and female count was not statistically significant by age group, ethnicity, and income level. However, education level and occupation significantly varied by gender (Table 1).

3.2. Prevalence of Hypertension.

The prevalence of hypertension in the study population was 32.5% (95% CI: 28.7–36.3). However, only 15.8% of participants were taking antihypertensive medication. Half of them (53.8% of hypertensive participants on treatment) were taking calcium channel blocker. A small proportion of the participants (2.2% of hypertensive participants on treatment) were also taking ayurvedic medicine for controlling hypertension. Of those on treatment, only half had controlled hypertension (<140/90 mmHg).

3.3. Sociodemographic Characteristics and Hypertension.

More males than females had high blood pressure (Table 2). Hypertension was also associated with age. Participants with lower educational status (primary and lower) were more likely to have hypertension. Ethnicity was also significantly associated with hypertension. However, there was no statistically significant association between occupation and hypertension.

3.4. Factors Associated with Hypertension

3.4.1. Smoking.

The proportion of current and past smokers was 19.9% and 17%, respectively. Both current smoking ($p = 0.009$) and past smoking ($p = 0.001$) participants were significantly associated with hypertension. The mean duration of smoking was also significantly higher ($p = 0.012$) in hypertensive participants than in normotensive participants (Table 3).

TABLE 1: Distribution of sociodemographic characteristics by gender.

Variables	Categories	Male N (%)	Female N (%)	Total N (%)	p value
Age groups	<30 years	49 (20.2)	69 (20.0)	118 (20.1)	
	30–39 years	47 (19.4)	90 (26.1)	137 (23.3)	
	40–49 years	69 (28.5)	81 (23.5)	150 (25.6)	0.147
	50–59 years	37 (15.3)	63 (18.3)	100 (17.0)	
	>60 years	40 (16.5)	42 (12.2)	82 (14.0)	
Education	No formal education	29 (12.0)	143 (41.4)	172 (29.3)	
	Primary and lower	30 (12.4)	53 (15.4)	83 (14.1)	
	Secondary	64 (26.4)	65 (18.8)	129 (22.0)	<0.01
	Higher Secondary	52 (21.5)	47 (13.6)	99 (16.9)	
	Bachelor and higher	67 (27.7)	37 (10.7)	104 (17.7)	
Ethnicity	Brahman	95 (39.3)	111 (32.2)	206 (35.1)	
	Chetri	68 (28.1)	103 (29.9)	171 (29.1)	0.246
	Newar	48 (19.8)	71 (20.6)	119 (20.3)	
	Others	31 (12.8)	60 (17.4)	91 (15.5)	
Occupation	Job	66 (27.3)	35 (10.1)	101 (17.2)	
	Self-employed	87 (36.0)	54 (15.7)	141 (24.0)	<0.01
	Homemaker	30 (12.4)	212 (61.4)	242 (41.2)	
	Others	59 (24.4)	44 (12.8)	103 (17.5)	
Marital status	Unmarried	36 (14.9)	32 (9.3)	68 (11.6)	
	Married	204 (84.3)	283 (82.0)	487 (83)	<0.01
	Others (separated or widow)	2 (0.8)	30 (8.7)	32 (5.5)	
Socioeconomic status	Below poverty line	115 (47.9)	170 (49.7)	285 (49.0)	0.671
	Above poverty line	125 (52.1)	172 (50.3)	297 (51.0)	

Note: primary and lower education, grade 1–5; secondary, grade 6–10; higher secondary, grade 11-12; job, governmental or nongovernmental employment; self-employed, working for oneself as a freelancer or the owner of a business or working in own farm; homemaker, a person, especially a housewife, who manages a home; other occupations, volunteer or student or unemployed or retired; below poverty line, income less than 40,933 Nepalese Rupees per annum.

3.4.2. Alcohol Consumption. More than one-quarter (27%) of participants reported current alcohol use. Alcohol consumption had a significant positive association ($p = 0.035$) with hypertension. The hypertensive participants reported drinking a significantly higher number of standard drinks in a single sitting ($p < 0.001$) than normotensive participants (Table 3).

3.4.3. Fruit and Vegetable Consumption. Approximately, 1 in every 10 participants (11.4%) reported consuming the recommended amount of fruit and vegetable daily. The daily median intake for total fruit and vegetables per person was 188.9 gm (interquartile range (IQR): 204 gm). For green leafy vegetable, only the median intake was 75 gm per day (IQR: 125 gm). Median daily fruit intake per person was 45 gm (IQR: 120 gm). Fruit and vegetable intake was not significantly associated ($p = 0.542$) with hypertension.

3.4.4. Physical Activity. More than three-quarters of participants (78.4%) had the sufficient physical activity level (≥600 METs/week). The median (IQR) of METs of moderate and vigorous physical activities per week was 1850 (IQR: 2853). Adequate physical activity was associated with normal blood pressure ($p = 0.038$).

3.4.5. Obesity. The mean of body mass index (BMI) among respondents was 24.8 kg/m². It was significantly different ($p < 0.001$) between people having high and normal blood pressure. Similarly, waist ($p < 0.001$) and hip ($p < 0.004$) circumferences were also significantly higher in hypertensive participants than in normotensive participants.

3.4.6. Diabetes and Other Factors. One in every ten participants (10.7%) reported that they had diabetes mellitus. Similarly, 12.6% of participants had the presence of cardiovascular disease (CVD) among their first-degree relatives and 31.6% of female participants had menopausal history. Diabetes ($p < 0.001$), cessation of menstruation ($p < 0.001$), and having family history of CVD ($p < 0.001$) were significantly associated with hypertension (Table 3).

3.5. Adjusted Associated Factors of Hypertension. In multivariable model, BMI ($\beta = 0.127$ and $p < 0.001$), smoking ($\beta = 0.671$ and $p = 0.005$), alcohol use ($\beta = 0.473$ and $p = 0.03$), insufficient physical activity ($\beta = 0.472$ and $p = 0.04$), and presence of diabetes ($\beta = 0.934$ and $p = 0.001$) were identified as significant factors associated with hypertension (Table 4). Every unit gain in BMI increased the likelihood of having hypertension by 13.5%. The chance of

TABLE 2: Association of sociodemographic characteristics with hypertension.

Variables	Categories	Hypertension		p value
		Yes	No	
		N (%)	N (%)	
Gender	Male	93 (38.4)	149 (61.6)	0.011
	Female	98 (28.4)	247 (71.6)	
Age groups	<30 years	7 (5.9)	111 (94.1)	<0.001
	30–39 years	22 (16.1)	115 (83.9)	
	40–49 years	71 (47.3)	79 (52.7)	
	50–59 years	45 (45.0)	55 (55.0)	
	≥60 years	46 (56.1)	36 (43.9)	
Education	No formal education	72 (41.9)	100 (58.1)	<0.01
	Primary and lower	33 (39.8)	50 (60.2)	
	Secondary	37 (28.7)	92 (71.3)	
	Higher secondary	22 (22.2)	77 (77.8)	
	Bachelor and higher	27 (26.0)	77 (74.0)	
Ethnicity	Brahman	54 (26.2)	152 (73.8)	0.049
	Chetri	55 (32.2)	116 (67.8)	
	Newar	46 (38.7)	73 (61.3)	
	Other	36 (50.0)	3 (50.0)	
Occupation	Job	32 (31.7)	69 (68.3)	0.725
	Self-employed	43 (30.5)	98 (69.5)	
	Homemaker	85 (35.1)	157 (64.9)	
	Others	31 (30.1)	72 (69.9)	
Marital status	Unmarried	8 (11.8)	60 (88.2)	<0.001
	Married	167 (34.3)	320 (65.7)	
	Others (separated or widow)	16 (50.0)	16 (50.0)	
Socioeconomic status	Below poverty line	95 (33.3)	190 (66.7)	0.665
	Above poverty line	94 (31.6)	203 (68.4)	

Note: primary and lower education, grade 1–5; secondary, grade 6–10; higher secondary, grade 11-12; job, governmental or nongovernmental employment; self-employed, working for oneself as a freelancer or the owner of a business or working in own farm; homemaker, a person, especially a housewife, who manages a home; other occupation, volunteer or student or unemployed or retired; below poverty line, income less than 40,933 Nepalese Rupees per annum.

being hypertensive among current smokers was 1.95 times higher than among nonsmokers. Similarly, current alcohol users had 60% higher chance of having hypertension than the participants who refrained from alcohol. After controlling for other factors, the odds of being hypertensive were about 60% higher for the participants who had insufficient physical activity compared to those who had sufficient physical activity. In the same way, presence of diabetes among study participants increased the odds of being hypertensive by 2.54 times compared to nondiabetic participants.

4. Discussion

Our study found a high prevalence of hypertension in people living in the newly declared municipalities of Kathmandu. The factors associated with hypertension in this study group were found to be smoking, BMI, alcohol use, poor physical activity, and diabetes. This was the first community-based study conducted to estimate the prevalence of hypertension and identify its associated factors in the area. However, this study could not examine causal relationship between

hypertension and its risk factors because of the nature of study design.

The prevalence of hypertension in the study population (32.5%) was higher than in those of noncommunicable disease (NCD) risk factor surveys in Nepal (21.5% in 2007; 25.7% in 2013) [21, 25]. This disparity in findings may be due to differences in the study populations as the NCD surveys were conducted both in urban and in rural areas, while the current study was conducted in a periurban setting. Rural Nepal has a lower burden of hypertension than urban areas [26]. Similarly, the finding was nearly the double of the hypertension prevalence (19.7%) reported by a study conducted in similar setting of Kathmandu in 2005 [27]. This almost twofold increase in hypertension prevalence in ten years may be due to changes in living conditions and lifestyle in that time. This is further supported by the findings from a study conducted in rural areas of Kathmandu that reported a threefold increase in hypertension prevalence in 25 years [26]. This increase was attributed to increasing BMI in the study population [28].

Although it is well established that smoking increases the risk of hypertension, the strength of this association may

TABLE 3: Association of behavioral, metabolic, and other factors with hypertension.

Variables	Categories	N	Hypertension Yes n (%) or mean ± SD or median (IQR)	Hypertension No n (%) or mean ± SD or median (IQR)	Total n or mean ± SD or median (IQR)	p value
Smoking (current)	Yes	587	50 (42.7)	67 (57.3)	117	0.009
	No		141 (30.0)	329 (70.0)	470	
Smoking (past)	Yes	470	36 (45.0)	44 (55.0)	80	0.001
	No		105 (26.9)	285 (73.1)	390	
Smoking duration among current smoker (years)	—	114	25 (24)	13.5 (20)	20 (26)	0.012*
Alcohol consumption (current)	Yes	587	62 (39.2)	96 (60.8)	158	0.035
	No		129 (30.1)	300 (69.9)	429	
Average standard alcohol intake in single sitting	—	156	4 (6)	2 (3)	3 (4)	<0.001*
Sufficient fruit and vegetable consumption	Yes	587	24 (35.8)	43 (64.2)	67	0.542
	No		167 (32.1)	353 (67.9)	520	
Sufficient physical activity	Yes	587	140 (30.4)	320 (69.6)	460	0.038
	No		51 (40.2)	76 (59.8)	127	
BMI (kg/m^2)	—	587	26.2 ± 4.5	24.1 ± 4.1	24.8 ± 4.4	<0.001
Waist circumference (cm)	—	587	84 ± 11.8	78 ± 10.1	83.9 ± 11	<0.001
Hip circumference (cm)	—	587	90.5 ± 9.9	88.1 ± 8.9	90.9 ± 9.3	0.004
Diabetes mellitus	Yes	587	34 (54.0)	29 (46.0)	63	<0.001
	No		157 (30.0)	367 (70.0)	524	
Menopause	Yes	281	41 (21.4)	151 (78.6)	192	<0.001
	No		43 (48.3)	46 (51.7)	89	
CVD family history	Yes	562	37 (52.1)	34 (47.9)	71	<0.001
	No		144 (29.3)	347 (70.7)	491	

*Mann-Whitney U test was used to compare nonnormally distributed data.
Note: sufficient fruit and vegetable consumption, intake of ≥400 gm of fruit and vegetable per day; sufficient physical activity, ≥600 METs of moderate and vigorous activity in a week; one standard drink, 10 grams of ethanol.
BMI, body mass index; CVD, cardiovascular disease.

TABLE 4: Multivariable analysis for hypertension.

Variables	Category	β	p value	AOR	95% CI for AOR Lower	95% CI for AOR Upper
Constant		−2.220	0.005	0.109		
BMI (kg/m^2)		0.127	<0.001	1.135	1.084	1.188
Smoking (current)	No			Reference		
	Yes	0.671	0.005	1.957	1.219	3.141
Alcohol user (current)	No			Reference		
	Yes	0.473	0.030	1.605	1.047	2.460
Physical activity	Sufficient			Reference		
	Nonsufficient	0.472	0.040	1.604	1.022	2.517
Diabetes mellitus-II	No			Reference		
	Yes	0.934	0.001	2.545	1.454	4.457

Note: sufficient physical activity, ≥600 METs of moderate and vigorous activity in a week.
BMI, body mass index.

differ between study settings and populations. Our study showed that smoking increased the likelihood of being hypertensive by twofold. This finding is consistent with previous studies conducted in India and China [29–31]. However, some observational studies reported smokers having a lower risk of hypertension than nonsmokers, which contrasted to our finding [32–37]. Our study also found that the median length of smoking duration was significantly higher among the hypertensive participants. Therefore, one of the reasons for the aforementioned inconsistency in findings could be the variations in frequency and total duration of smoking.

Our study found that the odds of having hypertension were increased by 1.6 times with the use of alcohol. The result was in line with the findings reported by Todkar et al. in India and Wei et al. in China [38, 39]. However, there are some studies that found protective effects of alcohol on hypertension [40, 41]. Some also failed to demonstrate any significant association between alcohol consumption and hypertension [30, 35]. These differences in findings might have occurred because of difference in amount and concentration of alcohol consumed. Sacco et al. and Kannel and Ellison concluded that protective effect of alcohol in hypertension and other cardiovascular diseases was mainly detected among the moderate alcohol users (up to two standard drinks per day). The effect was opposite among those consuming seven and more drinks per day [40, 41]. A meta-analysis of 15 randomized controlled trials observed a dose response relationship of alcohol reduction and on blood pressure [42]. This is supported by the current findings which demonstrated that the median number of standard drinks consumed was significantly higher among the hypertensive participants. Further research is required to explain the apparent bidirectional effects of alcohol intake on hypertension.

The current study revealed that one in every four participants reported being a current alcohol user. The proportion was higher than that of recent noncommunicable disease risk factor survey (17.4%) in Nepal [25]. This may be due to a higher social acceptance of alcohol use in the study areas compared to Nepal as a whole. The high rates of alcohol consumption in this population need to be considered when implementing programs to address hypertension.

Despite the well-recognized inverse relationship between fruit and vegetable consumption and hypertension [43, 44], our study showed no association between them. A study conducted in rural Nepal also reported a similar result [26]. A more detailed food frequency questionnaire in future studies may assist in confirming these findings. However, the fluctuating pattern of fruit and vegetable consumption in Nepal due to the seasonal availability of these foods may make clarifying the association with hypertension difficult [24]. The ideal measure of Nepalese fruit and vegetable consumption warrants further discussion.

This study found that sedentary lifestyle was an issue in this study population. The proportion of participants (21.6%) having insufficient physical activity (<600 METs/Week) was six times higher than that reported in a national survey (3.5%) [25]. Unplanned and rapid urbanization, high population density, increased use of motorized vehicles and,

modern technology could be predisposing factors for low physical activity among this population [45]. The increased risk of hypertension among study participants reporting low levels of physical activity was consistent with other studies [30, 32, 45]. These findings suggest that several cardiometabolic problems may arise in near future as the consequences of insufficient physical activity. Even though confirming the causal relationship between physical activity and cardiometabolic diseases, including hypertension, is beyond the scope of this study, several previous studies have demonstrated the association [46, 47]. Therefore, Nepal should not delay initiating interventions that improve physical activity through community-based strategies that incorporate informational, behavioral, social, policy-making, and environmental approaches [48].

Body mass index, waist circumference, and hip circumference, all measures related to overweight and obesity, were significantly higher in hypertensive participants than in normotensive participants. These findings were in line with results from previous studies conducted in Nepal [26, 28]. Like physical inactivity, obesity has also well-recognized independent relationship with a spectrum of cardiometabolic disorders including hypertension [49]. There are several mechanisms hypothesized to explain the link between obesity with hypertension [10, 11, 49, 50]. It is generally thought that the accumulation of visceral and ectopic fat in a number of tissues and organs alters the metabolic and hemodynamic pathways, leading to the development of hypertension in obese people [49, 50]. The reduction of overweight and obesity by improving nutrition and increasing regular physical activity is the best way to avoid or improve hypertension [51].

Diabetes was associated with twofold increased odds of being hypertensive. The finding was consistent with the results of the studies conducted in similar settings of Kathmandu, Nepal [52, 53], and internationally [54, 55]. Hypertension is often reported to be one of the most common comorbid conditions in those suffering from diabetes. For instance, around half of diabetic patients in Australia have hypertension [56]. Similarly, almost a quarter of hypertensive patients were found to have diabetes in China and India [57, 58]. The coexistence of hypertension and diabetes might be because of sharing common risk factors like smoking, alcohol consumption, unhealthy diets, and physical inactivity. Due to nature of this study, it is difficult to state with certainty whether diabetes led to hypertension or hypertension led to diabetes. This study only included self-reported diabetic cases, which would underestimate the rate of diabetes in the study population. Further research is required in this population to accurately estimate the impact of diabetes on hypertension.

Our study also found associations between hypertension and other recognized risk factors including menopause [59–61]. Similarly, presence of cardiovascular diseases including hypertension among first-degree relatives of the participants had a significant association with hypertension among study population. The familial pattern of hypertension was well established long before [62], and it is now considered as one of the major nonmodifiable risk factors for hypertension, like age and race [63].

This study identifies some of the major factors associated with hypertension in people living in the outer areas of Kathmandu. Several of these factors could be targeted to improve the health of the population in these areas. One example where improvements have been made is in relation to smoking. The proportion of current smoking in our study (19.9%) was similar to that of a national survey (18.5%) conducted in Nepal [25]. After signing the WHO Framework Convention on Tobacco Control (WHO FCTC), Nepal is implementing tobacco control initiatives such as health warnings on tobacco products, prohibition of smoking in public places, heavy taxation of the tobacco industry, and increasing public awareness of harmful effects of tobacco. Since these initiatives have been implemented there has been a decreasing trend in prevalence of smoking in Nepal [64, 65]. The presence of large proportion of past smokers (17%) in current study might also suggest the trend of quitting smoking in the study areas. These initiatives should also lead to an improvement in the health of people in Nepal, including a reduction in the risk of hypertension. Initiatives to improve factors like physical activity and alcohol consumption in these regions of Nepal would also be useful in reducing the risk of hypertension and improving overall health.

5. Conclusion

Overall, this study determined a high prevalence of hypertension in the study population. Hypertension was associated with smoking, alcohol consumption, low physical activity, obesity, and diabetes. Therefore, community-based approaches for reduction of hypertension and its risk factors are essential. Effective community-based preventive and control strategies might provide the best opportunities to avoid hypertension driven health and economic consequences in Nepal.

Ethical Approval

The study protocol was reviewed and approved by Ethical Review Board of the Nepal Health Research Council, Kathmandu. Written consent was obtained from all participants after detailed explanation of research purpose and assurance of maintaining privacy and confidentiality. Those who needed further treatment were referred to tertiary treatment centers.

Competing Interests

The authors declare that they have no competing interests.

Authors' Contributions

Raja Ram Dhungana provided concept, designed and executed the study, analyzed and interpreted the data, and prepared the first draft of the paper. Achyut Raj Pandey, Bihungum Bista, and Suira Joshi provided an input on statistical analysis, interpretation of study, and preparation of the draft. Surya Devkota contributed in study concept, design, and interpretation. All authors read and approved the final paper.

Acknowledgments

The authors want to express their gratitude and appreciation to Dr. Damien Cordery, Senior Epidemiologist, for providing the first review of the paper. They would like to thank field supervisor and data enumerator team: Dr. Savyata Panthi, Mr. Rajan Gyawali, Mr. Krishna Gyawali, Miss Santi Timalsina, Mr. Nawaraj Vetwal, Mr. BikasMaharjan, Mr. Deepen Devkota, Mr. Dependra Jung Rana, Miss Bibechana Pandey, Miss Amrita Paudel, Mr. Lokendra Karki, Mr. Santosh Singh Thapa, Miss Shila Sapkota, and Miss Jenny Roka. Also, special thanks are due to Kageshwari-Manohara and Nagarjun municipalities' members, FCHV team, and local leaders for helping in community mobilization. This study was funded by a research grant from Jayanti Memorial Trust, Kathmandu, Nepal.

References

[1] S. S. Lim, T. Vos, A. D. Flaxman et al., "A comparative risk assessment of burden of disease and injury attributable to 67 risk factors and risk factor clusters in 21 regions, 1990–2010: a systematic analysis for the Global Burden of Disease Study 2010," *The Lancet*, vol. 380, no. 9859, pp. 2224–2260, 2012.

[2] Global Health Observatory Data Repository, http://apps.who .int/gho/data/view.main.2540?lang=en.

[3] T. A. Gaziano, A. Bitton, S. Anand, and M. C. Weinstein, "The global cost of nonoptimal blood pressure," *Journal of Hypertension*, vol. 27, no. 7, pp. 1472–1477, 2009.

[4] World Health Organization, "A global brief on Hypertension, silent killer, global public health crisis. 2013," 2014, http://apps.who.int/iris/bitstream/10665/79059/1/WHO_DCO_WHD_2013.2_eng.pdf.

[5] WHO, *The World Health Report 2002: Reducing Risks, Promoting Healthy Life*, World Health Organization, Geneva, Switzerland, 2002.

[6] J. A. Ambrose and R. S. Barua, "The pathophysiology of cigarette smoking and cardiovascular disease: an update," *Journal of the American College of Cardiology*, vol. 43, no. 10, pp. 1731–1737, 2004.

[7] L. J. Beilin and I. B. Puddey, "Alcohol and hypertension: an update," *Hypertension*, vol. 47, no. 6, pp. 1035–1038, 2006.

[8] H. D. Sesso, N. R. Cook, J. E. Buring, J. E. Manson, and J. M. Gaziano, "Alcohol consumption and the risk of hypertension in women and men," *Hypertension*, vol. 51, no. 4, pp. 1080–1087, 2008.

[9] N. R. C. Campbell, D. T. Lackland, and M. L. Niebylski, "2014 dietary salt fact sheet of the world hypertension league, international society of hypertension, pan American health organization technical advisory group on cardiovascular disease prevention through dietary salt reduction, the world health organization collaborating centre on population salt reduction, and world action on salt & health," *Journal of Clinical Hypertension*, vol. 17, no. 1, pp. 7–9, 2015.

[10] L. Landsberg, "Diet, obesity and hypertension: an hypothesis involving insulin, the sympathetic nervous system, and adaptive thermogenesis," *Quarterly Journal of Medicine*, vol. 61, no. 236, pp. 1081–1090, 1986.

[11] F. Abbasi, B. W. Brown Jr., C. Lamendola, T. McLaughlin, and G. M. Reaven, "Relationship between obesity, insulin resistance, and coronary heart disease risk," *Journal of the American College of Cardiology*, vol. 40, no. 5, pp. 937–943, 2002.

[12] K.-H. Wagner and H. Brath, "A global view on the development of non communicable diseases," *Preventive Medicine*, vol. 54, pp. S38–S41, 2012.

[13] A. Contractor, B. K. Sarkar, M. Arora, and K. Saluja, "Addressing cardiovascular disease burden in low and middle income countries (LMICs)," *Current Cardiovascular Risk Reports*, vol. 8, no. 11, pp. 1–9, 2014.

[14] E. Muzzini and G. Aparicio, *Urban Growth and Spatial Transition in Nepal*, The World Bank, Washington, DC, USA, 2014.

[15] Government of Nepal, *National Population and Housing Census 2011*, vol. 2, Central Bureau of Statistics, Kathmandu, Nepal, 2012.

[16] World Health Organization, *WHO STEPS Surveillance Manual*, World Health Organization, Geneva, Switzerland, 2008.

[17] The WHO STEPwise approach to chronic disease risk factor surveillance (STEPS), http://www.who.int/chp/steps/STEPS_Instrument_v2.1.pdf.

[18] W. L. Haskell, I.-M. Lee, R. R. Pate et al., "Physical activity and public health: updated recommendation for adults from the American College of Sports Medicine and the American Heart Association," *Circulation*, vol. 116, no. 9, pp. 1081–1093, 2007.

[19] The 2011 Compendium of Physical Activities: Tracking Guide, https://sites.google.com/site/compendiumofphysicalactivities/tracking-guide.

[20] Central Bureau of Statistics and World Bank, Poverty in Nepal 2010-11: Findings from NLSS-III, 2012, http://un.org.np/data-coll/Demography-Publications/2011%20Key%20Findings(%20NLSS%20III).pdf.

[21] Ministry of Health and Population GoN and Society for Local Integrated Development Nepal (SOLID Nepal) and WHO, "WHO STEPS surveillance: non-communicable diseases risk factors survey," in *Kathmandu*, Ministry of Health and Population, Government of Nepal, Society for Local Integrated Development Nepal (SOLID Nepal) and WHO, 2008.

[22] J. N. Hall, S. Moore, S. B. Harper, and J. W. Lynch, "Global variability in fruit and vegetable consumption," *American Journal of Preventive Medicine*, vol. 36, no. 5, pp. 402–409.e405, 2009.

[23] C. Lenfant, A. V. Chobanian, D. W. Jones, and E. J. Roccella, "Seventh report of the joint national committee on the prevention, detection, evaluation, and treatment of high blood pressure (JNC 7): resetting the hypertension sails," *Hypertension*, vol. 41, no. 6, pp. 1178–1179, 2003.

[24] S. K. Wanga and S. Lemeshow, *Sample Size Determination in Health Studies. A Practical Manual Ginebra*, World Health Organization, Geneva, Switzerland, 1991.

[25] K. K. Aryal, S. Neupane, S. Mehata et al., *Non Communicable Disease Risk Factors: STEPS Survey Nepal 2013*, Nepal Health Research Council, 2013.

[26] R. R. Dhungana, S. Devkota, M. K. Khanal et al., "Prevalence of cardiovascular health risk behaviors in a remote rural community of Sindhuli district, Nepal," *BMC Cardiovascular Disorders*, vol. 14, article 92, 2014.

[27] D. Sharma, M. Bkc, S. Rajbhandari et al., "Study of prevalence, awareness, and control of hypertension in a suburban area of Kathmandu, Nepal," *Indian Heart Journal*, vol. 58, no. 1, pp. 34–37, 2005.

[28] A. Vaidya, R. P. Pathak, and M. R. Pandey, "Prevalence of hypertension in Nepalese community triples in 25 years: a repeat cross-sectional study in rural Kathmandu," *Indian Heart Journal*, vol. 64, no. 2, pp. 128–131, 2012.

[29] R. B. Singh, J. Fedacko, D. Pella et al., "Prevalence and risk factors for prehypertension and hypertension in five Indian cities," *Acta Cardiologica*, vol. 66, no. 1, pp. 29–37, 2011.

[30] C. S. Shanthirani, R. Pradeepa, R. Deepa, G. Premalatha, R. Saroja, and V. Mohan, "Prevalence and risk factors of hypertension in a selected South Indian population—the Chennai Urban Population Study," *Journal of Association of Physicians of India*, vol. 51, pp. 20–27, 2003.

[31] V. Mohan, M. Deepa, S. Farooq, M. Datta, and R. Deepa, "Prevalence, awareness and control of hypertension in Chennai—the Chennai Urban Rural Epidemiology study (CURES—52)," *Journal of Association of Physicians of India*, vol. 55, pp. 326–332, 2007.

[32] P. Malhotra, S. Kumari, R. Kumar, S. Jain, and B. K. Sharma, "Prevalence and determinants of hypertension in an un-industrialised rural population of North India," *Journal of Human Hypertension*, vol. 13, no. 7, pp. 467–472, 1999.

[33] S. Panesar, S. Chaturvedi, N. Saini, R. Avasthi, and A. Singh, "Prevalence and predictors of hypertension among residents aged 20–59 years of a slum-resettlement colony in Delhi, India," *WHO South-East Asia Journal of Public Health*, vol. 2, no. 2, pp. 83–87, 2013.

[34] J.-C. Katte, A. Dzudie, E. Sobngwi et al., "Coincidence of diabetes mellitus and hypertension in a semi-urban Cameroonian population: a cross-sectional study," *BMC Public Health*, vol. 14, article 696, 2014.

[35] J. Chataut, R. K. Adhikari, and S. Np, "The prevalence of and risk factors for hypertension in adults living in central development region of Nepal," *Kathmandu University Medical Journal*, vol. 9, no. 33, pp. 13–18, 2011.

[36] Z. Sun, L. Zheng, R. Detrano et al., "Incidence and predictors of hypertension among rural Chinese adults: results from Liaoning Province," *Annals of Family Medicine*, vol. 8, no. 1, pp. 19–24, 2010.

[37] G. D. Friedman, A. L. Klatsky, and A. B. Slegelaub, "Alcohol, tobacco, and hypertension," *Hypertension*, vol. 4, no. 5, part 2, pp. Iii143–Iii150, 1982.

[38] S. S. Todkar, V. V. Gujarathi, and V. S. Tapare, "Period prevalence and sociodemographic factors of hypertension in rural Maharashtra: a cross-sectional study," *Indian Journal of Community Medicine*, vol. 34, no. 3, pp. 183–187, 2009.

[39] Q. Wei, J. Sun, J. Huang et al., "Prevalence of hypertension and associated risk factors in Dehui City of Jilin Province in China," *Journal of Human Hypertension*, vol. 29, no. 1, pp. 64–68, 2015.

[40] R. L. Sacco, M. Elkind, B. Boden-Albala et al., "The protective effect of moderate alcohol consumption on ischemic stroke," *The Journal of the American Medical Association*, vol. 281, no. 1, pp. 53–60, 1999.

[41] W. B. Kannel and R. C. Ellison, "Alcohol and coronary heart disease: the evidence for a protective effect," *Clinica Chimica Acta*, vol. 246, no. 1-2, pp. 59–76, 1996.

[42] X. Xin, J. He, M. G. Frontini, L. G. Ogden, O. I. Motsamai, and P. K. Whelton, "Effects of alcohol reduction on blood pressure: a meta-analysis of randomized controlled trials," *Hypertension*, vol. 38, no. 5, pp. 1112–1117, 2001.

[43] J. M. Nuñez-Cordoba, A. Alonso, J. J. Beunza, S. Palma, E. Gomez-Gracia, and M. A. Martinez-Gonzalez, "Role of vegetables and fruits in Mediterranean diets to prevent hypertension,"

European Journal of Clinical Nutrition, vol. 63, no. 5, pp. 605–612, 2009.

[44] M. T. Utsugi, T. Ohkubo, M. Kikuya et al., "Fruit and vegetable consumption and the risk of hypertension determined by self measurement of blood pressure at home: the Ohasama study," *Hypertension Research*, vol. 31, no. 7, pp. 1435–1443, 2008.

[45] A. Vaidya and A. Krettek, "Physical activity level and its sociodemographic correlates in a peri-urban Nepalese population: a cross-sectional study from the Jhaukhel-Duwakot health demographic surveillance site," *International Journal of Behavioral Nutrition and Physical Activity*, vol. 11, no. 1, article 39, 2014.

[46] B. Arroll and R. Beaglehole, "Does physical activity lower blood pressure: a critical review of the clinical trials," *Journal of Clinical Epidemiology*, vol. 45, no. 5, pp. 439–447, 1992.

[47] S. P. Whelton, A. Chin, X. Xin, and J. He, "Effect of aerobic exercise on blood pressure: a meta-analysis of randomized, controlled trials," *Annals of Internal Medicine*, vol. 136, no. 7, pp. 493–503, 2002.

[48] C. Blanchard, T. Shilton, and F. Bull, "Global Advocacy for Physical Activity (GAPA): global leadership towards a raised profile," *Global Health Promotion*, vol. 20, no. 4, supplement, pp. 113–121, 2013.

[49] K. P. Davy and J. E. Halle, "Obesity and hypertension: two epidemics or one?" *American Journal of Physiology—Regulatory Integrative and Comparative Physiology*, vol. 286, no. 5, pp. R803–R813, 2004.

[50] P. Poirier, T. D. Giles, G. A. Bray et al., "Obesity and cardiovascular disease: pathophysiology, evaluation, and effect of weight loss," *Arteriosclerosis, Thrombosis, and Vascular Biology*, vol. 26, no. 5, pp. 968–976, 2006.

[51] B. H. Goodpaster, J. P. DeLany, A. D. Otto et al., "Effects of diet and physical activity interventions on weight loss and cardiometabolic risk factors in severely obese adults: a randomized trial," *The Journal of the American Medical Association*, vol. 304, no. 16, pp. 1795–1802, 2010.

[52] M. R. Chhetri and R. S. Chapman, "Prevalence and determinants of diabetes among the elderly population in the Kathmandu Valley of Nepal," *Nepal Medical College Journal*, vol. 11, no. 1, pp. 34–38, 2009.

[53] U. K. Shrestha, D. L. Singh, and M. D. Bhattarai, "The prevalence of hypertension and diabetes defined by fasting and 2-h plasma glucose criteria in urban Nepal," *Diabetic Medicine*, vol. 23, no. 10, pp. 1130–1135, 2006.

[54] A. Awoke, T. Awoke, S. Alemu, and B. Megabiaw, "Prevalence and associated factors of hypertension among adults in Gondar, Northwest Ethiopia: a community based cross-sectional study," *BMC Cardiovascular Disorders*, vol. 12, article 113, 2012.

[55] Y. Gao, G. Chen, H. Tian et al., "Prevalence of hypertension in China: a cross-sectional study," *PLoS ONE*, vol. 8, no. 6, Article ID e65938, 2013.

[56] G. E. Caughey, A. I. Vitry, A. L. Gilbert, and E. E. Roughead, "Prevalence of comorbidity of chronic diseases in Australia," *BMC Public Health*, vol. 8, article 221, 2008.

[57] J. Liu, R. Wang, K. Desai, and L. Wu, "Upregulation of aldolase B and overproduction of methylglyoxal in vascular tissues from rats with metabolic syndrome," *Cardiovascular Research*, vol. 92, no. 3, pp. 494–503, 2011.

[58] K. Venugopal and M. Z. Mohammed, "Prevalence of hypertension in type-2 diabetes mellitus," *CHRISMED Journal of Health and Research*, vol. 1, no. 4, pp. 223–227, 2014.

[59] J. A. Staessen, G. Ginocchio, L. Thijs, and R. Fagard, "Conventional and ambulatory blood pressure and menopause in a prospective population study," *Journal of Human Hypertension*, vol. 11, no. 8, pp. 507–514, 1997.

[60] A. S. Sapkota, A. Sapkota, K. Acharya, M. Raut, and B. Jha, "Study of metabolic syndrome in postmenopausal women," *Annals of Clinical Chemistry and Laboratory Medicine*, vol. 1, no. 1, pp. 6–11, 2015.

[61] M. Coylewright, J. F. Reckelhoff, and P. Ouyang, "Menopause and hypertension: an age-old debate," *Hypertension*, vol. 51, no. 4, pp. 952–959, 2008.

[62] C. B. Thomas, "Familial patterns in hypertension and coronary heart disease," *Circulation*, vol. 20, no. 1, pp. 25–29, 1959.

[63] K. Bell, J. Twiggs, and B. R. Olin, *Hypertension: The Silent Killer: Updated JNC-8 Guideline Recommendations*, Alabama Pharmacy Association, Montgomery, Ala, USA, 2015.

[64] MOHP, New ERA, and ICF International, "Nepal Demographic and Health Survey," in *Kathmandu*, MOHP, New ERA, ICF International, 2006.

[65] MOHP, New ERA, and ICF International, "Nepal demographic and health survey," in *Nepal: Demographic and Health Survey*, MOHP, New ERA, ICF International, 2011.

11

Provider Adherence to National Guidelines for Managing Hypertension

Jeanette Sessoms, Kathryn Reid, Ishan Williams, and Ivora Hinton

University of Virginia School of Nursing, McLeod Hall, P.O. Box 800782, Charlottesville, VA 22908-0782, USA

Correspondence should be addressed to Jeanette Sessoms; jms2cy@virginia.edu

Academic Editor: Roberto Pontremoli

Purpose. To evaluate provider adherence to national guidelines for the treatment of hypertension in African Americans. *Design.* A descriptive, preexperimental, quantitative method. *Methods.* Electronic medical records were reviewed and data were obtained from 62 charts. Clinical data collected included blood pressure readings, medications prescribed, laboratory studies, lifestyle modification, referral to hypertension specialist, and follow-up care. *Findings.* Overall provider adherence was 75%. Weight loss, sodium restriction, and physical activity recommendations were documented on 82.3% of patients. DASH diet and alcohol consumption were documented in 6.5% of participants. Follow-up was documented in 96.6% of the patients with controlled blood pressure and 9.1% in patients with uncontrolled blood pressure. Adherence in prescribing ACEIs in patients with a comorbidity of DM was documented in 70% of participants. Microalbumin levels were ordered in 15.2% of participants. Laboratory adherence prior to prescribing medications was documented in 0% of the patients and biannual routine labs were documented in 65% of participants. *Conclusion.* Provider adherence overall was moderate. Despite moderate provider adherence, BP outcomes and provider adherence were not related. Contributing factors that may explain this lack of correlation include patient barriers such as nonadherence to medication and lifestyle modification recommendations and lack of adequate follow-up. Further research is warranted.

1. Introduction

Hypertension (HTN) is a medical condition that is characterized by high or uncontrolled blood pressure. Inadequate control of HTN can lead to more serious vascular conditions affecting the major blood vessels in the heart, brain, and body. Additionally, HTN and diabetes mellitus (DM) frequently coexist, which further increases the risk of developing vascular complications. Vascular complications are a group of disorders that affects the heart and blood vessels. Hypertension is a major risk factor for vascular disease including heart attacks and strokes [1]. In 2008, an estimated 17.3 million people died from vascular complications. Of those 17.3 million vascular-associated deaths, 6.2 million were due to strokes [2]. It is predicted that, by the year 2030, an estimated 23.3 million will die from stroke and heart disease [2]. Addressing risk factors that contribute to HTN may help prevent vascular complications. According to the World Health Organization (WHO) [3], complications of

HTN such as strokes account for 9.4 million of the astounding 17 million vascular-associated deaths. Another consideration is the financial burden of HTN; according to the Centers for Disease Control and Prevention (CDC) [4], the annual cost of HTN treatment was 131 billion dollars.

The physical and financial burdens of HTN are not unique to any one group of individuals. However, it has been well documented that African Americans (AAs) have a disproportionate burden of morbidity and mortality compared to Caucasians [1]. Data collected from 2008 suggest that non-Hispanic blacks accounted for 31.7% of the 59.4 million people with HTN, whereas non-Hispanic whites accounted for only 26.8% [2]. Despite research and interventions to decrease both the physical and financial burdens of uncontrolled HTN, specifically in the AA population, HTN remains a national problem [5].

Numerous interventions have been documented to improve control of HTN in AAs. The aims of such interventions have been to reduce the barriers to better control.

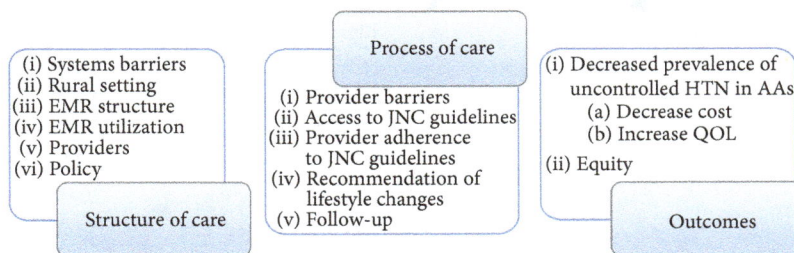

FIGURE 1: Application of Donabedian's quality of care.

Provider-centered barriers are the focus of this study and include limited patient-provider communication regarding lifestyle changes, lack of adherence to established guidelines for HTN management, and resistance to change. In addition, systems barriers were assessed and include access to care, medication costs, and lack of healthcare coverage [6]. Racial disparities related to geographical areas in healthcare lead to disproportionate mortality and morbidity in rural areas.

Patients often seek medical attention for chronic conditions from their primary care providers. Geographic location of this population and clinic locations can influence patient outcomes [7]. Rurality adds to the burden of HTN in AAs. Healthcare disparities such as ethnicity, poverty, and access to care are all associated with rurality and contribute to the higher incidence of HTN in AAs. For example, barriers to healthcare in rural communities include transportation, lack of health insurance, and lack of healthcare facilities and providers, all of which contribute to limited access to healthcare. As a result, rural communities have a higher incidence of chronic diseases such as HTN [7] and have poorer outcomes [8].

As previously mentioned, a major problem for rural communities is access to healthcare. Improving access to healthcare for rural America is a priority. The National Rural Health Association [9] has developed a timeline for the Affordable Care Act, which is designed to address the issues pertaining to access to healthcare. Provisions on the timeline include workforce improvement, payment reimbursement, and requirement of the electronic health record requirements, to name a few. Student loan repayment programs for those working in rural or underserved areas and improving Medicare and Medicaid reimbursement in rural practices are some specific provisions that have been implemented to improve access to healthcare in rural communities [9].

2. Methods

2.1. Theoretical Framework. The theoretical framework of Avedis Donabedian was used as a tool to guide this research. His framework was used to assess the quality of care provided in healthcare. The three components that form the foundation of this theory are (1) structure of care, (2) process of care, and

(3) outcomes. The concept is grounded on the principle of healthcare outcomes as a result of the medical care provided by medical professionals [10].

Donabedian (as cited in McDonald et al. [11]) describes structure of care as any process that relates to the organizational and physical aspects of care settings. A few specific examples of this process are facilities, equipment, and operational and financial processes supporting medical care. The second component of this framework is process of care. Process of care is dependent upon the structures of care to supply resources and methods that are necessary for participants to carry out patient care activities. Patient-provider communication, practice habits, and care management are all examples of process of care. Further, the goal of process of care is to improve patient health by promoting recovery, patient survival, and even patient satisfaction [10]. The final concept of this model, outcomes, is simply the patient outcomes based on medical health after the application of the two previous components [10]. Figure 1 depicts the components of Donabedian's theory and how it is applicable to this study.

2.2. Study Design. A retrospective review of the EMR was conducted to identify hypertensive AA patients in a rural clinic who were seen from July 1, 2014, to August 31, 2014. A descriptive, preexperimental, quantitative method was used to evaluate the degree of provider adherence to national HTN guidelines in AAs living in a rural community. Inclusion criteria for the patients included (Figure 2) (a) age 20 to 80 years, (b) AAs with a diagnosis of HTN, and (c) receiving antihypertensive medications. Exclusion criteria included (a) specific end organ damage (i.e., CKD, stroke, cardiomyopathy, or myocardial infarctions), (b) age younger than 20 or greater than 80 years, (c) no office visits during research dates or office visits for reasons other than HTN, (d) no established relationship with a single primary care provider (PCP), (e) diagnosis of medical nonadherence, (f) race other than AA, and (g) deceased patients.

A sample of 62 participants met the inclusion criteria.

2.3. Study Setting and Sample. The study was conducted at a multiphysician practice located in a rural community. The practice serves a population of 45,273, 63.8% of which are

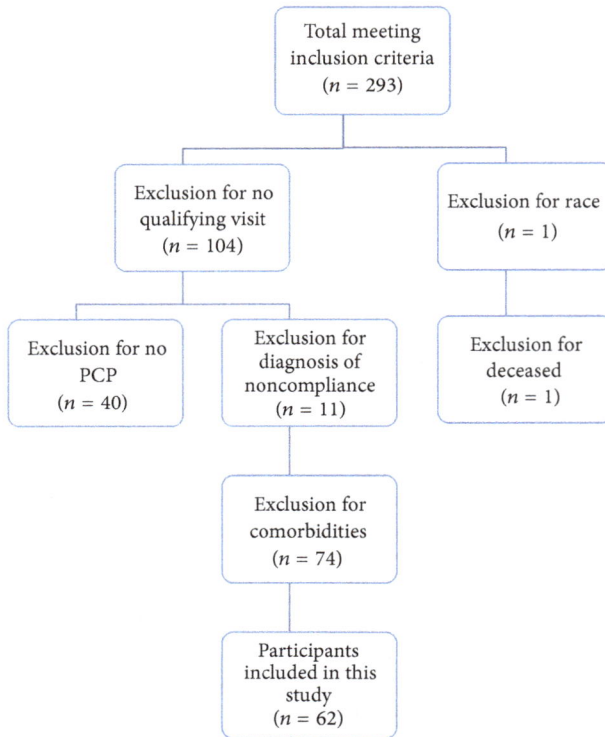

FIGURE 2: Participant selection algorithm.

TABLE 1: Joint National Committee Classification of blood pressure for adults.

Blood pressure classification	Systolic blood pressure (mmHg)	Diastolic blood pressure (mmHg)
Normal	<120	and <80
Prehypertension	120–139	or 80–89
Hypertension	≥140	≥90
Stage 1 hypertension	140–159	or 90–99
Stage 2 hypertension	≥160	or ≥100

AAs [12]. The practice accepts Medicare, Medicaid, private insurances, and the indigent. The practice serves pediatric to geriatric patients. There are four primary care providers, one cardiologist, two pulmonologists, one neurologist, and one podiatrist. Primary care providers were the focus of this study. The study aims to assess healthcare provider adherence to JNC hypertensive guidelines in AAs.

2.4. Data Collection and Procedures. The primary source data were selected from the EMR Centricity developed by General Electric Healthcare. An EMR is a digital or electronic version of a paper chart that contains the patient's medical history. A report was populated using the following criteria: (1) the practice site location, (2) race specified as black or African American, (3) birthdate on or after 01/01/1949 but before 01/01/1995, (4) appointment date on or after 07/01/2014 but before 09/01/2014, and (5) active International Classification of Diseases, Ninth Revision (ICD-9) codes containing 401 for hypertension. The EMR was reviewed to identify onset of HTN if feasible, provider selection of antihypertensive drugs for initial treatment, and additional drug choices. HTN was defined as a blood pressure ≥140/90 mmHg in the general population and >130/80 mmHg in hypertensive individuals with a comorbidity of DM in accordance with JNC 7 or patients taking antihypertensive medications. Patients who met the inclusion criteria were selected by convenience sample. A list of those patients was composed and each was assigned a research identifier. Potential participants were consecutively recruited and a sample size of 62 participants met the inclusion criteria. Demographic variables assessed included age, gender, marital status, and insurance coverage. Other variables that were considered include the following antihypertensive drug classes: (a) thiazide diuretics, (b) angiotensin-converting-enzyme inhibitors (ACEIs), (c) angiotensin II receptor blockers (ARBs), and (d) calcium channel blockers (CCBs). Evaluation of monotherapy and combination therapy was also performed.

2.5. Measures. JNC 7 (as cited in Chobanian et al. [13]) describes HTN as a systolic blood pressure ≥140 mmHg or a diastolic blood pressure of ≥90 mmHg in the general population, including AAs. If the patient has a comorbidity such as DM, a systolic blood pressure >130 mmHg and a diastolic blood pressure of >80 mmHg are considered suboptimal in the treatment of HTN. The coexistence of HTN and DM further increases the risk of vascular complications such as strokes and renal disease, which is why the optimal blood pressure goal is lower [13].

Diagnostic measurements for the classification of HTN were performed based on JNC 7 guidelines (Table 1). According to JNC 7, two consecutive readings in contralateral arms at least 5 minutes apart while sitting are categorized as HTN. By auscultation, blood pressures were manually obtained by nurses using the appropriate size cuff with a sphygmomanometer. Patients were in a seated position with feet on the floor and arm positioned at the level of the heart. They had been seated for at least 5 minutes or longer. The providers performed repeat BPs in suboptimal readings after at least 5 minutes. JNC 7 describes the stages of HTN. A normal blood pressure is a systolic blood pressure of <140 mmHg and a diastolic blood pressure of <90 mmHg. Stage 1 is a systolic blood pressure reading of 140 to 159 mmHg or a diastolic BP reading of 90 to 99 mmHg. Stage 2 is classified as a systolic blood pressure ≥160 mmHg and a diastolic reading of ≥100 mmHg. In the general AA population, initial monotherapy with diuretics, specifically thiazide diuretics (TDs), or CCBs should be used for stage 1 HTN or a diuretic in combination with other drug classes for combination drug therapy regimen for stage 2 HTN. JNC 7 recommends specialty referrals if blood pressure is not controlled after maximizing three medication classes, with one being a TD. Lastly, for those with compelling indications, such as those with a comorbidity of DM, ACEIs are recommended to reduce strokes and other vascular complications [13].

With regard to follow-up, JNC 7 recommends a monthly follow-up office visit if blood pressure is not at goal and a follow-up office visit every 3 to 6 months if BP is at goal. Laboratory values for potassium and creatinine should be obtained 1 to 2 times annually and patients with a comorbidity of DM should have their urine microalbumin levels measured at least annually. Patients newly diagnosed with HTN should have a urinalysis, blood glucose, hematocrit, potassium, creatinine, calcium, and lipid profile drawn prior to beginning pharmacological treatment.

JNC 7 recommends lifestyle modification education. Better outcomes have been found when lifestyle modification is incorporated into the plan of care. The following are the areas recommended for lifestyle modification: (a) weight loss, (b) following the Dietary Approaches to Stop Hypertension (DASH) diet, which consists of a diet rich in fruit and vegetables, low fat dairy products, and reduced intake of saturated and total fat, (c) adhering to sodium restrictions, (d) regular physical activity, and (e) limiting alcohol consumption.

2.6. Data Analysis. Statistical analyses were performed on the outcomes of blood pressure control in participants who were prescribed antihypertensive medications based on JNC 7 guidelines compared to those who were not and also on blood pressures that were at goal and those that were not. Additionally, outcomes of provider adherence to the guidelines were measured based on adherence to medication choice recommendations, documented lifestyle modification recommendations, laboratory studies, and follow-up for patients with HTN and HTN with a comorbidity of DM. Descriptive analysis was conducted using crosstabs, frequencies, and means comparison and reported as percentages to describe the results. Crosstabs were used to determine the number of times the recommended combination of a thiazide diuretic was used in combination with an ACEI or ARB. Frequencies were conducted to identify the percentage of patients not prescribed a TD or CCB as monotherapy. Further, the use of means comparison was to compare differences in BP outcomes in patients prescribed ACEIs compared to TDs as monotherapy. Additionally, a chi square analysis was performed to determine if there is a relationship between provider adherence and blood pressure outcomes.

3. Results

3.1. Providers. Physicians accounted for 64.5% ($n = 40$) of the providers in this study. Nurse practitioners (NPs) accounted for 35.5% ($n = 22$). Of the 29 patients with blood pressure at goal, a physician was the provider in 75.9% ($n = 22$) of the office visits while NPs provided care in 24.1% ($n = 7$) of the visits.

The demographic characteristics of the 62 participants are described in Table 2. Of the 62 patients studied, 41.9% were male and 58.1% were female. Patient age was divided into 2 categories: less than 65 years and 65 years and older. There were 50% patients in each age group. The mean age was 62.8 years. The most frequent stage of uncontrolled HTN was stage 1 accounting for 84.4% of the 32 patients. Stage 2 HTN was detected in 15.6% of the patients. There were 16 nondiabetic patients whose BP was not at goal. Of those 16, 81% had stage 1 HTN and the remaining 19% had stage 2 HTN. In patients

TABLE 2: Demographics.

Characteristic	Frequency	Percent
Gender		
Male	26	41.9
Female	36	58.1
Total	62	100.0
Age		
<65 years	31	50.0
≥65	31	50.0
Total	62	100.0
Stages of hypertension		
Stage 1	5	8.1
Stage 2	27	43.5
Controlled	30	48.4
Total	32	100.0
Marital status		
Married	19	30.6
Divorced	6	9.7
Single	14	22.6
Widowed	8	12.9
Undetermined	15	24.2
Total	62	100.0
Insurance		
Medicare	35	56.5
Medicaid	4	6.5
BCBS	15	24.2
Self-pay	4	6.5
Private	4	6.5
Total	62	100.0

aged less than 65 years, 45.2% of the 31 patients had stage 1 HTN and 12.9% had stage 2 HTN. In the age group of 65 and over, stage 1 accounted for 41.9% of patients and stage 2 HTN accounted for 3.2%. Medicare coverage accounted for 56.5% of the study participants. Blue Cross Blue Shield (BCBS) accounted for the second most utilized health insurance with 24.2% of the patients enrolled. Medicaid, self-pay, and private insurances each accounted for 6.5% of the patients.

3.2. Pharmacologic Treatment. Drug therapy regimens are reported in Table 3. Of the 62 patients studied, 12.9% ($n = 8$) were on monotherapy and 87.1% ($n = 54$) were on combination therapy. Combination therapy is described as taking two or more medications. Those with a comorbidity of DM accounted for 53.2% ($n = 33$) of the 62 patients. JNC 7 guidelines suggest that patients with a comorbidity of DM should take ACEIs to decrease morbidity and mortality. Of the 33 diabetic patients, only 69.7% ($n = 23$) were taking ACEIs as recommended. TDs or CCBs were not prescribed in any of the eight patients on monotherapy. Of the 54 patients taking combination therapy, 87% ($n = 47$) were taking either a TD or CCB. In the patients studied, 53.2% ($n = 33$) of the 62 warranted medication adjustments as a result of uncontrolled blood pressure. Only 15.2% ($n = 5$) had

TABLE 3: Medication regimen.

On TD or CCB	Frequency (*n*)	Percent
Monotherapy with TD or CCB (*n* = 8)		
Yes	0	0
No	8	100
Total	8	100.0
Combination therapy with TD or CCB (*n* = 54)		
Yes	47	87.0
No	7	13.0
Total	54	100.0
ACEI if there is comorbidity of DM (*n* = 33)		
Yes	23	69.7
No	10	30.3
Total	33	100.0

TD: thiazide diuretic; CCB: calcium channel blocker; ACEI: angiotensin converting enzyme inhibitor; DM: diabetes mellitus.

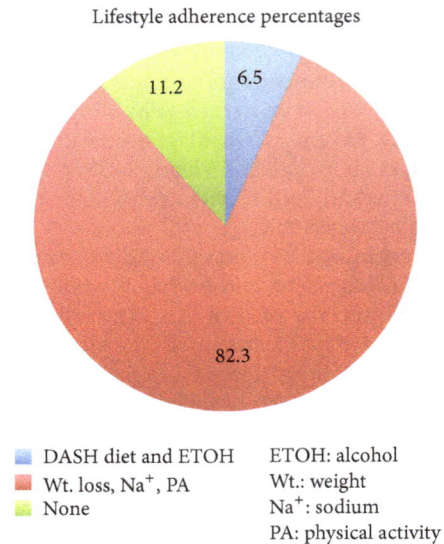

Lifestyle adherence percentages

- DASH diet and ETOH ETOH: alcohol
- Wt. loss, Na$^+$, PA Wt.: weight
- None Na$^+$: sodium
  PA: physical activity

FIGURE 3: Lifestyle adherence.

medication adjustments, leaving 84.8% (*n* = 28) inadequately treated. One patient (1.6%) required a referral to a HTN specialist as a result of maximizing three different medication classes, including a TD. That patient was not referred.

In the eight patients on monotherapy, 37.5% (*n* = 3) of them met their blood pressure goal despite not being on a TD or CCB. Of the 54 patients on combination therapy, 87% (*n* = 47) were on a TD or CCB as recommended by JNC 7. Of those 47 patients, 55.3% (*n* = 26) achieved goal blood pressures. A chi square test was used to determine if there is a relationship between being prescribed JNC 7 medication regimen and blood pressure outcomes. There was no significant relation between taking the recommended TD or CCB and blood pressure control (χ^2 = 0.0; P = 0.99).

3.3. Lifestyle Modifications. The categories examined under lifestyle modifications included DASH diet, weight loss, sodium restrictions, physical activity (PA), and alcohol consumption (see Figure 3). Only 6.5% (*n* = 4) of the 62 patients had documentation of provider recommendations for the DASH diet and alcohol consumption. The DASH diet includes recommendations for limiting alcohol consumption. Weight loss, sodium restriction, and PA recommendations were documented in 82.3% (*n* = 51) of the patients.

3.4. Follow-Up Care. JNC 7 recommends follow-up every 3 to 6 months if BP is controlled. Providers were adherent to follow-up recommendations 96.6% (*n* = 28) of the time in the 29 patients with controlled blood pressure. In the remaining 33 patients who required monthly follow-up due to uncontrolled blood pressure, providers were only 9.1% (*n* = 3) adherent to the recommendations.

3.5. Laboratory Recommendations. Providers were adherent to obtaining laboratory tests prior to initiating treatment in 0% of the two patients with new diagnoses of HTN. The adherence rate for biannual laboratory tests in patients with historical diagnosis of HTN was 65% (*n* = 39) of the 60

qualifying patients. In patients with a comorbidity of DM, JNC 7 recommends measuring annual urine microalbumin levels. Providers were 15.2% (*n* = 5) adherent to the guidelines in the 33 diabetic patients.

4. Discussion

Endless and organized activities that result in measurable improvement in healthcare services and targeted patient outcomes have been described as QI [14]. The way care is delivered is related to quality. The US Department of Health and Human Services [14] identified the 4 principles of quality improvement (QI) as (1) QI work as systems and processes, (2) focus on patients, (3) focus on being part of the team, and (4) focus on use of data. QI work as systems and processes refers to resources and activities that are carried out and are evaluated simultaneously to improve quality of care or outcomes [14]. This is modeled after Donabedian's framework for quality improvement. This study focused on the systems or structural components of systems barriers such as the rural setting the study was conducted in, EMR structure, EMR utilization, providers, and policy. Activities assessed included provider barriers, access to JNC 7 guidelines, provider adherence to those guidelines, recommendation of lifestyle changes, laboratory assessment, and follow-up.

Evaluation of the first 2 components is necessary to produce or improve patient outcomes. Outcome goals include decreasing the prevalence of uncontrolled HTN in AAs, decreasing cost associated with HTN, increasing quality of life, and equity. This study was conducted to assess what is currently being done in this rural primary care setting to address the increased prevalence and mortality of HTN in AAs. Using the methodical framework of Donabedian, both quantitative (frequencies) and qualitative (descriptive) data were collected and analyzed to assess the current system and to identify areas for improvement. The practice guidelines of JNC 7 were used as performance measures for comparison.

The JNC conducts and analyzes evidence-based studies periodically. Subsequently, JNC formulates recommendations based on those findings. The National Heart Lung and Blood Institute (NHLBI) traditionally has endorsed previous versions. Controversy surrounding the Eighth Report of the Joint National Committee (JNC 8) has led to NHLBI not endorsing JNC 8 [15]. Other federal organizations have also declined to endorse the new recommendations. The controversy surrounds the increased BP goal of <150/90 in patients aged >60 and a goal of <140/90 for those aged 18 to 60, including those having comorbidities of DM and CKD. JNC 8 guidelines were avoided for this study due to this controversy and its relatively new release.

There are several main findings of this study. First, the first-line drug choice as monotherapy in the treatment of HTN in AAs should be TDs or CCBs, as recommended by JNC 7. While there were only eight patients receiving monotherapy, none of them were on TDs or CCBs, which indicates 100% nonadherence to the guidelines regarding monotherapy. In fact, the majority of the patients on monotherapy were on ACEIs, while the remaining were on ARBs. However, studies have found that ACEIs and ARBs are less effective in the AA population. These findings are consistent with the studies reviewed in the literature review for this study. One such study compared the effectiveness of ACEIs as monotherapy between AAs and Whites [16]. Whites had a greater systolic (mean difference of 4.64) and diastolic (mean difference of 2.82) reduction in BP compared to AAs. In contrast, providers were more consistent with the guideline recommendations in AAs on combination drug therapy. Provider adherence was documented in 87% of the patients receiving combination therapy. This finding is consistent with previous studies. One of the goals of a previous study was to determine provider adherence to national guidelines including a TD in combination therapy in AAs of Nigerian decent [17]. The majority (88.8%) of the study sample was prescribed combination therapy inclusive of a TD. In addition, combination therapy was more effective than monotherapy in reducing both systolic and diastolic BP (32.64 mmHg compared to 15.43 mmHg and 18.56 mmHg compared to 6.96 mmHg, resp.).

Less than half of the 62 patients in this study have at goal BP readings at the level recommended by JNC 7 despite moderate provider adherence. Similar findings were found in a previous study. Provider adherence to the guidelines overall was 76%. Mean BP values decreased but insignificantly concluding no correlation with provider adherence and attaining BP goals [18]. In this study, medication adjustments were not made in 18% of the 33.2% that required adjustments. This could be a contributing factor to patients not meeting their BP goal. However, adjusting medications is not always associated with attaining BP goals [18]. Additionally, provider adherence in prescribing ACEIs in patients with a comorbidity of DM was seen in 70% of the population. Similar results were found in a previous study. Provider adherence to prescribing an ACEI or ARB in patients with comorbidities such as DM was seen in 88% of the population [18]. Studies have shown that the use of ACEIs in this population decreases mortality and morbidity by decreasing end organ damage and cardiovascular incidents.

Lifestyle modification, as an adjunct to pharmacologic therapy, has been associated with better BP control. Provider adherence to alcohol consumption and DASH diet recommendations was poorly documented. Detailed recommendations for the DASH diet and alcohol were only documented in 4 of the 62 EMRs. Adherence was high in the recommendations for physical activity, weight loss, and sodium restrictions. The smart plan is inclusive of these 3 recommendations, which was documented in 51 of the 62 patients.

Patient adherence with adequate office visit follow-up has been known to yield better BP control. JNC 7 recommends an office visit follow-up every 3 to 6 months in patients with BP at goal and monthly visits for those who are not at goal. Provider adherence was evident in the 3-to-6-month follow-up population (97%). A monthly follow-up recommendation for those with uncontrolled BP was poorly represented in this study.

Uncontrolled BP can lead to end organ damage such as renal insufficiency or failure, heart attacks, or strokes. Further, the medications used to treat HTN can have adverse effects on other organs. JNC 7 recommendations include a urinalysis, blood glucose, hematocrit, potassium, creatinine, calcium, and lipids in patients newly diagnosed with HTN before initiating therapy. Due to the limitations of the EMR, only 2 patients were identified as newly diagnosed. Of these patients, neither of them had laboratory testing performed prior to starting treatment. Diabetics should have their urine microalbumin level measured annually. Only 15% of diabetics had documented microalbumin levels within the preceding 6 months.

There are several limitations to this study. Due to small sample size, variability and vagueness should be noted as limitations. For example, the finding of no documentation of patients receiving labs prior to the initiation of drug therapy may provide a greater impact and consistency in a larger sample size. A larger sample size would produce more detailed, robust, and explanatory assessments. Secondly, the study was conducted during only the summer months and over a short duration. Extending the study period and expanding the study to include fall or winter months may provide input for comparison to determine if seasons impact BP control.

5. Conclusions

Despite evidence-based recommendations by JNC 7, provider adherence in AAs has room for improvement. Provider pharmacologic choices and lifestyle modification recommendations are major components to blood pressure control in this population. Thiazide diuretics are recommended as initial monotherapy and in combination therapy for African Americans. CCBs are recommended as an acceptable alternative to thiazide diuretics. CCBs are preferred over ACEIs because of the increased risk of stroke, myocardial infarctions, and other vascular conditions associated with ACEIs. Conversely, providers have demonstrated a preference in prescribing ACEIs and ARBS in monotherapy. Better adherence in prescribing a TD or CCB is seen in prescribing patterns for patients on combination therapy. Providers are not adherent to the monthly follow-up recommendations required for medication adjustment or specialist referrals when BP is not at goal. Lack of lifestyle modification documentation, specifically the DASH diet and alcohol consumption, is consistent with nonadherence to the JNC 7 guidelines. Although there appears to be no relationship between receiving the recommended medications and BP outcomes, more than half of the population did not meet BP goals.

The principal factor assessed in the process of care was provider barriers. Specific components impacting provider barriers include access to JNC 7 guidelines, provider adherence to JNC 7 guidelines, recommendation of lifestyle changes, and follow-up. Provider adherence to the guidelines overall was poor. Lack of documentation, provider-prescribing habits, and lack of knowledge of up-to-date, evidence-based guidelines may be contributing factors. While there is a gap between evidence-based national guidelines and clinical practice to controlling HTN, all contributing factors, including physician, patient, and systems barriers [19], require further exploration if successful interventions are to be developed.

References

[1] H. B. Bosworth, T. Dudley, M. K. Olsen et al., "Racial differences in blood pressure control: potential explanatory factors," *The American Journal of Medicine*, vol. 119, no. 1, pp. 70.e9–70.e15, 2006.

[2] W. Carroll, *Hypertension in America: Estimates for the U. S. Civilian Noninstitutionalized Population, Age 18 and Older, 2008*, Agency for Healthcare Research and Quality, Rockville, Md, USA, 2011, http://meps.ahrq.gov/mepsweb/data_files/publications/st315/stat315.pdf.

[3] World Health Organization, "A global brief on hypertension," Tech. Rep. WHO/DCO/WHD/2013.2, World Health Organization, 2013, http://apps.who.int/iris/bitstream/10665/79059/1/WHO_DCO_WHD_2013.2_eng.pdf?ua=1.

[4] Center for Disease Control and Prevention, "Vital signs: awareness and treatment of uncontrolled hypertension among adults—United States, 2003–2010," *Morbidity and Mortality Weekly Report*, vol. 61, no. 35, pp. 703–709, 2012, http://www.cdc.gov/mmwr/preview/mmwrhtml/mm6135a3.htm.

[5] US Department of Health and Human Services and Health Resources and Services Administration, "Hypertension control," 2011, http://www.hrsa.gov/quality/toolbox/measures/hypertension/index.html.

[6] R. Khatib, J.-D. Schwalm, S. Yusuf et al., "Patient and healthcare provider barriers to hypertension awareness, treatment and follow up: a systematic review and meta-analysis of qualitative and quantitative studies," *PLoS ONE*, vol. 9, no. 1, Article ID e84238, 2014.

[7] R. W. Durant, G. Parmar, F. Shuaib et al., "Awareness and management of chronic disease, insurance status, and health professional shortage areas in the reasons for geographic and racial differences in stroke (regards): a cross-sectional study," *BMC Health Services Research*, vol. 12, article 208, 2012.

[8] G. K. Murphy, F. A. McAlister, D. L. Weir, L. Tjosvold, and D. T. Eurich, "Cardiovascular medication utilization and adherence among adults living in rural and urban areas: a systematic review and meta-analysis," *BMC Public Health*, vol. 14, article 544, 2014.

[9] National Rural Health Association and Office of Government Affairs, "Health care reform timeline," 2007, http://www.rural-healthweb.org/go/left/government-affairs/health-reform-and-you/health-care-reform-timeline.

[10] A. Donabedian, "The quality of care: how can it be assessed?" *The Journal of the American Medical Association*, vol. 260, no. 12, pp. 1743–1748, 1988.

[11] K. M. McDonald, V. Sundaram, D. M. Bravata et al., *Closing the Quality Gap: A Critical Analysis of Quality Improvement Strategies*, vol. 7 of *Care Coordination*, 2007, http://www.ncbi.nlm.nih.gov/books/NBK44015/.

[12] US Department of Commerce and United States Census Bureau, "State & county quickfacts," 2014, http://quickfacts.census.gov/qfd/states/51000.html.

[13] A. V. Chobanian, G. L. Bakris, H. R. Black et al., "The seventh report of the Joint National Committee on Prevention, Detection, Evaluation, and Treatment of high blood pressure: the JNC 7 report," *The Journal of the American Medical Association*, vol. 289, no. 19, pp. 2560–2571, 2003.

[14] US Department of Health and Human Services and Health Resources and Services Administration, "Quality improvement," 2011, http://www.hrsa.gov/quality/toolbox/methodology/qualityimprovement/part4.html.

[15] H. Bauchner, P. B. Fontanarosa, and R. M. Golub, "Updated guidelines for management of high blood pressure recommendations, review, and responsibility," *The Journal of the American Medical Association*, vol. 311, no. 5, pp. 477–478, 2014.

[16] R. N. Peck, L. R. Smart, R. Beier et al., "Difference in blood pressure response to ACE-Inhibitor monotherapy between black and white adults with arterial hypertension: a meta-analysis of 13 clinical trials," *BMC Nephrology*, vol. 14, article 201, 2013.

[17] E. U. Etuk, S. A. Isezuo, A. Chika, J. Akuche, and M. Ali, "Prescription pattern of anti-hypertensive drugs in a tertiary health institution in Nigeria," *Annals of African Medicine*, vol. 7, no. 3, pp. 128–132, 2008.

[18] R. M. Peters, R. Benkert, K. Butler, and N. Brunelle, "Provider adherence to JNC 7 guidelines and blood pressure outcomes in African Americans," *Journal of Clinical Outcomes Management*, vol. 14, no. 1, 2007, http://www.turner-white.com/pdf/jcom_jan07_blood.pdf.

[19] T. Odedosu, A. Schoenthaler, D. L. Vieira, C. Agyemang, and G. Ogedegbe, "Overcoming barriers to hypertension control in African Americans," *Cleveland Clinic Journal of Medicine*, vol. 79, no. 1, pp. 46–56, 2012.

12

Prevalence, Awareness, Treatment, and Control of Hypertension among Chinese First-Generation Migrants and Italians

Pietro A. Modesti,[1] **Maria Calabrese,**[2] **Ilaria Marzotti,**[1] **Hushao Bing,**[3] **Danilo Malandrino,**[1] **Maria Boddi,**[1] **Sergio Castellani,**[1] **and Dong Zhao**[4]

[1]*Department of Experimental and Clinical Medicine, University of Florence, Florence, Italy*
[2]*Diabetology Unit, Ospedale Misericordia e Dolce, Prato, Italy*
[3]*Associazione Culturale Cinese di Fujian in Italia, Prato, Italy*
[4]*Department of Epidemiology, Capital Medical University Beijing Anzhen Hospital and National Institute of Heart, Lung & Blood Disease, Beijing, China*

Correspondence should be addressed to Pietro A. Modesti; pa.modesti@unifi.it

Academic Editor: Tomohiro Katsuya

Data on health needs of Chinese living in the South of Europe are lacking. To compare prevalence, awareness, treatment, control, and risk factors for hypertension between Chinese migrants and Italian adults, a sample of 1200 first-generation Chinese migrants and 291 native Italians aged 35–59 years living in Prato (Italy) was recruited in a community-based participatory cross-sectional survey. Primary outcome measure was hypertension, diagnosed for blood pressure values ≥ 140/90 mmHg or current use of antihypertensive medications. Associations with exposures (including age, gender, body mass index, waist, education level, total cholesterol, and triglycerides) were examined using logistic regression. When compared with Italians, Chinese had higher hypertension prevalence (27.2% versus 21.3%, $p < 0.01$), with comparable levels of awareness (57.4% and 48.4%) but lower treatment rates (70.6% and 90.0%, resp.). In both ethnic groups age and parental history of hypertension were predictors of awareness and treatment, body mass index being predictor of hypertension diagnosis. In Chinese participants, where the optimum cut-off point for body mass index was ≥23.9 kg/m^2, the sensibility and specificity prediction for hypertension were 61.7% and 59.8%, respectively (area under the ROC curve = 0.629). Implementation of specific, culturally adapted health programs for the Chinese community is now needed.

1. Introduction

The distribution of cardiovascular risk factors, as well as the benefits of advances in prevention and treatment of chronic disease, are not shared equally across economic and ethnic groups either in the United States [1] or in Europe [2–4]. Cultural factors seem to play a primary role in limiting the efficacy of prevention strategies conceived for the native population in reaching first-generation migrants. This issue is now relevant for most EU countries where immigration flows importantly grew in recent decades [2]. As recently stated by the European Society of Cardiology [5], information

on health needs of minority groups living in Europe is now available for subjects originating from Sub-Saharan African countries and South Asia [6, 7], whereas data for Chinese are still limited [8]. In recent decades China experienced a rapid increase in stroke incidence [9] and the control of hypertension and other risk factors is now recognized as a public health priority [10–12].

In the last decades migration flows from China to Europe have been mainly directed towards Italy and Spain [13], and Chinese are now the third largest overseas-born population in Italy [14]. In particular, Prato has the highest proportion of Chinese immigrants of any Italian province, subjects being mainly occupied in the textiles industry of the area [15]. Risk factor distribution in the Chinese community of Prato was recently investigated in the CHIP (CHinese In Prato) survey which enrolled Chinese first-generation migrants aged 18 to 59 years [16, 17]. However, data on the differences in hypertension burden between Chinese and Europid adults are lacking. This information is essential for health policies, strategies, and plans [18].

The present study was thus performed (1) to compare the prevalence of hypertension and other main risk factors between first-generation Chinese immigrants and Italian adults in the age group 35 to 59 years; (2) to investigate the relationship of hypertension with obesity indices; and (3) to identify the optimal BMI cut-off value to be adopted for screening purposes.

2. Methods

2.1. Setting, Study Design, and Participants. Located in Tuscany, 30 Km far from Florence, Prato has a population of more than 180,000 with a number of Chinese regular residents in the area constantly growing from 169 in 1990 to 15,957 in 2014 [19]. In 2014 the CHIP survey, incorporating principles of community-based participatory research [20, 21], was performed. More precisely a community-academic partnership, composed of the Consulate General of Florence, the four local community-based Chinese organizations, and the Chinese and Italian Universities, was built to develop a sensitive, culturally appropriate, no coercive recruitment, and enrolment process [19]. A network sampling procedure was adopted [16, 17, 22]. To be eligible for the present analysis, participants recruited in 2014 had (1) to self-identify to be born in continental China and to have grandparents born in that country; (2) to be between 35 and 59 years of age; and (3) to live permanently in Prato. In 2014 a cohort composed of native Italian population was randomly sampled from General Practice lists stratified by age and gender using an extraction program. Each subject was initially sent a letter informing them about the study, followed by an invitation to attend for screening. Subjects were replaced after two invitations. Those with whom no contact was established after three invitations were sent a letter by recorded delivery mail. Response rate of the eligible Italian subjects approached during recruitment was 67%. Exclusion criteria included pregnant women, critically ill individuals, and impaired cognitive ability as judged by clinical staff members.

2.2. Ethics, Consent, and Permissions. The study was approved by the Ethical Committee of the Azienda Ospedaliero-Universitaria Careggi (Ref. OSS.14.089). Written informed consent was obtained from all participants. Subjects were provided with a written description of the study in their choice of Chinese or Italian and written consent was obtained at time of entry from each participant. Participants with untreated clinical diseases identified during the examinations were advised to see their general practitioner or referred to the Hospital of Prato. No other incentives were offered to study participants. Data collected were anonymous and deidentified. The screening phase was performed between June 2014 and April 2015.

2.3. Data Collection. All participants were instructed to fast overnight before the day of survey. In the early morning (between 07.00 and 10.00 am) individuals attended the Research Centre where trained Chinese and Italian staff members administered a questionnaire and performed physical (blood pressure and anthropometry) and biochemical blood measurements (glucose, total cholesterol, and triglycerides).

Questionnaire gathered information on participant sociodemographic data, tobacco use, alcohol consumption, medical and reproductive history, medication use, and migration [17].

Blood pressure (BP) was measured three times using a clinically validated semiautomatic digital sphygmomanometer (M6; Omron Matsusaka Co. Ltd., Japan) with appropriate cuff size according to current guidelines [23]. The average of the last two readings was used for analysis. Body weight, height, and waist and hip circumferences were measured according to standardized protocols [24]. Waist-to-hip ratio was calculated as waist circumference (cm) divided by hip circumference (cm). Waist-to-height ratio was calculated as waist circumference (cm) divided by height (cm). Biochemical measurements were performed on finger-prick blood samples using validated dry chemistry methods (AccuChek AVIVA, Roche Diagnostics S.p.A., Mannheim, Germany for glucose and MultiCare-in, HPS, Italy, for total cholesterol and triglycerides) [25, 26]. Nonfasting participants were asked to return at fast for blood tests. Participants with fasting glucose ≥ 126 mg/dL were also asked to return for confirmatory testing. All requested participants attended the second visit.

2.4. Diagnostic Criteria. The primary outcome variable was the prevalence of hypertension, defined as systolic BP ≥ 140 mmHg, or diastolic BP ≥ 90 mmHg, or being on antihypertensive medication [23]. Awareness of hypertension was defined as self-report of any previous diagnosis of hypertension by a healthcare professional among participants with hypertension. Treatment of hypertension was defined as self-reported use of a prescription medication for management of hypertension at the time of survey. Control of hypertension was defined as antihypertensive treatment associated with average systolic and diastolic BP values < 140 mmHg and < 90 mmHg, respectively. Blood pressure was stratified according to the recommendations of the 2013 ESH-ESC guidelines (grades ESH-ESC) [23].

Diagnosis of diabetes mellitus (DM) was based on fasting plasma glucose criteria (≥126 mg/dL confirmed by repeat testing) and/or current treatment with glucose-lowering drugs [27]. High cholesterol was classified for total cholesterol levels ≥ 240 mg/dL [28, 29] and high triglycerides for triglycerides levels ≥ 200 mg/dL [29].

Other exposures included education level (no studies, primary and secondary school, high school, college, or more), alcohol use, smoking (current smokers and noncurrent smokers defined as those who never smoked and former smokers who quit smoking), health insurance (none, registration to

TABLE 1: Demographic data and selected clinical and laboratory findings in Italian and Chinese participants.

Variables	Chinese $n = 1200$	Italians $n = 291$	p value	Difference (95% CI)
Age (years)	46.2 ± 7.1	47.6 ± 7.5	0.004	-1.4 (-2.3 to -0.4)
Height (cm)	163.1 ± 7.9	171.3 ± 10.7	0.001	-8.1 (-9.2 to -7.0)
Weight (kg)	63.3 ± 10.7	74.8 ± 12.2	0.001	-11.5 (-12.9 to -10.1)
Body mass index (kg/m^2)	23.7 ± 3.1	25.4 ± 3.2	0.001	-1.7 (-2.2 to -1.3)
Hip circumference (cm)	95.4 ± 6.4	98.3 ± 12.2	0.001	-2.8 (-3.9 to -1.8)
Waist circumferences (cm)	82.7 ± 9.5	88.3 ± 13.3	0.001	-5.6 (-6.9 to -4.2)
Waist to hip ratio	0.866 ± 0.070	0.898 ± 0.077	0.001	-0.032 (-0.042 to -0.023)
Systolic BP (mmHg)	120.5 ± 19.2	120.4 ± 13.9	0.889	0.2 (-2.2 to 2.5)
Diastolic BP (mmHg)	80.3 ± 11.7	77.8 ± 10.9	0.001	2.5 (1.0 to 4.0)
Heart rate (bpm)	71.7 ± 10.2	70.9 ± 8.8	0.235	0.8 (-0.5 to 2.0)
Fasting glucose (mg/dL)	118.3 ± 33.4	103.6 ± 12.9	0.001	14.7 (10.8 to 18.7)
Total cholesterol (mg/dL)	233.1 ± 62.0	190.3 ± 55.5	0.001	42.8 (35.0 to 50.6)
Triglycerides (mg/dL)	194.9 ± 105.9	163.1 ± 86.8	0.001	31.8 (18.6 to 44.9)

Values are mean ± SD.

National Health System, or private), Italian speaking (yes, no), BMI, and waist. For occupational classification of workers (excluding retired and unemployed), "blue collars" (workers who perform manual labors) and "white collar" (workers who perform professional job duties in an office setting) were considered.

2.5. Statistical Analysis. The sample size for comparison of Italian and Chinese groups aged 35–59 years was based on an estimated hypertension prevalence of 20% in Italian and 29% in Chinese populations. Considering a 5% confidence level (alpha error) and 80% statistical power (beta error), the estimated sample size was at least 281 individuals. Values are expressed as mean ± standard deviation (SD) or n cases (%). Analyses were stratified by 5-year age groups (35–39 years; 40–44 years; 45–49 years; 50–54 years; 55–59 years). Age standardized rates were based on direct standardization using the WHO World Standard Population [30]. Associations of hypertension with exposures were explored with logistic regression analysis. Exposures included age, sex, education categories, current smoking, high total cholesterol, high triglycerides, BMI, and waist-hip ratio tertiles (defined separately for each sex and ethnic group). When appropriate, test of hypothesis was done at significance level 0.05 two-sided. For regression analysis ORs and 95% CI were calculated. Receiver operating characteristics (ROC) curves for hypertension or undiagnosed hypertension and the areas under the curve were then calculated for BMI with corresponding 95% confidence intervals. The largest sensitivity-specificity product value obtained from each ROC curve was calculated. IBM SPSS software (version 22.0, SPSS Inc., Chicago, Illinois, USA) was used for analysis.

3. Results

3.1. Characteristics of Participants. Overall, 1200 Chinese and 291 Italian participants were investigated for the present study. Chinese participants had left China at an average age

of 34.6 ± 8.2 years. Only 17.0% had lived in China urban areas, the large majority (83.0%) coming from rural China. In the Chinese cohort 201 subjects did not complete primary education, this condition being more prevalent among women than men (OR 2.35; 95% CI 1.69 to 3.27). Participants able to speak Italian were 29% with no differences by gender. Only 23% of investigated subjects had access to health services on a par with Italian citizens (subscription to the Regional Health System) with no differences by gender. Other 19% of participants self-reported the attribution of the Temporary Present Foreigner code with free temporary access (1 year) to healthcare. However, the large majority (58%) had no free access to the healthcare (private or public). Chinese participants were mainly occupied in light manual works in the textile industry ($n = 1119$, 93%), only a minority being housekeepers ($n = 29$; 2.4%), or manager or self-employed professionals ($n = 18$; 1.5%). Conversely, in the Italian cohort, only 60 participants (21%) were manual workers, 126 were manager or self-employed professionals (43.3%), and 87 (29.9%) were white-collar office worker. Participants unemployed and seeking work were 2 (0.2%) and 6 (2.1%) in the Chinese and Italian cohort, respectively. Overall, 450 out of the 635 women (71%) in the Chinese cohort had at least one previous abort for unwanted pregnancy versus 27 out of the 149 women (18%) of the Italian cohort (chi-square test, $p < 0.001$).

Main measurements in Italian and Chinese study participants are reported in Table 1. Chinese were significantly shorter and lighter and had lower BMIs than the Italian participants. Waist and hip circumferences and waist-to-hip ratio were also significantly smaller in Chinese. However, mean levels of diastolic BP, fasting glucose, total cholesterol, and triglycerides were significantly higher in Chinese than in Italian participants (Table 1).

3.2. Hypertension Burden in the Chinese and Italian Cohorts. Overall, hypertension was diagnosed in 326 and 62 subjects among Chinese and Italian participants (27.2% and 21.3%,

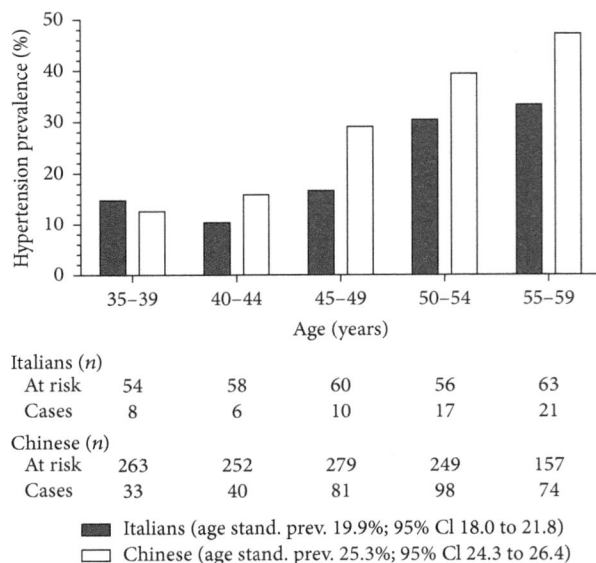

FIGURE 1: Age specific and age standardized (to WHO population 2001) prevalence of hypertension in the CHIP study population aged 35 to 59 years.

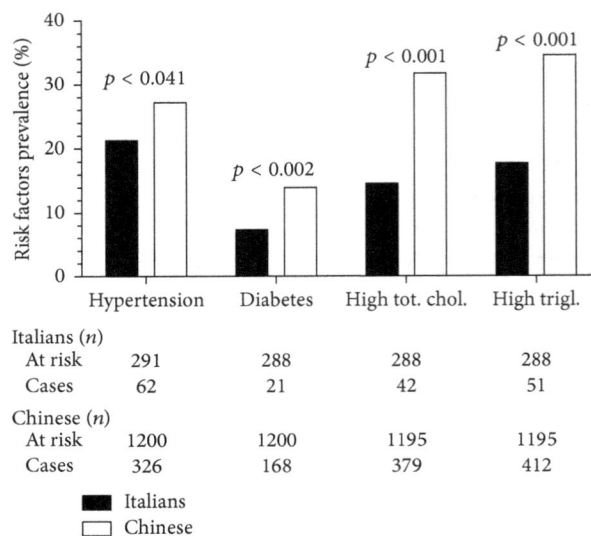

FIGURE 2: Prevalence of hypertension, diabetes, hypercholesterolemia (total cholesterol $\geq$ 240 mg/dL), and hypertriglyceridemia (triglycerides $\geq$ 200 mg/dL) in the Chinese and Italian cohorts.

resp.). Age specific hypertension prevalence is reported in Figure 1. Age standardized prevalence was 25.3% (95% Cl 24.3 to 26.4) and 19.9% (95% Cl 18.0 to 21.8) in the Chinese and Italian cohorts, respectively. In the Italian cohort all the 62 participants with hypertension had Grade 1 HT whereas, in the Chinese cohort, 66 (24%) and 20 participants (7%) had Grade 2 and Grade 3 HT, respectively. Participants with hypertension aware of their condition were 187 (57.4%) in the Chinese and 30 (48.4%) in the Italian cohort (age- and sex-adjusted OR 1.53; 95% Cl 0.88 to 2.66). Although Chinese with hypertension aware of their condition were less frequently treated with drugs than native Italians ($n = 132$; 70.6% and $n = 27$; 90.0%, resp.; age- and sex-adjusted OR 0.23; 95% Cl 0.06 to 0.85), the rate of BP control did not differ between the two groups ($n = 56$, 42% and $n = 12$, 44% in the Chinese and Italian Cohort, resp.; age- and sex-adjusted OR 0.91; 95% Cl 0.39 to 2.13). Among subjects with hypertension belonging to the Chinese cohort, the use of antihypertensive drugs was independent from the registration to the Regional Healthcare system.

Prevalence of all main risk factors was higher in the Chinese than in the Italian cohort (Figure 2) (Table 2). The OR for hypertension (Chinese versus Italians) further increased when education and work categories were included in the model (Model 2). When controlling also for obesity indices and other exposures a further increase was observed (Model 3) (Table 2).

At adjusted multivariable logistic regression only body mass index was associated with hypertension in both ethnic groups (Table 3). The overall ability of body mass index to correctly identify Chinese subjects with both hypertension and undiagnosed hypertension in the Chinese cohort was finally assessed with ROC curves. In the whole Chinese cohort, where the optimum cut-off points for body mass index were $\geq$23.9 kg/m^2, the sensibility and specificity prediction for

hypertension were 61.7% and 59.8%, respectively (Table 4). The areas under the ROC curves of body mass index for hypertension prediction were 0.629 and 0.597 in the whole Chinese cohort and among Chinese unaware of hypertension, respectively.

4. Discussion

According to the present findings, first-generation Chinese immigrants have a higher prevalence of hypertension and main risk factors than the Italian population independently from socioeconomic conditions. Around 2.8 million Chinese citizens currently reside legally in Council of Europe member States, with the largest groups being in Italy, France, Russia, and the United Kingdom. In the last two decades the presence of Chinese remained almost stable in Northern Europe whereas it importantly increased in Italy, mostly in the textile industry area near Florence. The limited studies comparing health needs of Chinese and Europid populations highlight the strength of the present study. In the Health Survey for England [31] the Chinese community living in UK had a prevalence of hypertension which was comparable to values we found in Chinese living in Italy. The characteristics of the two communities may differ, because the Chinese community now living in Prato is mainly composed of subjects born in China whereas most Chinese participants investigated in UK were born in Europe. On the other hand hypertension in the Europid cohort was more prevalent in UK than in Italy, so that, differently from what observed in UK [31], Chinese in Prato had higher prevalence of hypertension than native Italian population. These findings might let us hypothesize that Chinese migrants do not alter their original habits to follow the habits of the host country. In the same line it is to be considered that, among subjects with hypertension belonging to the Chinese cohort, the use of antihypertensive drugs was

TABLE 2: Odds ratios (95% CI) for different factors (Chinese versus Italians).

	Model 1 OR (95% Cl)	Model 2 OR (95% Cl)	Model 3 OR (95% Cl)
Smoke (past or current)	0.62 (0.43 to 0.89)	0.64 (0.38 to 1.10)	0.74 (0.41 to 1.35)
Alcohol (yes)	0.37 (0.28 to 0.50)	0.45 (0.28 to 0.71)	0.38 (0.22 to 0.66)
Body mass index	0.86 (0.82 to 0.89)	0.85 (0.79 to 0.91)	0.93 (0.90 to 0.97)
Waist	0.95 (0.93 to 0.96)	0.94 (0.92 to 0.96)	1.03 (0.91 to 1.17)
Total cholesterol $\geq$ 240 mg/dL	3.07 (2.13 to 4.42)	2.36 (1.32 to 4.20)	1.65 (0.87 to 3.13)
Triglycerides $\geq$ 200 mg/dL	2.84 (2.01 to 4.00)	2.97 (1.70 to 5.19)	2.20 (1.18 to 4.09)
Hypertension	1.61 (1.16 to 2.24)	2.65 (1.47 to 4.76)	3.44 (1.71 to 6.94)

Model 1 adjusted for age and sex.
Model 2 adjusted for age, sex, education, and work.
Model 3 adjusted for age, sex, education, work, and all exposures included in the table.

TABLE 3: Association between exposures and hypertension at multivariate logistic regression (adjusted for all exposures reported in the table) performed among Chinese and Italian participants.

Ethnicity	Exposures	All subjects OR (95% Cl)	$p <$	Not aware of hypertension OR (95% Cl)	$p <$
Chinese	Age (years)	1.09 (1.07 to 1.12)	0.001	1.06 (1.03 to 1.10)	0.001
	Gender (male)	1.00 (0.73 to 1.37)	0.988	1.04 (0.68 to 1.58)	0.873
	Education level	1.01 (0.83 to 1.23)	0.960	1.01 (0.78 to 1.32)	0.935
	Work (white collar)	1.94 (0.95 to 3.97)	0.070	3.00 (1.34 to 6.75)	0.008
	Body mass index (kg/m^2)	1.11 (1.04 to 1.19)	0.002	1.09 (1.00 to 1.20)	0.050
	Waist (cm)	1.02 (1.00 to 1.05)	0.091	1.01 (0.98 to 1.05)	0.460
Italians	Age (years)	1.03 (0.99 to 1.08)	0.184	1.00 (0.93 to 1.06)	0.865
	Gender (male)	1.23 (0.63 to 2.40)	0.546	1.53 (0.63 to 3.73)	0.348
	Education level	0.75 (0.41 to 1.38)	0.358	0.83 (0.36 to 1.90)	0.657
	Work (white collar)	1.10 (0.49 to 2.47)	0.817	0.63 (0.24 to 1.69)	0.363
	Body mass index (kg/m^2)	1.26 (1.13 to 1.41)	0.001	1.28 (1.11 to 1.47)	0.001
	Waist (cm)	0.99 (0.96 to 1.01)	0.323	0.97 (0.94 to 1.00)	0.056

TABLE 4: Areas (with 95% confidence intervals) under the receiver operating curves and cut-off values for body mass index, for identifying hypertension in the whole Chinese cohort and in Chinese participants unaware of hypertension.

Sex	All Chinese participant				Chinese participants unaware of hypertension			
	Area	SE	(Area 95% CI)	Cut-off	Area	SE	(Area 95% CI)	Cut-off
Men	0.621	0.027	(0.568 to 0.673)	24.0	0.570	0.039	(0.494 to 0.646)	23.8
Women	0.634	0.024	(0.586 to 0.681)	23.9	0.619	0.033	(0.554 to 0.685)	23.6
All	0.629	0.018	(0.593 to 0.664)	23.9	0.597	0.025	(0.548 to 0.647)	23.7

independent from the registration to the Regional Healthcare system or the capability to speak Italian. In particular rate of treatment was lower in the Chinese than in the Italian cohort, despite comparable levels of hypertension awareness. Specific prevention strategies have thus to be implemented in the Chinese community. Investing in a multiethnic perspective is thus necessary for eliminating inequities in risk factor control because prevention programs addressed to resident population might be inefficient for ethnic minorities [18, 32].

It has been consistently reported that risk factor distribution and health needs among different populations are markedly influenced by socioeconomic conditions [1]. The socioeconomic differences of the two investigated populations might influence observed results. In the present study Chinese participants were manual workers with low education level, mostly coming from rural China. The Italian sample is mainly composed of middle-class citizens. The two samples can be considered representatives of the two ethnic groups living in Prato. However, when socioeconomic indicators (education level and work) were included in the model the OR of Chinese for hypertension further increased. It is therefore conceivable that additional factors might play a role. Specific investigations on nutritional habits and sodium consumption are needed.

Overweight and obesity are established risk factors for hypertension [33, 34]. In the present survey BMI rather than central obesity was independently associated with hypertension in both Chinese and Italian cohort. Most importantly, notwithstanding the significantly higher prevalence of hypertension and other risk factors in Chinese than in the Italian cohort, Chinese participants were found to have markedly lower mean BMIs than the Italians. It is noteworthy that in Chinese participants the higher BMI was associated with hypertension with a cut-off value of $24 \, \text{kg/m}^2$. The WHO consultation group indeed recommended a lower cut-off of BMI for Asian with respect to native European populations [35] and the identified diagnostic cut-off for overweight in Chinese was $24 \, \text{kg/m}^2$ [36]. This information is important in the light of prevention because the different cut-off value for obesity have to be adopted by physicians who are facing the new patients [37]. The existence of a distinct cut-off value is also to be communicated within the Chinese community because the emulation of native population might lead migrants to increased risk.

5. Study Limitations

This study has several potential limitations.

First, the study design was cross-sectional, so we cannot conclude the cause-effect relationship.

Second, we are aware that the inclusion of undocumented migrants in the present surveys bears limitations. This group is usually excluded from epidemiological studies and surveys because the ability to go back to a list of individuals in some form is lacking. This is the reason why the sampling method of the study subjects differed between Chinese immigrants and Italian inhabitants. On this basis, it would be inappropriate to compare the two groups. However, in consideration of the limited availability of data regarding Chinese migration to the South of Europe, of the high presence of this ethnic group in the area, and of the fact that most EU countries currently offer emergency care to undocumented migrants, current insight on specific health needs of Chinese population in Italy might be important to offer health authority the opportunity to launch specific health programs [18]. The direct participation of the whole Chinese Community in the present shared project following the principles of a participatory research is to be acknowledged representing a proof of their willingness to collaborate in future actions of screening within the community.

Third, the sample size of Italians was limited to fully investigate age- and sex-stratified associations. In addition present survey investigated subjects in work ages of 35 to 59 years. We are aware that additional studies with larger sample sizes are needed to evaluate ethnic differences in hypertension burden, particularly at older ages. However, the creation of a cohort composed by young and middle aged subjects may offer the opportunity to follow these subjects in the future and to investigate the transition to the process of care in the Chinese community.

6. Conclusions

This study shows a high prevalence of hypertension and other main risk factors among young and middle-aged first-generation Chinese migrants settled in Italy. Present findings provide health authority useful information to respond to health needs of Chinese community and develop upstream specific preventive strategies.

Disclosure

The design and conduct of the study; collection, management, analysis, and interpretation of the data; preparation, review, and approval of the manuscript; and decision to submit the manuscript for publication were the responsibilities of the authors alone and independent of the funder.

Authors' Contributions

Pietro A. Modesti conceived, designed, and coordinated the study, performed data analysis, and drafted the manuscript; Maria Calabrese, Ilaria Marzotti, Sergio Castellani, Maria Boddi, and Dong Zhao were involved in conception and design of the study and contributed to the interpretation of data; Dong Zhao oversaw the Chinese version of the questionnaire and provided substantial contribution in data analysis and interpretation of findings. All authors had full access to all the data in the study, revised the manuscript critically for important intellectual content, and gave the final approval of the version to be published. Pietro A. Modesti is the guarantor.

Acknowledgments

The authors thank all the Chinese individuals who participated in the study; Dr. Wang Fuguo (Consul General of the People's Republic of China), Dr. Wang Jian (Consul), and Mr. Chen Hong Sheng (Friendship Association of Chinese in Prato) for providing the necessary support to interact with the Chinese Community; and Eleonora Perruolo, Jing Yang, Wang Xiaoling, Zhang Mengyue, Yang Zihua, Guo Jia, Lara Bini, Maira Camera, and Sonia Fligor for their contribution in the acquisition of data. This study was supported by grant from the Regione Toscana.

References

[1] E. P. Havranek, M. S. Mujahid, D. A. Barr et al., "Social determinants of risk and outcomes for cardiovascular disease: a scientific statement from the American Heart Association," *Circulation*, vol. 132, no. 9, pp. 873–898, 2015.

[2] B. Rechel, P. Mladovsky, D. Ingleby, J. P. Mackenbach, and M. McKee, "Migration and health in an increasingly diverse Europe," *The Lancet*, vol. 381, no. 9873, pp. 1235–1245, 2013.

[3] R. Bhopal, L. Hayes, M. White et al., "Ethnic and socio-economic inequalities in coronary heart disease, diabetes and risk

factors in Europeans and South Asians," *Journal of Public Health Medicine*, vol. 24, no. 2, pp. 95–105, 2002.

[4] J. Lindstrom, A. Neumann, K. E. Sheppard et al., "Take action to prevent diabetes—the IMAGE toolkit for the prevention of type 2 diabetes in Europe," *Hormone and Metabolic Research*, vol. 42, pp. S37–S55, 2010.

[5] M. F. Piepoli, AW. Hoes, S. Agewall et al., "2016 European Guidelines on cardiovascular disease prevention in clinical practice: The Sixth Joint Task Force of the European Society of Cardiology and Other Societies on Cardiovascular Disease Prevention in Clinical Practice (constituted by representatives of 10 societies and by invited experts)Developed with the special contribution of the European Association for Cardiovascular Prevention & Rehabilitation (EACPR)," *European Heart Journal*, vol. 37, pp. 2315–2381, 2016.

[6] P. A. Modesti, G. Reboldi, F. P. Cappuccio et al., "Panethnic differences in blood pressure in Europe: a systematic review and meta-analysis," *PLoS ONE*, vol. 11, no. 1, Article ID e0147601, 2016.

[7] K. A. C. Meeks, D. Freitas-Da-Silva, A. Adeyemo et al., "Disparities in type 2 diabetes prevalence among ethnic minority groups resident in Europe: a systematic review and meta-analysis," *Internal and Emergency Medicine*, vol. 11, no. 3, pp. 327–340, 2016.

[8] Z. Gong and D. Zhao, "Cardiovascular diseases and risk factors among Chinese immigrants," *Internal and Emergency Medicine*, vol. 11, no. 3, pp. 307–318, 2016.

[9] D. Zhao, J. Liu, W. Wang et al., "Epidemiological transition of stroke in China: twenty-oneyear observational study from the sino-MONICA-Beijing project," *Stroke*, vol. 39, no. 6, pp. 1668–1674, 2008.

[10] W. Yang, J. Lu, J. Weng et al., "Prevalence of diabetes among men and women in China," *The New England Journal of Medicine*, vol. 362, no. 12, pp. 1090–1101, 2010.

[11] Y. Xu, L. Wang, J. He et al., "Prevalence and control of diabetes in Chinese adults," *JAMA*, vol. 310, no. 9, pp. 948–959, 2013.

[12] D. Zhao, J. Liu, W. Xie, and Y. Qi, "Cardiovascular risk assessment: a global perspective," *Nature Reviews Cardiology*, vol. 12, no. 5, pp. 301–311, 2015.

[13] K. Latham and B. Wu, *Chinese Immigration into the EU: New Trends, Dynamics and Implications*, Europe China Research and Advice Network, London, UK, 2013.

[14] R. Testa, A. R. Bonfigli, S. Genovese, and A. Ceriello, "Focus on migrants with type 2 diabetes mellitus in European Countries," *Internal and Emergency Medicine*, vol. 11, no. 3, pp. 319–326, 2016.

[15] Y. Gao, *Concealed Chains: Labour Exploitation and Chinese Migrants in Europe*, International Labour Office, Geneva, Switzerland, 2010.

[16] P. A. Modesti, M. Calabrese, D. Malandrino, A. Colella, G. Galanti, and D. Zhao, "New findings on type 2 diabetes in first-generation Chinese migrants settled in Italy: Chinese in Prato (CHIP) cross-sectional survey," *Diabetes/Metabolism Research and Reviews*, vol. 33, no. 2, 2017.

[17] P. A. Modesti, M. Calabrese, E. Perruolo et al., "Sleep history and hypertension burden in first-generation Chinese migrants settled in Italy: the CHIinese in prato cross-sectional survey," *Medicine*, vol. 95, no. 14, Article ID e3229, 2016.

[18] P. A. Modesti, F. Perticone, G. Parati, E. Agabiti Rosei, and D. Prisco, "Chronic disease in the ethnic minority and migrant groups: time for a paradigm shift in Europe," *Internal and Emergency Medicine*, vol. 11, no. 3, pp. 295–297, 2016.

[19] P. A. M. Modesti, Y. Han, Y. Jing et al., "Design and arrangement of the CHIP (CHinese In Prato) study," *Epidemiologia e Prevenzione*, vol. 38, no. 6, pp. 357–363, 2014.

[20] C. R. Horowitz, M. Robinson, and S. Seifer, "Community-based participatory research from the margin to the mainstream are researchers prepared?" *Circulation*, vol. 119, no. 19, pp. 2633–2642, 2009.

[21] C. R. Horowitz, B. L. Brenner, S. Lachapelle, D. A. Amara, and G. Arniella, "Effective recruitment of minority populations through community-led strategies," *American Journal of Preventive Medicine*, vol. 37, no. 6, pp. S195–S200, 2009.

[22] J. Font and M. Méndez, *Surveying Ethnic Minorities and Immigrant Populations. Methodological Challenges and Research Strategies*, Amsterdam University Press, Amsterdam, The Netherlands, 2013.

[23] G. Mancia, R. Fagard, K. Narkiewicz et al., "2013 ESH/ESC Guidelines for the management of arterial hypertension: the Task Force for the management of arterial hypertension of the European Society of Hypertension (ESH) and of the European Society of Cardiology (ESC)," *Journal of Hypertension*, vol. 31, pp. 1281–1357, 2013.

[24] P. A. Modesti, P. Agostoni, C. Agyemang et al., "Cardiovascular risk assessment in low-resource settings: a consensus document of the European Society of Hypertension Working Group on Hypertension and Cardiovascular Risk in Low Resource Settings," *Journal of Hypertension*, vol. 32, no. 5, pp. 951–960, 2014.

[25] S. Rapi, C. Bazzini, C. Tozzetti, V. Sbolci, and P. A. Modesti, "Point-of-care testing of cholesterol and triglycerides for epidemiologic studies: evaluation of the multicare-in system," *Translational Research*, vol. 153, no. 2, pp. 71–76, 2009.

[26] G. Freckmann, C. Schmid, S. Pleus et al., "System accuracy evaluation of systems for pointof- care testing of blood glucose: a comparison of a patient-use system with six professional-use systems," *Clinical Chemistry and Laboratory Medicine*, vol. 52, no. 7, pp. 1079–1086, 2014.

[27] American Diabetes Association, "2. Classification and Diagnosis of Diabetes," *Diabetes Care*, vol. 39, supplement 1, pp. S13–S22, 2016.

[28] J. He, D. Gu, K. Reynolds et al., "Serum total and lipoprotein cholesterol levels and awareness, treatment, and control of hypercholesterolemia in China," *Circulation*, vol. 110, no. 4, pp. 405–411, 2004.

[29] National Cholesterol Education Program (NCEP) Expert Panel on Detection, Evaluation, and Treatment of High Blood Cholesterol in Adults (Adult Treatment Panel III), "Third Report of the National Cholesterol Education Program (NCEP) Expert Panel on Detection, Evaluation, and Treatment of High Blood Cholesterol in Adults (Adult Treatment Panel III) final report," *Circulation*, vol. 106, no. 25, pp. 3143–3421, 2002.

[30] O. B. Ahmad, C. Boschi-Pinto, A. D. Lopez, C. J. L. Murray, R. Lozano, and M. Inoue, *Age Standardization of Rates: A New WHO Standard*, World Health Organization, 2001.

[31] P. Zaninotto, J. Mindell, and V. Hirani, "Prevalence of cardiovascular risk factors among ethnic groups: results from the Health Surveys for England," *Atherosclerosis*, vol. 195, no. 1, pp. e48–e57, 2007.

[32] D. Shi, J. Li, Y. Wang et al., "Association between health literacy and hypertension management in a Chinese community: a retrospective cohort study," *Internal and Emergency Medicine*, 2017.

[33] J. A. Cutler, P. D. Sorlie, M. Wolz, T. Thom, L. E. Fields, and E. J. Roccella, "Trends in hypertension prevalence, awareness, treatment, and control rates in United States adults between 1988–1994 and 1999–2004," *Hypertension*, vol. 52, no. 5, pp. 818–827, 2008.

[34] T. A. Kotchen, "Obesity-related hypertension: epidemiology, pathophysiology, and clinical management," *American Journal of Hypertension*, vol. 23, no. 11, pp. 1170–1178, 2010.

[35] WHO, "Appropriate body-mass index in Asian populations and its implications for policy and intervention strategies," *Lancet*, vol. 363, p. 902, 2004.

[36] Z. Bei-Fan, "Predictive values of body mass index and waist circumference for risk factors of certain related diseases in Chinese adults: study on optimal cut-off points of body mass index and waist circumference in Chinese adults," *Asia Pacific Journal of Clinical Nutrition*, vol. 11, pp. S685–S693, 2002.

[37] P. A. Modesti, G. Galanti, P. Cala', and M. Calabrese, "Lifestyle interventions in preventing new type 2 diabetes in Asian populations," *Internal and Emergency Medicine*, vol. 11, no. 3, pp. 375–384, 2016.

13

Cardiovascular Risk Assessment in Angolan Adults

João M. Pedro ⓘ,[1,2] **Miguel Brito**,[1,3] **and Henrique Barros** ⓘ[2,4]

[1]*Centro de Investigação em Saúde de Angola (CISA), Caxito, Angola*
[2]*EPIUnit, Instituto de Saúde Pública, Universidade do Porto, Rua das Taipas, No. 135, 4050-600 Porto, Portugal*
[3]*Health and Technology Research Center, Escola Superior de Tecnologia da Saúde de Lisboa, Instituto Politécnico de Lisboa,*
  Av. D. João II, Lote 4.69.01, 1990-096 Lisboa, Portugal
[4]*Faculdade de Medicina, Universidade do Porto, Al. Prof. Hernâni Monteiro, 4200-319 Porto, Portugal*

Correspondence should be addressed to João M. Pedro; joao.almeidapedro@cisacaxito.org

Academic Editor: Franco Veglio

From a community-based survey conducted in Angola, 468 individuals aged 40 to 64 years and not using drug therapy were evaluated according to the World Health Organisation STEPwise Approach to Chronic Disease Risk Factor Surveillance. Using data from tobacco use, blood pressure, blood glucose, and total cholesterol levels, we estimated the 10-year risk of a fatal or nonfatal major cardiovascular event and computed the proportion of untreated participants eligible for pharmacological treatment according to clinical values alone and total cardiovascular risk. The large majority of participants were classified as having a low (<10%) 10-year cardiovascular risk (87.6%), with only 4.5% having a high (≥ 20%) cardiovascular risk. If we consider the single criteria for hypertension, 48.7% of the population should be considered for treatment. This value decreases to 22.0% if we apply the risk prediction chart. The use of hypoglycaemic drugs does not present any differences (19.0% in both situations). The use of lipid-lowering drugs (3.8%) is only recommended by the risk prediction chart. This study reveals the need of integrated approaches for the treatment of cardiovascular disorders in this population. Risk prediction charts can be used as a way to promote a better use of limited resources.

1. Introduction

Cardiovascular diseases (CVD) caused 17.9 million deaths worldwide in 2015, a number that has increased globally by 12.5% since 2005, with almost 80% of these deaths occurring in low and middle-income countries [1]. Their common occurrence and associated mortality, loss of independence and productivity, impaired quality of life, and social and economic costs are compelling reasons for public health concern globally [2].

The epidemiology of CVD is distinctly different in sub-Saharan Africa (SSA), compared to the rest of the world, where an unprecedented decline in mortality and a corresponding increase in the life expectancy at birth are shifting the epidemiological landscape of the region [3]. Countries in this region, where Angola is located, face a double burden as they struggle to cope with noncommunicable and infectious diseases associated with lack of socioeconomic development [3].

In 1990 the percentage of deaths by CVD in the region was 7.5% (the fourth cause of death), rising to 11.2% in 2015, being the third cause of mortality [4]. Myocardial infarctions, together with strokes, were responsible for 10.8% of deaths among females and 8.6% in males, in 2015 in SSA [4]. This represents an increase in mortality of 38.0% for stroke and 52.1% for myocardial infarction in both sexes, since 1990 [4], revealing a rising trend of CVD in SSA. The estimates made for Angola follow the same pattern, with strokes being responsible for 5.4% and myocardial infarction for 4.7% of all deaths, in 2015, the fourth and sixth cause of mortality in Angola, respectively [4].

Risk factors for CVD are shared with the majority of noncommunicable diseases and are due to exposure to behavioural risk factors: tobacco and alcohol consumption, unhealthy diet, and physical inactivity, individually modifiable. These unhealthy behaviours influence metabolic pathways and ultimately result in intermediate risk factors: obesity, hypertension, diabetes, and dyslipidaemia [5–7].

Common approaches that address behavioural and metabolic risk factors, which often coexist in the same person and act synergistically to increase an individual's total risk, are proven effective for prevention [6, 7], but in some settings, the risk factors are tackled one-by-one, without a common strategy. To design the right strategy for an individual, it is important to realise his/her "global risk" of developing CVD [7–9]. The World Health Organization (WHO) and the International Society of Hypertension (ISH) created a risk prediction chart [8], which can be applied in different populations.

In this short report, we aimed to quantify the proportion of individuals eligible for pharmacological treatment for hypertension, diabetes, and hypercholesterolemia according to single risk factor and total cardiovascular risk approaches, according to the WHO-ISH risk prediction chart.

2. Materials and Methods

The present report is a subset analysis from CardioBengo, a community-based study conducted in the catchment area of the Dande-Health Demographic Surveillance System (Dande-HDSS), located in the Dande Municipality, in Bengo Province, Angola [10]. This survey, done between September 2013 and March 2014, constitutes a larger baseline on cardiovascular risk factors [11], using the methodology proposed by the WHO STEPwise approach to Surveillance (STEPS) to Chronic Disease Risk Factor manual (core and expanded version 3.0) [12].

2.1. Sample Characterization. The subset of individuals from the CardioBengo study considered for this analysis follows the WHO-ISH risk prediction chart criteria of application [8]. The initial CardioBengo sample was made by 2,484 individuals (15 to 64 years old), drawn as a representative sex- and age-stratified random sample from the Dande-HDSS population database as previously described [11, 13].

The WHO-ISH risk prediction chart criteria of application [8] only consider individuals aged 40 or older. In the initial set, only 688 participants are aged above 40 years. From this group, 123 were excluded due to missing information in any of the parameters considered in the WHO-ISH risk prediction chart (current smoking status, systolic blood pressure, total blood cholesterol, and diabetes), and another 97 were excluded because they were already receiving pharmacological treatment for any of the three conditions (hypertension, diabetes, and hypercholesterolaemia). In this way, the final sample consists of 468 participants.

2.2. Data Collection. Participants were evaluated by trained interviewers and certified health professionals. As previously described in the CardioBengo study protocol [11],

information on age and tobacco consumption was collected through an interview, and blood pressure and all clinical measurements (measured only in participants with overnight fasting) were obtained with the use of point of care devices, namely, automatic sphygmomanometer OMRON M6 Comfort (OMRON Healthcare Europe BV, Hoofddorp, Netherlands); blood glucose meter ACCU-CHEK Aviva (Roche Diagnostic, Indianapolis, USA); and ACCUTREND Plus (Roche Diagnostic, Indianapolis, USA) with ACCUTREND CHOLESTEROL reactive strips (Roche Diagnostic, Indianapolis, USA) [11].

2.3. Prediction Methods and Eligibility for Pharmacological Treatment. The WHO-ISH prediction chart for the Africa D region was used to classify each participant regarding the individual absolute cardiovascular risk [8], based on sex (male or female), age (40–49, 50–59 and ≥ 60 years), current smoking status (nonsmoker or smoker), systolic blood pressure (SBP) (120-139, 140–159, 160–179, and ≥ 180 mmHg), total blood cholesterol (4, 5, 6, 7, and 8 mmol/l), and diabetes (presence or absence, considering the WHO cut point of 6.9 mmol/l [14]).

The WHO-ISH prediction charts estimate the 10-year risk of a fatal or nonfatal major cardiovascular event (myocardial infarction or stroke) expressed in five categories—≤10% (low), 10–19% (moderate), 20–29% (high), and ≥30% (very high)—in people who do not have established cardiovascular diseases [8].

The eligibility for treatment with antihypertensive, hypoglycaemic, or lipid-lowering drugs was defined according to the WHO guidelines for assessment and management of cardiovascular risk [8]. Also, eligibility for treatment according to the single risk factor approach was considered: for antihypertensive drug use SBP of ≥140 mmHg [15, 16]; for hypoglycaemic drug use fasting blood glucose >6.9 mmol/l [14]; and for lipid-lowering drugs use a total blood cholesterol level ≥8 mmol/l [9].

2.4. Statistical Analysis. Data were double entered into a PostgreSQL® database and imported into SPSS® version 23 (IBM, New York, USA) for data analysis. Descriptive data are reported as absolute frequencies and percentages. We estimated the proportion of participants classified in different categories of total cardiovascular risk, as well as the proportion of subjects eligible for pharmacological treatment (according to the different criteria), by sex. We consider a 95% confidence interval (95% CI) for all proportions calculated.

2.5. Ethical Approval. All procedures performed in this study were in accordance with the standards of the Ethics Committee of the Angolan Ministry of Health and with the 1964 Helsinki declaration and its later amendments. Written informed consent was obtained from all participants.

3. Results

The majority of the population in this study was female (69.7%) following the structure of the Dande-HDSS [10], with 17.9% of the population aged above 60 years. Smoking was

TABLE 1: Characteristics of the participants and prevalence by sex.

	Total (*n* = 468) % (95% CI)	Female (*n* = 326) % (95% CI)	Male (*n* = 142) % (95% CI)
Age (years)			
40-49	36.3 (32.1-40.8)	35.0 (30.0-40.3)	39.4 (31.7-47.6)
50-59	45.7 (41.2-50.2)	47.9 (42.5-53.3)	40.8 (33.1-49.0)
≥ 60	17.9 (14.7-21.6)	17.2 (13.5-21.7)	19.7 (14.0-27.0)
Current smoking status			
Non-smoker	89.3 (86.2-91.8)	92.6 (89.2-95.0)	81.7 (74.5-87.2)
Smoker	10.7 (8.2-13.8)	7.4 (5.0-10.8)	18.3 (12.8-25.5)
Systolic blood pressure (mmHg)			
120-139	51.3 (46.8-55.8)	47.5 (42.1-52.9)	59.9 (51.7-67.6)
140-159	26.7 (22.9-30.9)	26.7 (22.2-31.8)	26.8 (20.2-34.6)
160-179	14.3 (11.4-17.8)	16.6 (13.0-21.0)	9.2 (5.5-15.1)
≥ 180	7.7 (5.6-10.4)	9.2 (6.5-12.8)	4.2 (1.9-8.9)
Total blood cholesterol (mmol/l)			
4	55.6 (51.1-60.0)	52.1 (46.7-57.5)	63.4 (55.2-70.9)
5	27.1 (23.3-31.3)	26.7 (22.2-31.8)	28.2 (21.4-36.1)
6	13.0 (10.3-16.4)	15.0 (11.5-19.3)	8.5 (4.9-14.2)
7	4.3 (2.8-2.8)	6.1 (4.0-9.2)	0
8	0	0	0
Diabetes[a]			
Absence	81.0 (77.2-84.3)	81.6 (77.0-85.4)	79.6 (72.2-85.4)
Presence	19.0 (15.7-22.8)	18.4 (14.6-23.0)	20.4 (14.6-27.8)
With SBP >140 mmHg and Diabetes	9.8 (7.4-12.8)	9.5 (6.8-13.2)	10.6 (6.5-16.7)

[a]Fasting blood glucose ≥6.9 mmol/l.

more frequent among men (18.3% versus 7.4% in women) with almost half the population (48.7%) presenting a SBP ≥140 mmHg, with a higher occurrence in women (52.5% versus 40.1% in men). None of the individuals presented total blood cholesterol >8 mmol/l, with only women presenting values >7 mmol/l (6.1%). The prevalence of diabetes was similar among men and women (18.4% in women and 20.4% in men), with almost 10% of the population having both SBP ≥140 mmHg and diabetes (Table 1).

Most of the participants (87.6%) were classified as having low (<10%) 10-year cardiovascular risk. The frequencies were 7.9%, 2.6%, and 1.9% for the cardiovascular risk categories 10–19 (moderate), 20–29 (high), and ≥30% (very high), respectively. Women presented higher frequencies than men in all cardiovascular risk categories above the moderate level and the total cardiovascular risk increased with age (Table 2).

Considering only the criteria of SBP ≥140 mmHg, 48.7% of the population should be considered for treatment with antihypertensive drugs, but if we apply the WHO/ISH criteria based on the prediction chart, this number will decrease by more them half to 22.0%. On the other hand, the use of lipid-lowering drugs is not considered for any individual by the singular criteria, but if we apply the prediction chart, this number rises to 3.8% (Table 3).

4. Discussion

Only 4.5% of the population was classified as having at least a high (≥20%) cardiovascular risk. These results are in accordance with those described in other populations of the continental sub-Saharan Africa, namely, 3.7% in Mozambique [17] and 5% in Nigeria [18], or in other low and middle-income countries in Asia (4.9% in rural India, 1.3% in Cambodia, 2.3% in Malaysia, and 6% in Mongolia) [19, 20]. In all these surveys, the accumulation of risk factors exists in different levels. In this analysis, almost one-tenth of the population accumulates at least two major risk factors (hypertension and diabetes).

This raises additional concerns when we analyse this subset of results together with the values found in the CardioBengo population aged 16 to 64 years: a prevalence of hypertension of 18.0%, diabetes of 9.2%, and hypercholesterolaemia of 4.0%, with a low awareness and control levels [13]. The CVD are present in this population, but this does not imply that the health systems in the region are ready to face with this growing reality.

According to the WHO guidelines for assessment and management of cardiovascular diseases [8], at least one-quarter of the participants in this report would be eligible for treatment with antihypertensive drugs, whereas if only the single criteria were applied for hypertension, almost half would be considered for pharmacological treatment. Even if some discussion is possible about the applicability of pharmacological treatment with a SBP of 140, the specific behaviour of blood pressure in black individuals (as the population observed) should be considered [16].

TABLE 2: Distribution of 10-year risk of a fatal or nonfatal major cardiovascular event, according to sex and age.

	Total, % (95% CI)			
	≤10% Low	10-19% Moderate	20-29 % High	≥30% Very High
40-49 years	34.2 (30.0-38.6)	1.3 (0.6-2.8)	0.6 (0.2-1.9)	0.2 (0.0-1.2)
50-59 years	40.6 (36.2-45.1)	3.6 (2.3-5.7)	0.6 (0.2-1.9)	0.9 (0.3-2.2)
≥ 60 years	12.8 (10.1-16.2)	3.0 (1.8-5.0)	1.3 (0.6-2.8)	0.9 (0.3-2.2)
Total	**87.6 (84.3-90.3)**	**7.9 (5.8-10.7)**	**2.6 (1.5-4.4)**	**1.9 (1.0-3.6)**
	Female, % (95% CI)			
	≤10% Low	10-19% Moderate	20-29 % High	≥30% Very High
40-49 years	32.5 (27.7-37.8)	1.5 (0.7-3.5)	0.6 (0.2-2.2)	0.3 (0.1-1.7)
50-59 years	41.7 (36.5-47.1)	4.0 (2.3-6.7)	0.9 (0.3-2.7)	1.2 (0.5-3.1)
≥ 60 years	11.7 (8.6-15.6)	3.1 (1.7-5.6)	1.8 (0.8-4.0)	0.6 (0.2-2.2)
Total	**85.9 (81.7-89.3)**	**8.6 (6.0-12.1)**	**3.4 (1.9-5.9)**	**2.1 (1.0-4.4)**
	Male, % (95% CI)			
	≤10% Low	10-19% Moderate	20-29 % High	≥30% Very High
40-49 years	38.0 (30.5-46.2)	0.7 (0.1-3.9)	0.7 (0.1-3.9)	-[a]
50-59 years	38.0 (30.5-46.2)	2.8 (1.1-7.0)	-[a]	-[a]
≥ 60 years	15.5 (10.5-22.3)	2.8 (1.1-7.0)	-[a]	1.4 (0.4-5.0)
Total	**91.5 (85.8-95.1)**	**6.3 (3.4-11.6)**	**0.7 (0.1-3.9)**	**1.4 (0.4-5.0)**

[a]No individuals in this category.

TABLE 3: Frequencies of individuals who require pharmacological treatment by sex.

	Single risk criteria			Considering WHO/ISH[a] risk prediction		
	Total, % (95% CI)	Female, % (95% CI)	Male, % (95% CI)	Total, % (95% CI)	Female, % (95% CI)	Male, % (95% CI)
Antihypertensive drugs	48.7 (44.2-53.2)	52.5 (47.0-57.8)	40.1 (32.4-48.4)	22.0 (18.5-26.0)	25.8 (21.3-30.8)	13.4 (8.7-20.0)
Lipid-lowering drugs	-[b]	-[b]	-[b]	3.8 (2.4-6.0)	4.9 (3.0-7.8)	1.4 (0.4-5.0)
Hypoglycaemic drugs	19.0 (15.7-22.8)	18.4 (14.6-23.0)	20.4 (14.6-27.8)	19.0 (15.7-22.8)	18.4 (14.6-23.0)	20.4 (14.6-27.8)

[a]World Health Organization/International Society of Hypertension.
[b]No individuals in this category.

The use of the WHO-ISH risk prediction chart has already been proven as more cost effective than other approaches that make treatment decisions based on individual risk factor thresholds only, especially for hypertension management [7, 21–23]. In a South-African study, different strategies for initiation of drug treatment were tested, and the conclusion points to the fact that hypertension treatment based on the total cardiovascular risk is more effective at saving lives and less costly than those based only on the BP level [24].

In this prediction chart, we included the total cholesterol measurement; however, the WHO-ISH chart offers the possibility of not using this measurement [8]. The use of laboratory (or point of care) assessment in low-resource settings is dispensable, avoiding additional costs to the system without losing a significant predictive power or introducing

an overconsumption of drugs, allowing for a better targeting of resources to those who are more likely to develop CVD [25, 26].

The high percentage of individuals that requires pharmacological treatment for diabetes (19.0%, very similar between gender) is alarming, considering the fact that diabetes alone is a very important health condition, but also an important risk factor for CVD; adults with diabetes have a two or three times higher rate of CVD than adults without diabetes [8, 27].

Health promotion initiatives such as smoking cessation and individual advisement on specific lifestyle and diet control are also strategies necessary to align with the use of pharmacological treatments. Even if some of the proposed methodologies (statins for hypercholesterolemia, for example) cannot be easily applied due to the steady supply of drugs, changes to personal lifestyle should be encouraged, with good results in the decrease of the global cardiovascular risk [18, 21, 22].

The focus of targeting high-risk people through a total cardiovascular risk approach instead of a single risk factor approach reduces health care expenditure by reducing drug costs [18]. However, to diminish CVD burden in the entire population in a sustainable way, wider interventions are needed. The focus should be on the primary healthcare, where the majority of the individuals have access, allowing for the promotion of opportunistic screening of CVD risk factors and patient registration and tracking, with a better use of available resources [23].

The findings in this report should be interpreted cautiously. The study was conducted only at a district-level, and due to the criteria of application of the WHO-ISH risk prediction chart the sample size was small. Even with these limitations, this report adds evidence to the emerging public health issue of CVD, especially in older individuals, and provides additional information on the impact of the use of risk prediction charts.

5. Conclusion

The use of the WHO-ISH guidelines for cardiovascular risk prediction reduces the population eligible for pharmacological treatment, giving prominence to an integrated approach based on lifestyle changes. This may sound appropriate to a low-resource setting, but the low education level of this population and the lower ability in older individuals for altering behaviours are factors to consider in future interventions. The training of health professionals and raising awareness may be the starting point to tackle CVD in this population, where the use of these charts can have a role to play in the wise use of resources available.

Disclosure

The funders had no role in study design, data collection and analysis, decision to publish, or preparation of the manuscript. The authors alone are responsible for the views expressed in this publication and they do not necessarily represent the decisions, policy, or views of any of the funders.

Acknowledgments

The authors wish to thank the clinical staff of the Bengo General Hospital for establishing and supporting the follow-up consultation. They thank all Dande-HDSS staff for their continuing support during fieldwork, namely, Joana Paz and Ana Oliveira for their field supervision roles, Eduardo Saraiva for data entry supervision and database management, and Edite Rosário for the training of field-workers and assistance in data collection procedures, and most importantly, the local administration and all of the individuals who accepted to take part in the study. The promoters of CISA funded this study as follows: Camões, Institute of Cooperation and Language, Portugal; the Calouste Gulbenkian Foundation, Portugal; the Government of Bengo Province and the Angolan Ministry of Health. Also the Eduardo dos Santos Foundation, Angola, funded this study.

References

[1] H. Wang, M. Naghavi, and C. Allen, "Global, regional, and national life expectancy, all-cause mortality, and cause-specific mortality for 249 causes of death, 1980–2015: a systematic analysis for the Global Burden of Disease Study 2015," *Lancet*, vol. 388, pp. 1459–1544, 2016.

[2] D. Labarthe, *Epidemiology And Prevention of Cardiovascular Diseases: A Global Challenge*, Jones and Bartlett Publishers, Sudbury, MD, USA, 2nd edition, 2011.

[3] D. T. Jamison, R. G. Feachem, M. W. Makgoba et al., *Disease and Mortality in Sub-Saharan Africa*, World Bank, Washington, DC, USA, 2nd edition, 2006.

[4] Institute for Health Metrics and Evaluation. GBD compare - Viz Hub, 2018, http://vizhub.healthdata.org/gbd-compare/.

[5] World Health Organization, *Global status report on Noncommunicable diseases. Geneva: World Health Organization*, 2014, http://apps.who.int/iris/bitstream/10665/148114/1/9789241564854_eng.pdf.

[6] World Health Organization, *Global Atlas on Cardiovascular Disease Prevention And Control*, World Health Organization, Geneva, Switzerland, 2011.

[7] World Health Organization, *Global health risks: Mortality and burden of disease attributable to selected major risks. Geneva: World Health Organization*, 2009, http://www.who.int/healthinfo/global_burden_disease/GlobalHealthRisks_report_Front.pdf.

[8] World Health Organization, *Prevention of Cardiovascular Disease: Guidelines for Assessment And Management of Cardiovascular Risk. Geneva: World Health Organization*, 2007, http://www.who.int/cardiovascular_diseases/guidelines/Full%20text.pdf.

[9] World Health Organization, *Global Action Plan for The Prevention And Control of Noncommunicable Diseases 2013-2020. Geneva: World Health Organization*, 2013, http://apps.who.int/iris/bitstream/10665/94384/1/f9789241506236_eng.pdf.

[10] M. J. Costa, E. Rosário, A. Langa, G. António, A. Bendriss, and S. V. Nery, "Setting up a demographic surveillance system in Northern Angola," *Etude de la Population Africaine*, vol. 26, no. 2, pp. 133–146, 2012.

[11] J. M. Pedro, E. Rosário, M. Brito, and H. Barros, "CardioBengo study protocol: A population based cardiovascular longitudinal study in Bengo Province, Angola," *BMC Public Health*, vol. 16, no. 1, 2016.

[12] World Health Organization, *The STEPS Instrument and Support Materials*, 2013, http://www.who.int/chp/steps/instrument/en/.

[13] J. M. Pedro, M. Brito, and H. Barros, "Prevalence, awareness, treatment and control of hypertension, diabetes and hypercholesterolaemia among adults in Dande municipality, Angola," *Cardiovascular Journal of Africa*, vol. 29, no. 2, pp. 73–81, 2018.

[14] World Health Organization, *Definition and diagnosis of diabetes mellitus and intermediate hyperglycaemia: report of a WHO/IDF consultation*, World Health Organization, Geneva, Switzerland, 2006.

[15] M. A. Weber, E. L. Schiffrin, W. B. White et al., "Clinical Practice Guidelines for the Management of Hypertension in the Community," *The Journal of Clinical Hypertension*, vol. 16, no. 1, pp. 14–26, 2014.

[16] J. M. Flack, D. A. Sica, G. Bakris et al., "Management of high blood pressure in Blacks: an update of the International Society on Hypertension in Blacks consensus statement," *Hypertension*, vol. 56, no. 5, pp. 780–800, 2010.

[17] A. Damasceno, P. Padrão, C. Silva-Matos, A. Prista, A. Azevedo, and N. Lunet, "Cardiovascular risk in Mozambique: Who should be treated for hypertension?" *Journal of Hypertension*, vol. 31, no. 12, pp. 2348–2355, 2013.

[18] S. Mendis, L. H. Lindholm, S. G. Anderson et al., "Total cardio-vascular risk approach to improve efficiency of cardiovascular prevention in resource constrain settings," *Journal of Clinical Epidemiology*, vol. 64, no. 12, pp. 1451–1462, 2011.

[19] A. G. Ghorpade, S. R. Shrivastava, S. S. Kar, S. Sarkar, S. M. Majgi, and G. Roy, "Estimation of the cardiovascular risk using world health organization/international society of hypertension (WHO/ISH) risk prediction charts in a rural population of South India," *International Journal of Health Policy and Management*, vol. 4, no. 8, pp. 531–536, 2015.

[20] D. Otgontuya, S. Oum, B. S. Buckley, and R. Bonita, "Assessment of total cardiovascular risk using WHO/ISH risk prediction charts in three low and middle income countries in Asia," *BMC Public Health*, vol. 13, no. 1, p. 539, 2013.

[21] World Health Organization, *Prevention and control of noncommunicable diseases: guidelines for primary health care in low-resource settings. Geneva: World Health Organization*, 2012, http://apps.who.int/iris/bitstream/10665/76173/1/9789241548397_eng.pdf.

[22] P. A. Modesti, P. Agostoni, C. Agyemang et al., "Cardiovascular risk assessment in low-resource settings: a consensus document of the European Society of Hypertension Working Group on Hypertension and Cardiovascular Risk in Low Resource Settings," *Journal of Hypertension*, vol. 32, no. 5, pp. 951–960, 2014.

[23] P. Bovet, A. Chiolero, F. Paccaud, and N. Banatvala, "Screening for cardiovascular disease risk and subsequent management in low and middle income countries: Challenges and opportunities," *Public Health Reviews*, vol. 36, no. 1, 2015.

[24] T. A. Gaziano, K. Steyn, D. J. Cohen, M. C. Weinstein, and L. H. Opie, "Cost-effectiveness analysis of hypertension guidelines in South Africa: Absolute risk versus blood pressure level," *Circulation*, vol. 112, no. 23, pp. 3569–3576, 2005.

[25] A. Pandya, M. C. Weinstein, J. A. Salomon, D. Cutler, and T. A. Gaziano, "Who needs laboratories and who needs statins? Comparative and cost-effectiveness analyses of non-laboratory-based, laboratory-based, and staged primary cardiovascular disease screening guidelines," *Circulation: Cardiovascular Quality and Outcomes*, vol. 7, no. 1, pp. 25–32, 2014.

[26] P. R. Nordet, S. Mendis, A. Dueñas et al., "Total cardiovascular risk assessment and management using two prediction tools, with and without blood cholesterol," *MEDICC Review*, vol. 15, no. 4, pp. 36–40, 2013.

[27] *Global Report on Diabetes. Geneva: World Health Organization*, 2016, http://apps.who.int/iris/bitstream/10665/204871/1/9789241565257_eng.pdf.

14

Association of Serum Bisphenol A with Hypertension in Thai Population

Wichai Aekplakorn,[1] La-or Chailurkit,[2] and Boonsong Ongphiphadhanakul[2]

[1]*Department of Community Medicine, Faculty of Medicine, Ramathibodi Hospital, Mahidol University, Bangkok 10400, Thailand*
[2]*Department of Medicine, Faculty of Medicine, Ramathibodi Hospital, Mahidol University, Bangkok 10400, Thailand*

Correspondence should be addressed to Wichai Aekplakorn; wichai.aek@mahidol.ac.th

Academic Editor: B. Waeber

Objective. The present study aimed to examine the association between serum BPA and hypertension and evaluated whether it was influenced by estradiol level. *Methods.* A subsample of 2588 sera randomly selected from the Thai National Health Examination Survey IV, 2009, was measured for serum BPA and estradiol. Logistic regression was used to examine the association controlling for age, sex, diabetes, body mass index, and estradiol level. *Results.* Compared with the lowest quartile, the adjusted odds ratio (AOR) of hypertension for the fourth quartile of serum BPA was 2.16 (95% CI 1.31, 3.56) in women and 1.44 (0.99, 2.09) in men. There was no interaction between serum BPA and estradiol level. For analysis using log(BPA) as a continuous variable, the AOR per unit change in log(BPA) was 1.09 (95% CI 1.02, 1.16). Among postmenopausal women, the AOR for the fourth quartile of BPA was 2.33 (95% CI 1.31, 4.15) and, for premenopausal women, it was 2.12 (95% CI 0.87, 5.19). *Conclusion.* Serum BPA was independently associated with hypertension in women and was not likely to be affected by estrogen; however, its mechanism related to blood pressure needs further investigation.

1. Introduction

Bisphenol A (BPA) is a widely used chemical in the production of plastic food containers in many consumer products and of epoxy resins in dental fillings. Exposure to BPA is very common in almost all US adults [1], Asian population [2], and about 80% of Thai population [3]. Recently, this chemical has received much attention for its association with many health impacts [4]. BPA, a xenoestrogen, might mimic estrogen and disrupt the function of estrogen through estrogen receptor [5]. So far, health effects associated with exposure to BPA as reported in the literature include estrogenic activity, thyroid hormone disruption [6], pancreatic beta cell function disturbance, and increased risk of diabetes [3]. Epidemiological studies have shown that BPA in urine and serum is associated with diabetes [7–11], obesity [12], and self-reported cardiovascular diseases [13–15]. Bae et al. reported an association of urinary BPA with hypertension, especially among those not previously known to have hypertension [16].

Shankar and Teppala reported the association of urinary BPA with hypertension independent of other risk factors [17].

Globally, high blood pressure is the most common risk factor for cardiovascular diseases death. It contributed to 40% of cardiovascular deaths in 2010 [18]. Although conventional risk factors for hypertension such as salt intake and obesity were described [19], knowledge of other environmental risk factors and their role in hypertension might be useful in prevention and control of the condition. As estrogen has vasorelaxation effect [20, 21], it is not clear whether exposure to BPA is associated with high blood pressure and in what direction. Previous study has reported an association between urinary BPA and hypertension; however, there has been no prior study using serum BPA as exposure indicator. It is less clear whether high BP is related to BPA and the effect is influenced by estrogen level. The objective of the present study was to determine the association between serum BPA and blood pressure and if so whether the effect was related to estrogen level or menopausal status.

2. Methods

Data were from Thai National Health Examination Survey (NHES) 2009. Details of sampling methods were described previously elsewhere [22]. In brief, a subsample of 2588 sera from the NHES IV was randomly selected and measured for the level of bisphenol A and estradiol. The sample was randomly selected according to sex and 6 age groups (15–29, 30–44, 45–59, 60–69, 70–79, and 80–89). 25 samples were selected from each stratum, and a total of 2588 samples were available.

The NHES was approved by the Ethics Committee of Ministry of Public Health, and written informed consent was obtained from all participants. This study was also approved by the Ethics Committee of Ramathibodi Hospital, Faculty of Medicine, Mahidol University.

Demographic data such as age and sex were included. Body mass index (BMI) was calculated as weight in kilograms divided by the square of height in meters. Serum BPA levels were measured by competitive ELISA (IBL International GmH, Hamburg, German) with an intra-assay and interassay precision of 11.8% and 13.6%, respectively. Serum levels of 17β-estradiol (E2) were determined by electrochemiluminescence immunoassay on a Cobase 411 analyzer (Roche Diagnostics GmbH). The intra-assay precision was 4.3%.

Measurements of blood pressure were performed by trained field research assistants using automatic sphygmomanometer Microlife model A100 (Microlife AG, Widnau, Switzerland) with appropriate arm cuffs. Prior to measurement, participants rested for 5 min in a sitting position according to the standard protocol [23]. Three measurements of blood pressure were obtained from each participant. An average of the second and third values was calculated and used in the analysis.

Alcohol drinking is defined as self-reported alcohol beverage consumption in the past 12 months. Smoking is defined as follows: current cigarette smokers were defined as individuals who had smoked ≥100 cigarettes during their lifetime and at the time of interview responded that they smoked every day or some days [24].

2.1. Definition of Hypertension. Hypertension is defined as mean systolic blood pressure (SBP) equal to or greater than 140 mmHg or mean diastolic blood pressure (DBP) equal to or greater than 90 mmHg or on medication to lower blood pressure in the past two weeks. Unaware hypertension is defined as individuals with hypertension, who have never been told by health professionals that they had hypertension. In the analysis, we also examined the association with those who treated hypertension in the past two weeks and for those who were diagnosed but did not receive medication to lower their blood pressure.

2.2. Statistical Analysis. All analyses took into account the complex survey design by weighting for the total population. Descriptive statistical analyses of percentages, means, and standard variation (SD) were performed. Student's unpaired *t*-test was used to compare means between groups. Geometric mean of BPA was calculated and used due to the skewness of BPA distribution. BPA level was categorized into quartile. Means and proportions of several clinical variables including pulse pressure, SBP, DBP, fasting plasma glucose, serum estrogen level, diabetes, and several hypertension status variables were calculated according to quartile of BPA and then compared. Logistic regression was used to examine the association between BPA and blood pressure and hypertension status. First, each hypertension status variable was regressed on the log(BPA) as a continuous variable in the model. Potential confounding variables that were adjusted included age, sex, BMI, alcohol drinking, smoking and diabetes status, and estradiol level. We tested for the interaction between BPA and estrogen level by adding an interaction term between log(BPA) and estradiol level in the model. To handle the problem of missing values of log(BPA) for undetected BPA level as zero, individuals with zero BPA level were assigned to 0.005 (an average of the lowest value and zero). We also ran logistic regression using quartile of BPA as categorical variable in the model. To determine whether the effects of BPA or hypertension status varied by menopausal status, an additional stratified analysis for the association of BPA and hypertension was performed separately for premenopausal and postmenopausal status. There were 19 postmenopausal women having history of taking hormone supplement; however, excluding this group of women did not change the results, so we did not exclude them from the analysis. All the analyses were performed using Stata software version 10.1 (StataCorp. College Station, Texas, USA). Statistical significance was set at a *P* value of <0.05.

3. Results

Table 1 gives the basic characteristics of the 2,558 participants. Mean age of the participants was 40.37 (SD 16.81) years. Overall geometric mean of BPA was 0.34 (SD 0.02) ng/mL with a slightly higher value but was not significant in men compared to that in women. Prevalence of hypertension in men and women was relatively similar at 18%. The pronounced differences were the significantly higher prevalence of smoking and alcohol drinking in men compared to women. Mean of estradiol level in women was significantly higher than that in men (*P* < 0.001). Women had a higher BMI compared with men.

Table 2 shows the weighted geometric mean BPA by sex and several clinical conditions. Mean BPA was significantly higher in individuals with hypertension than in those with normotension (*P* < 0.01), especially in women (*P* < 0.01). Geometric means of BPA were also higher among other hypertension variables designated for high blood pressure such as those with unaware hypertension and among those with high SBP ≥ 140 mmHg. There were no significant differences in BPA levels between smokers and nonsmokers as well as between alcohol drinkers and nondrinkers.

Table 3 shows the distribution of several blood pressure variables as varied by quartiles of BPA. Overall, SBP and DBP were not significantly varied by BPA quartiles. Compared with the lowest quartile, prevalence of all hypertension, unaware hypertension, and those treated or not treated

TABLE 1: Basic characteristics of the study samples.

	Men ($n = 1275$)	Women ($n = 1283$)	Total ($n = 2558$)	P value
Age, yr[a]	39.58 (16.95)	41.12 (16.64)	40.37 (16.81)	0.02
BPA, ng/mL[a]	0.35 (0.02)	0.33 (0.02)	0.34 (0.02)	0.22
SBP, mm Hg[a]	122.81 (16.01)	118.99 (17.46)	120.86 (16.89)	<0.001
DBP, mm Hg[a]	75.70 (10.93)	73.49 (10.23)	74.57 (10.63)	<0.001
Diabetes[b]	121 (5.01)	143 (6.17)	264 (5.60)	0.13
All HT[b]	440 (18.62)	422 (17.46)	862 (18.03)	0.51
Unaware HT[b]	204 (11.62)	152 (6.92)	356 (9.22)	0.001
HT with treatment[b]	195 (5.22)	235 (8.82)	430 (7.06)	<0.001
HT without treatment[b]	245 (13.39)	187 (8.63)	432 (10.98)	<0.01
Smoking[b]	416 (39.61)	46 (1.60)	462 (20.18)	<0.001
Alcohol drinking[b]	663 (67.96)	267 (25.46)	930 (46.27)	<0.001
BMI, kg/m^2 [a]	22.74 (3.99)	24.44 (4.87)	23.61 (4.55)	<0.001
BMI ≥ 25 kg/m^2 [b]	331 (24.05)	481 (40.75)	812 (32.59)	<0.001
E2, pg/mL[a]	36.83 (22.55)	70.08 (97.81)	53.79 (74.20)	<0.001

[a]Mean (SD), [b]number (percentage).
BPA: bisphenol A, SBP: systolic blood pressure, DBP: diastolic blood pressure, HT: hypertension, BMI: body mass index, and E2: estradiol.

TABLE 2: Geographic mean (SE) of serum BPA by blood pressure status and selected factors among Thai men and women.

	Geometric mean of BPA (ng/mL)								
Condition	Men ($n = 1275$)			Women ($n = 1283$)			Total ($n = 2558$)		
	No	Yes	P value	No	Yes	P value	No	Yes	P value
All HT	0.34 (0.02)	0.43 (0.04)	0.05	0.30 (0.02)	0.47 (0.04)	<0.001	0.32 (0.02)	0.45 (0.03)	<0.001
Unaware HT	0.35 (0.02)	0.37 (0.06)	0.76	0.32 (0.02)	0.49 (0.05)	<0.001	0.34 (0.02)	0.41 (0.04)	0.07
SBP ≥ 140 mmHg	0.35 (0.02)	0.40 (0.06)	0.34	0.31 (0.02)	0.50 (0.04)	<0.001	0.33 (0.02)	0.45 (0.04)	<0.01
DBP ≥ 90 mmHg	0.35 (0.02)	0.43 (0.05)	0.14	0.32 (0.02)	0.43 (0.05)	0.05	0.34 (0.02)	0.43 (0.04)	0.04
HT with treatment	0.35 (0.02)	0.51 (0.05)	<0.01	0.32 (0.02)	0.49 (0.04)	<0.001	0.33 (0.01)	0.50 (0.03)	<0.001
BMI ≥ 25 kg/m^2	0.35 (0.02)	0.36 (0.04)	0.05	0.33 (0.02)	0.33 (0.03)	0.82	0.34 (0.02)	0.34 (0.02)	0.83
Smoking	0.34 (0.02)	0.38 (0.03)	0.28	0.33 (0.02)	0.38 (0.07)	0.41	0.33 (0.02)	0.38 (0.03)	0.13
Alcohol drinking	0.43 (0.3)	0.32 (0.02)	<0.01	0.33 (0.02)	0.33 (0.03)	0.90	0.36 (0.02)	0.32 (0.02)	0.11
Menopause	—	—	—	0.32 (0.02)	0.36 (0.02)	0.09	—	—	—

BPA: bisphenol A, HT: hypertension, and BMI: body mass index.

were significantly highest in the fourth quartile. To explore whether the association of BPA with hypertension was related to level of estrogen or menopausal status, an interaction term was added in the logistic regression models. Figure 1 shows the age-adjusted percentages of hypertension with and without treatment according to quartile of BPA level in men and women. Compared to the first quartile, the age-adjusted hypertension prevalence significantly increased in the fourth quartile for women for both hypertension with treatment and hypertension without treatment ($P = 0.03$ and 0.04, resp.), but not in men.

Table 4 gives odds ratios of association between log(BPA) and hypertension status controlling for age, BMI, diabetes, smoking, and estradiol level among females with an interaction between log(BPA) and estradiol level. Log(BPA) was significantly associated with hypertension with an odds ratio of 1.09 (1.02, 1.16). Using several definitions for hypertension status (unaware hypertension (HT), SBP ≥ 140 mmHg, DBP ≥ 90 mmHg, treated HT, or untreated HT) yielded similar

results of no interaction between BPA and estradiol. Table 5 gives the association between BPA quartile and a number of different definitions of hypertension. Overall, compared with the first quartile, those in the highest quartile of BPA had a significant 76% higher chance of hypertension. The association appeared to be stronger among women with an adjusted odds ratio of 2.16 (95% CI 1.31, 3.56) for the highest quartile. The association was even slightly stronger for unaware hypertension (adjusted OR 2.54, 95% CI 1.11, 6.83). We further performed a stratified analysis according to menopausal status. Table 6 shows the significant associations of hypertension status with the highest quartile of BPA among postmenopausal women, but not among premenopausal women (2.33, 95% CI 1.31, 4.15, and 2.12, 95% CI 0.87, 5.19, resp.). An additional analysis using log(BPA) as continuous variable as shown in Table 7 yielded consistent results of significant associations with hypertension status with AORs ranging from 1.02 to 1.15.

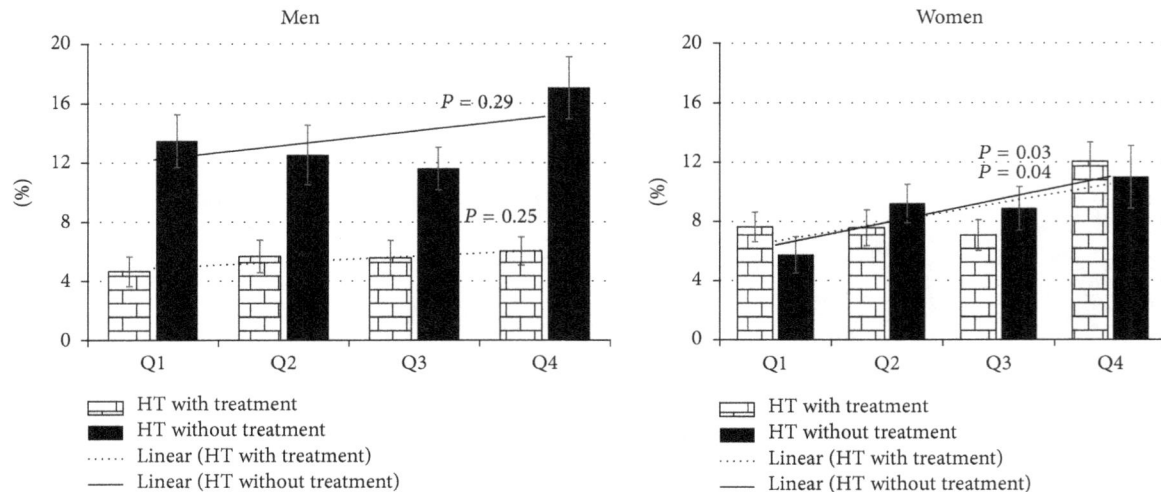

FIGURE 1: Age-adjusted percentages of hypertension with and without treatment by quartile of BPA level in men and women.

4. Discussion

The present study revealed that serum BPA was independently associated with hypertension. The positive association was found for all hypertension and unaware HT among women. The association was not likely to be confounded by age, sex, BMI, diabetes, and estrogen level. Although there was no clear interaction between BPA and estrogen level, the association between BPA and hypertension appeared to be stronger among postmenopausal women. The positive association between serum BPA and hypertension was consistent with studies using urinary BPA as surrogate. Bae and colleagues reported that urinary BPA was positively associated with blood pressure but negatively associated with heart rate variability [16]. Shankar and colleague analyzed data from NHANES 2003-2004 and found the association of urinary BPA with hypertension [17].

Mechanism of action of BPA on cardiovascular system is complex and the mode of action on blood pressure is unclear; however, there are several pathways that might be possible. A study suggests that exposure to BPA is related to insulin resistance and its role in weight gain and obesity [25]. Activation of ERβ can reduce systematic arterial pressure via autonomic influence [26]. Hypertension and vascular dysfunction have been shown in whole body ERβ knockout mice [27, 28]. BPA is associated with decrease in free thyroid hormone [6], and hypothyroid has been reported to be associated with hypertension [29]. Endothelial cell injury induced by BPA through oxidative stress has been reported [30]. Insulin resistance is closely related to hypertension [31].

Effects of BPA binding to estrogen receptors on cardiovascular system might be different from those of estrogen. BPA has dual actions as an agonist and antagonist of estrogen for estrogen receptor alpha (ERα) but acts only as an agonist for estrogen receptor beta (ERβ) [5]. Estrogen is important for maintaining and repairing endothelium mediated by ERα through increase in eNOS and cyclooxygenase resulting in vasorelaxation [20, 21]. The higher prevalence of hypertension among postmenopausal women might be attributed to the decline in estrogen level; however, it is not likely to affect the differences by menopausal status in the magnitude of association between BPA and hypertension. The effect of BPA as estrogen disruptor might be stronger in postmenopausal women when natural estrogen declines and is replaced with BPA. The significant association in postmenopausal but not in premenopausal women should be interpreted with caution. The greater and significant association in postmenopausal women might be due to the larger sample size in this age group. However, it is possible that this group of women had lower level of estrogen and the effect of BPA on estrogen receptor became dominant. The association was not related to hormone replacement, as the analysis with exclusion of women with history of taking hormone supplement did not change the results.

The different degrees of association according to criteria for hypertension were observed. The association was strongest for all hypertension but was weaker for high SBP and high DBP. This could be due to the fact that some individuals with hypertension were treated medically to lower BP level leading to an attenuated magnitude of association. For treated or untreated hypertension, the associations were relatively consistent suggesting that the medication for hypertension was not likely to affect the association.

There are some limitations in the present study. First, the present study used serum BPA as surrogate for BPA exposure which may have low sensitivity to reflect the burden of BPA in the body compared to urine BPA [32]. However, serum BPA reflected true level of BPA that is active [33]. Nonetheless, the underestimation of BPA levels might attenuate the association between BPA and hypertension. Second, the prevalence of hypertension (18.0%) in this population is not so high which might limit the power of the test for comparison among some subgroups and the nonsignificant findings in men or in premenopausal women might be due to the small sample size. It is possible that the association of BPA and hypertension might be confounded by other

TABLE 3: Age-adjusted mean (SE) and proportions (%) of selected characteristics in Thai population according to quartile of serum BPA in Thai population.

	All (n = 2558)					Men (n = 1275)					Women (n = 1283)				
	Q1	Q2	Q3	Q4	P for trends	Q1	Q2	Q3	Q4	P for trends	Q1	Q2	Q3	Q4	P for trends
Age, yr[a]	38.83 (0.56)	38.62 (0.52)	40.82 (0.64)	44.52 (0.83)	<0.001	38.05 (0.72)	36.23 (0.67)	40.51 (0.84)	44.79 (1.01)	<0.001	39.47 (0.70)	41.07 (0.72)	41.09 (0.94)	44.20 (1.04)	<0.01
BMI, kg/m^2[a]	23.66 (0.15)	23.80 (0.20)	23.56 (0.22)	23.34 (0.22)	0.24	22.64 (0.24)	22.89 (0.25)	23.13 (0.29)	22.35 (0.24)	0.68	24.49 (0.20)	24.68 (0.31)	23.94 (0.29)	24.53 (0.37)	0.57
SBP mmHg[a]	120.68 (0.54)	120.74 (0.43)	120.56 (0.51)	121.62 (0.79)	0.36	122.84 (0.84)	123.13 (0.61)	122.31 (0.62)	123.99 (1.08)	0.47	118.83 (0.74)	117.81 (0.68)	118.90 (0.79)	118.94 (1.17)	0.80
DBP mmHg[a]	74.58 (0.35)	74.56 (0.34)	74.33 (0.36)	74.83 (0.49)	0.83	75.11 (0.60)	75.94 (0.49)	75.64 (0.51)	76.75 (0.81)	0.13	74.17 (0.39)	73.18 (0.49)	73.14 (0.59)	72.54 (0.64)	0.04
Diabetes[b]	4.44 (0.79)	4.12 (0.78)	6.90 (0.93)	7.15 (0.88)	0.01	3.14 (0.68)	4.93 (1.54)	6.45 (1.37)	6.18 (1.02)	0.03	5.42 (1.12)	3.37 (0.53)	7.26 (1.13)	8.29 (1.34)	0.03
All HT[b]	15.44 (0.94)	17.59 (1.3)	16.63 (1.31)	23.22 (1.49)	0.001	18.11 (1.81)	18.31 (2.0)	17.18 (1.8)	23.11 (2.1)	0.07	13.3 (1.5 6)	16.77 (1.76)	16.00 (1.83)	23.32 (1.56)	<0.01
Unaware HT[b]	7.97 (0.77)	9.40 (1.15)	7.91 (1.03)	11.95 (1.38)	0.028	12.90 (1.82)	11.03 (2.07)	9.90 (1.44)	13.52 (1.87)	0.94	4.04 (1.04)	7.83 (1.04)	6.08 (1.24)	0.96 (2.01)	0.03
HT with treatment[b]	6.37 (0.70)	6.70 (0.87)	6.36 (0.80)	8.78 (0.77)	0.02	4.66 (1.0)	5.69 (1.10)	5.57 (1.19)	6.04 (0.95)	0.29	7.64 (1.0)	7.57 (1.20)	7.08 (1.04)	12.06 (1.30)	0.03
HT without treatment[b]	9.17 (0.72)	10.83 (1.11)	10.19 (1.00)	14.30 (1.51)	<0.001	13.49 (1.79)	12.53 (2.03)	11.60 (1.44)	17.05 (2.07)	0.25	5.75 (1.22)	9.21 (1.29)	8.87 (1.45)	10.98 (2.12)	0.04
SBP ≥ 140 mmHg[b]	10.68 (0.86)	12.37 (0.95)	9.52 (0.89)	15.12 (1.62)	0.06	13.4 (1.63)	13.65 (1.70)	9.11 (1.44)	16.08 (1.98)	0.60	8.49 (1.49)	11.10 (1.34)	9.79 (1.32)	13.94 (2.35)	0.05
DBP ≥ 90 mmHg[b]	7.73 (1.00)	7.99 (0.98)	8.42 (1.13)	9.24 (1.17)	0.36	11.92 (1.72)	9.08 (1.39)	8.14 (1.36)	11.86 (1.94)	0.88	4.46 (1.02)	7.09 (1.33)	8.69 (1.67)	6.07 (1.40)	0.15
Smoking[b]	20.00 (1.56)	20.83 (1.99)	16.86 (1.58)	23.37 (2.28)	0.62	43.05 (2.89)	39.89 (3.09)	33.41 (2.54)	41.70 (3.69)	0.43	1.45 (0.55)	1.67 (0.43)	1.73 (0.67)	1.33 (0.43)	0.92
Alcohol drinking[b]	6.75 (0.70)	12.09 (1.98)	6.88 (1.03)	7.64 (1.16)	0.79	14.21 (1.58)	21.05 (3.25)	13.58 (1.89)	13.62 (2.16)	0.35	0.57 (0.17)	2.42 (0.68)	0.60 (0.25)	0.28 (0.17)	0.10
E2, (pg/mL)[a]	56.51 (3.64)	48.02 (2.37)	57.32 (3.66)	53.41 (2.91)	0.92	39.66 (2.81)	35.08 (0.63)	35.08 (0.74)	37.52 (0.90)	0.38	71 (5.69)	65.73 (4.85)	78.52 (5.81)	70.67 (5.91)	0.60

[a]Mean (SE) and [b] percentage (SE).
BPA: bisphenol A, BMI: body mass index, SBP: systolic blood pressure, DBP: diastolic blood pressure, HT: hypertension, E2: estradiol, and Q: quartile.

TABLE 4: Adjusted odds ratios for high blood pressure associated with log (BPA) and E2 level with interaction term of log (BPA) and E2 level among women.

Variables	All HT	P value	Unaware HT	P value	SBP ≥ 140 mm Hg	P value
Age	1.07 (1.05, 1.08)	<0.001	1.04 (1.03, 1.05)	<0.001	1.07 (1.05, 1.08)	<0.001
BMI	1.10 (1.06, 1.14)	<0.001	1.08 (1.04, 1.13)	<0.001	1.10 (1.07, 1.14)	<0.001
Diabetes	2.22 (1.46, 3.39)	0.001	0.81 (0.46, 1.42)	0.43	1.75 (1.11, 2.77)	0.02
Smoking	1.38 (0.62, 3.08)	0.41	1.20 (0.43, 3.31)	0.71	0.71 (0.27, 1.84)	0.46
log (BPA)	1.09 (1.02, 1.16)	0.01	1.11 (1.00, 1.22)	0.06	1.04 (0.95, 1.13)	0.42
E2	0.99 (0.99, 1.00)	0.037	0.99 (0.99, 1.00)	0.05	0.99 (0.99, 1.00)	0.19
log (BPA) × E2	1.0 (1.0, 1.0)	0.20	1.0 (1.0, 1.00)	0.79	1.00 (0.99, 1.00)	0.68

BPA: bisphenol A, BMI: body mass index, HT: hypertension, SBP: systolic blood pressure, and E2: estradiol.

TABLE 5: Adjusted odds ratios for high blood pressure according to quartile of serum BPA.

		Odds ratios (95% CI)		
	Q1	Q2	Q3	Q4
All				
All HT	1	1.15 (0.92, 1.44)	1.08 (0.79, 1.47)	1.76 (1.33, 2.33)
Unaware HT	1	1.13 (0.78, 1.66)	0.97 (0.65, 1.45)	1.49 (1.05, 2.12)
SBP ≥ 140 mm Hg	1	1.14 (0.84, 1.54)	0.84 (0.59, 1.19)	1.52 (1.05, 2.21)
DBP ≥ 90 mm Hg	1	0.94 (0.64, 1.36)	1.09 (0.70, 1.70)	1.17 (0.74, 1.84)
HT with treatment	1	1.09 (0.69, 1.71)	0.95 (0.62, 1.47)	1.48 (1.07, 2.04)
HT without treatment	1	1.13 (0.84, 1.52)	1.11 (0.80, 1.53)	1.62 (1.16, 2.25)
Men				
All HT	1	0.93 (0.59, 1.45)	0.82 (0.51, 1.32)	1.44 (0.99, 2.09)
Unaware HT	1	0.79 (0.43, 1.46)	0.71 (0.43, 1.17)	1.09 (0.69, 1.71)
SBP ≥ 140 mm Hg	1	0.93 (0.53, 1.63)	0.57 (0.34, 0.94)	1.30 (0.83, 2.06)
DBP ≥ 90 mm Hg	1	0.65 (0.41, 1.04)	0.61 (0.34, 1.09)	1.04 (0.59, 1.84)
HT with treatment	1	1.28 (0.65, 2.52)	1.07 (0.47, 2.42)	1.26 (0.71, 2.21)
HT without treatment	1	0.84 (0.49, 1.47)	0.79 (0.49, 1.28)	1.39 (0.91, 2.12)
Women				
All HT	1	1.41 (0.92, 2.15)	1.35 (0.80, 2.28)	2.16 (1.31, 3.56)
Unaware HT	1	2.03 (1.05, 3.94)	1.61 (0.74, 3.49)	2.54 (1.11, 6.83)
SBP ≥ 140 mm Hg	1	1.41 (0.81, 2.46)	1.21 (0.71, 2.05)	1.81 (0.96, 3.42)
DBP ≥ 90 mm Hg	1	1.61 (1.13, 4.46)	2.24 (1.13, 4.46)	1.28 (0.60, 2.71)
HT with treatment	1	1.01 (0.58, 1.73)	0.86 (0.48, 1.52)	1.65 (1.05, 2.58)
HT without treatment	1	1.66 (0.93, 2.97)	1.71 (0.92, 3.16)	1.99 (0.94, 4.19)

Model adjusted for sex, age, BMI, diabetes, smoking, and alcohol drink.
BPA: bisphenol A, HT: hypertension, SBP: systolic blood pressure, DBP: diastolic blood pressure, and BMI: body mass index.

nutritional intakes such as salt intake as it is a risk factor for hypertension and it is possible that those who consumed a large amount of water or food contaminated with BPA also had high Na intake; however, the results were not likely to be confounded by common risk factors such as age, sex, alcohol intake, and diabetes status. The present study lacked data on medication used and was unable to look at the effect of antihypertension drugs and this issue needs further study. However, this study had strength as the sample was randomly selected as representative of general population.

In conclusion, the present study revealed that exposure to BPA was positively associated with hypertension and the results were not confounded by common risk factors. Effect of BPA on high blood pressure might be stronger in postmenopausal women; however, its mechanism related to estrogen on blood pressure needs further investigation.

Authors' Contribution

Wichai Aekplakorn designed the project, analyzed data, and prepared the paper. La-or Chailurkit performed laboratory analysis and data management. Boonsong Ongphiphadhanakul interpreted data and reviewed/edited the paper. All

TABLE 6: Adjusted odds ratio (AOR) for high blood pressure according to quartile of serum BPA among premenopausal and postmenopausal women.

		Odds ratios (95% CI)		
	BPA Q1	BPA Q2	BPA Q3	BPA Q4
Premenopause ($n = 512$)				
All HT	1	1.43 (0.69, 2.94)	1.55 (0.55, 4.34)	2.12 (0.87, 5.19)
Unaware HT	1	1.54 (0.54, 4.41)	1.96 (0.53, 7.31)	3.01 (0.81, 11.22)
SBP ≥ 140 mm Hg	1	1.72 (0.70, 4.20)	2.11 (0.68, 6.52)	2.75 (0.93, 8.10)
DBP ≥ 90 mm Hg	1	1.59 (0.57, 4.45)	2.94 (1.11, 7.8)	1.03 (0.32, 3.35)
HT with treatment	1	2.34 (0.73, 7.48)	0.15 (0.02, 1.35)	1.66 (0.59, 4.71)
HT without treatment	1	1.02 (0.40, 2.61)	2.25 (0.86, 5.91)	1.98 (0.59, 6.58)
Postmenopause ($n = 771$)				
All HT	1	1.56 (0.94, 2.57)	1.44 (0.88, 2.37)	2.33 (1.31, 4.15)
Unaware HT	1	2.94 (1.42, 6.07)	1.80 (0.91, 3.59)	2.47 (0.92, 6.58)
SBP ≥ 140 mm Hg	1	1.43 (0.78, 2.62)	1.10 (0.62, 1.95)	1.47 (0.73, 2.94)
DBP ≥ 90 mm Hg	1	2.05 (0.78, 5.38)	2.47 (0.87, 7.01)	1.92 (0.53, 6.99)
HT with treatment	1	0.77 (0.44, 1.36)	1.18 (0.64, 2.17)	1.74 (0.99, 3.07)
HT without treatment	1	3.02 (1.55, 5.90)	1.69 (0.90, 3.18)	2.26 (0.95, 5.42)

Postmenopause status was defined as self-reported of no menstruation or women aged ≥ 60 years.
BPA: bisphenol A, HT: hypertension, SBP: systolic blood pressure, and DBP: diastolic blood pressure.

TABLE 7: Adjusted odds ratio (AOR) for high blood pressure associated with log (BPA) in premenopausal and postmenopausal women.

	Premenopausal ($n = 512$)	Postmenopausal ($n = 771$)
All HT	1.06 (0.97, 1.17)	1.08 (1.01, 1.06)
Unaware HT	1.07 (0.92, 1.23)	1.15 (1.03, 1.28)
SBP ≥ 140 mm Hg	1.07 (0.95, 1.21)	1.04 (0.96, 1.13)
DBP ≥ 90 mm Hg	1.07 (0.96, 1.20)	1.10 (0.93, 1.29)
HT with treatment	1.00 (0.88, 1.15)	1.02 (0.94, 1.11)
HT without treatment	1.07 (0.96, 1.20)	1.13 (1.03, 1.25)

Model adjusted for age, BMI, diabetes, smoking, and E2.
BPA: bisphenol A, HT: hypertension, and E2: estradiol.

the authors participated in approving the final draft of the paper.

Acknowledgments

The 4th Thai National Health Examination Survey (NHESIV) was conducted by the National Health Examination Survey Office, Health Systems Research Institute, Thailand. The NHESIV study group includes National Health Examination Survey Office: Wichai Aekplakorn, Rungkarn Inthawong, Jiraluck Nonthaluck, Supornsak Tipsukum, and Yawarat Porrapakkham; Northern region: Suwat Chariyalertsak, Kanittha Thaikla (Chiang Mai University), Wongsa Laohasiriwong, Wanlop Jaidee, Sutthinan Srathonghon, Ratana Phanphanit, Jiraporn Suwanteerangkul, and Kriangkai Srithanaviboonchai; Northeastern region: Pattapong Kessomboon, Somdej Pinitsoontorn, Piyathida Kuhirunyaratn, Sauwanan Bumrerraj, Amornrat Rattanasiri, Suchad Paileeklee, Bangornsri Jindawong, Napaporn Krusun, and Weerapong Seeupalat (Khon Kaen University); Southern region: Virasakdi Chongsuvivatwong, Rassamee Sangthong, and Mafausis Dueravee (Prince of Songkla University); Central region: Surasak Taneepanichskul, Somrat Lertmaharit, Vilai Chinveschakitvanich, Onuma Zongram, Nuchanad Hounnaklang, and Sukarin Wimuktayon (Chulalongkorn University); Bangkok region: Panwadee Putwatana, Chalermsri Nuntawan, and Karn Chaladthanyagid (Mahidol University). The Thai National Health Examination Survey IV was supported by the Health Systems Research Institute; Bureau of Policy and Strategy, Ministry of Public Health; Thai Health Promotion Foundation; and the National Health Security Office, Thailand. The authors thank Professor Dr. Amnuay Thithapandha for his help in editing the paper.

References

[1] A. M. Calafat, X. Ye, L.-Y. Wong, J. A. Reidy, and L. L. Needham, "Exposure of the U.S. population to Bisphenol A and 4-*tertiary*-octylphenol: 2003-2004," *Environmental Health Perspectives*, vol. 116, no. 1, pp. 39–44, 2008.

[2] Z. Zhang, H. Alomirah, H.-S. Cho et al., "Urinary bisphenol a concentrations and their implications for human exposure in several Asian countries," *Environmental Science and Technology*, vol. 45, no. 16, pp. 7044–7050, 2011.

[3] W. Aekplakorn, L. O. Chailurkit, and B. Ongphiphadhanakul, "Relationship of serum bisphenol A with diabetes in the Thai population, National Health Examination Survey IV, 2009," *Journal of Diabetes*, vol. 7, no. 2, pp. 240–249, 2014.

[4] F. S. vom Saal, B. T. Akingbemi, S. M. Belcher et al., "Chapel Hill bisphenol A expert panel consensus statement: integration of mechanisms, effects in animals and potential to impact human health at current levels of exposure," *Reproductive Toxicology*, vol. 24, no. 2, pp. 131–138, 2007.

[5] H. Hiroi, O. Tsutsumi, M. Momoeda, Y. Takai, Y. Osuga, and Y. Taketani, "Differential interactions of bisphenol A and 17beta-estradiol with estrogen receptor α (ERalpha) and ERbeta," *Endocrine Journal*, vol. 46, no. 6, pp. 773–778, 1999.

[6] C. Sriphrapradang, L.-O. Chailurkit, W. Aekplakorn, and B. Ongphiphadhanakul, "Association between bisphenol A and abnormal free thyroxine level in men," *Endocrine*, vol. 44, no. 2, pp. 441–447, 2013.

[7] R. Ahmadkhaniha, M. Mansouri, M. Yunesian et al., "Association of urinary bisphenol a concentration with type-2 diabetes mellitus," *Journal of Environmental Health Science and Engineering*, vol. 12, no. 1, p. 64, 2014.

[8] K. Kim and H. Park, "Association between urinary concentrations of bisphenol A and type 2 diabetes in Korean adults: a population-based cross-sectional study," *International Journal of Hygiene and Environmental Health*, vol. 216, no. 4, pp. 467–471, 2013.

[9] A. Shankar and S. Teppala, "Relationship between urinary bisphenol A levels and diabetes mellitus," *Journal of Clinical Endocrinology and Metabolism*, vol. 96, no. 12, pp. 3822–3826, 2011.

[10] G. Ning, Y. Bi, T. Wang et al., "Relationship of urinary bisphenol A concentration to risk for prevalent type 2 diabetes in Chinese adults: a cross-sectional analysis," *Annals of Internal Medicine*, vol. 155, no. 6, pp. 368–374, 2011.

[11] C. Sabanayagam, S. Teppala, and A. Shankar, "Relationship between urinary bisphenol A levels and prediabetes among subjects free of diabetes," *Acta Diabetologica*, vol. 50, no. 4, pp. 625–631, 2013.

[12] R. R. Newbold, E. Padilla-Banks, and W. N. Jefferson, "Environmental estrogens and obesity," *Molecular and Cellular Endocrinology*, vol. 304, no. 1-2, pp. 84–89, 2009.

[13] D. Melzer, N. J. Osborne, W. E. Henley et al., "Urinary bisphenol A concentration and risk of future coronary artery disease in apparently healthy men and women," *Circulation*, vol. 125, no. 12, pp. 1482–1490, 2012.

[14] D. Melzer, N. E. Rice, C. Lewis, W. E. Henley, and T. S. Galloway, "Association of urinary bisphenol A concentration with heart disease: evidence from NHANES 2003/06," *PLoS ONE*, vol. 5, no. 1, Article ID e8673, 2010.

[15] I. A. Lang, T. S. Galloway, A. Scarlett et al., "Association of urinary bisphenol A concentration with medical disorders and laboratory abnormalities in adults," *The Journal of the American Medical Association*, vol. 300, no. 11, pp. 1303–1310, 2008.

[16] S. Bae, J. H. Kim, Y.-H. Lim, H. Y. Park, and Y.-C. Hong, "Associations of bisphenol A exposure with heart rate variability and blood pressure," *Hypertension*, vol. 60, no. 3, pp. 786–793, 2012.

[17] A. Shankar and S. Teppala, "Urinary bisphenol A and hypertension in a multiethnic sample of US adults," *Journal of Environmental and Public Health*, vol. 2012, Article ID 481641, 5 pages, 2012.

[18] The Global Burden of Metabolic Risk Factors for Chronic Diseases Collaboration, "Cardiovascular disease, chronic kidney disease, and diabetes mortality burden of cardiometabolic risk factors from 1980 to 2010: a comparative risk assessment," *The Lancet Diabetes & Endocrinology*, vol. 2, no. 8, pp. 634–647, 2014.

[19] G. Mancia, R. Fagard, K. Narkiewicz et al., "2013 ESH/ESC Guidelines for the management of arterial hypertension: the Task Force for the management of arterial hypertension of the European Society of Hypertension (ESH) and of the European Society of Cardiology (ESC)," *Journal of Hypertension*, vol. 31, no. 7, pp. 1281–1357, 2013.

[20] M. E. Mendelsohn and R. H. Karas, "Molecular and cellular basis of cardiovascular gender differences," *Science*, vol. 308, no. 5728, pp. 1583–1587, 2005.

[21] E. Murphy, "Estrogen signaling and cardiovascular disease," *Circulation Research*, vol. 109, no. 6, pp. 687–696, 2011.

[22] W. Aekplakorn, R. Sangthong, P. Kessomboon et al., "Changes in prevalence, awareness, treatment and control of hypertension in Thai population, 2004–2009: Thai National Health Examination Survey III-IV," *Journal of Hypertension*, vol. 30, no. 9, pp. 1734–1742, 2012.

[23] T. G. Pickering, J. E. Hall, L. J. Appel et al., "Recommendations for blood pressure measurement in humans: an AHA scientific statement from the Council on High Blood Pressure Research Professional and Public Education Subcommittee," *Journal of Clinical Hypertension (Greenwich)*, vol. 7, no. 2, pp. 102–109, 2005.

[24] Centers for Disease Control and Prevention (CDC), "Cigarette smoking among adults—United States, 1992, and changes in the definition of current cigarette smoking," *MMWR. Morbidity and Mortality Weekly Report*, vol. 43, pp. 342–346, 1992.

[25] B. S. Rubin and A. M. Soto, "Bisphenol A: perinatal exposure and body weight," *Molecular and Cellular Endocrinology*, vol. 304, no. 1-2, pp. 55–62, 2009.

[26] X.-J. Du, R. A. Riemersma, and A. M. Dart, "Cardiovascular protection by oestrogen is partly mediated through modulation of autonomic nervous function," *Cardiovascular Research*, vol. 30, no. 2, pp. 161–165, 1995.

[27] T. Pelzer, V. Jazbutyte, K. Hu et al., "The estrogen receptor-α agonist 16α-LE2 inhibits cardiac hypertrophy and improves hemodynamic function in estrogen-deficient spontaneously hypertensive rats," *Cardiovascular Research*, vol. 67, no. 4, pp. 604–612, 2005.

[28] I. Nikolic, D. Liu, J. A. Bell, J. Collins, C. Steenbergen, and E. Murphy, "Treatment with an estrogen receptor-beta-selective agonist is cardioprotective," *Journal of Molecular and Cellular Cardiology*, vol. 42, no. 4, pp. 769–780, 2007.

[29] D. H. P. Streeten, G. H. Anderson Jr., T. Howland, R. Chiang, and H. Smulyan, "Effects of thyroid function on blood pressure. Recognition of hypothyroid hypertension," *Hypertension*, vol. 11, no. 1, pp. 78–83, 1988.

[30] H. Ooe, T. Taira, S. M. M. Iguchi-Ariga, and H. Ariga, "Induction of reactive oxygen species by bisphenol A and abrogation of bisphenol A-induced cell injury by DJ-1," *Toxicological Sciences*, vol. 88, no. 1, pp. 114–126, 2005.

[31] J. R. Sowers, "Insulin resistance and hypertension," *The American Journal of Physiology—Heart and Circulatory Physiology*, vol. 286, no. 5, pp. H1597–H1602, 2004.

[32] J. G. Teeguarden, A. M. Calafat, X. Ye et al., "Twenty-four hour human urine and serum profiles of bisphenol A during high-dietary exposure," *Toxicological Sciences*, vol. 123, no. 1, pp. 48–57, 2011.

[33] J. Teeguarden, S. Hanson-Drury, J. W. Fisher, and D. R. Doerge, "Are typical human serum BPA concentrations measurable and sufficient to be estrogenic in the general population?" *Food and Chemical Toxicology*, vol. 62, pp. 949–963, 2013.

15

Predictors of Noncompliance to Antihypertensive Therapy among Hypertensive Patients Ghana: Application of Health Belief Model

Yaa Obirikorang,[1] Christian Obirikorang ⓘ,[2] Emmanuel Acheampong ⓘ,[2,3]
Enoch Odame Anto ⓘ,[2,3] Daniel Gyamfi,[4] Selorm Philip Segbefia,[2]
Michael Opoku Boateng,[1,5] Dari Pascal Dapilla,[1,5] Peter Kojo Brenya,[2]
Bright Amankwaa ⓘ,[2] Evans Asamoah Adu,[4] Emmanuel Nsenbah Batu,[2]
Adjei Gyimah Akwasi,[6] and Beatrice Amoah[2]

[1]Department of Nursing, Faculty of Health and Allied Sciences, Garden City University College (GCUC), Kenyasi, Kumasi, Ghana
[2]Department of Molecular Medicine, School of Medical Science, Kwame Nkrumah University of Science and Technology (KNUST), Kumasi, Ghana
[3]School of Medical and Health Science, Edith Cowan University, Joondalup, Australia
[4]Department of Medical Laboratory Technology, Faculty of Allied Health Sciences, KNUST, Ghana
[5]Department of Nursing, Kintampo Municipal Hospital, Kintampo, Ghana
[6]Department of Community Health, School of Medical Sciences, KNUST, Ghana

Correspondence should be addressed to Emmanuel Acheampong; emmanuelacheal990@yahoo.com

Academic Editor: Tomohiro Katsuya

This study determined noncompliance to antihypertensive therapy (AHT) and its associated factors in a Ghanaian population by using the health belief model (HBM). This descriptive cross-sectional study conducted at Kintampo Municipality in Ghana recruited a total of 678 hypertensive patients. The questionnaire constituted information regarding sociodemographics, a five-Likert type HBM questionnaire, and lifestyle-related factors. The rate of noncompliance to AHT in this study was 58.6%. The mean age (SD) of the participants was 43.5 (±5.2) years and median duration of hypertension was 2 years. Overall, the five HBM constructs explained 31.7% of the variance in noncompliance to AHT with a prediction accuracy of 77.5%, after adjusting for age, gender, and duration of condition. Higher levels of perceived benefits of using medicine [aOR=0.55(0.36-0.82),p=0.0001] and cue to actions [aOR=0.59(0.38-0.90),p=0.0008] were significantly associated with reduced noncompliance while perceived susceptibility [aOR=3.05(2.20-6.25), p<0.0001], perceived barrier [aOR=2.14(1.56-2.92), p<0.0001], and perceived severity [aOR=4.20(2.93-6.00),p<0.0001] were significantly associated with increased noncompliance to AHT. Participant who had completed tertiary education [aOR=0.27(0.17-0.43), p<0.0001] and had regular source of income [aOR=0.52(0.38-0.71), p<0.0001] were less likely to be noncompliant. However, being a government employee [aOR=4.16(1.93-8.96), p=0.0002)] was significantly associated increased noncompliance to AHT. Noncompliance to AHT was considerably high and HBM is generally reliable in assessing treatment noncompliance in the Ghanaian hypertensive patients. The significant predictors of noncompliance to AHT were higher level of perceived barriers, susceptibility, and severity. Intervention programmes could be guided by the association of risk factors, HBM constructs with noncompliance to AHT in clinical practice.

1. Background

Hypertension (HTN) is a major risk factor for cardiovascular diseases such as heart failure, myocardial infarction, and stroke [1–4]. Cardiovascular diseases are the major cause of mortality among adults globally [1] of which about 50% can be ascribed to complications of HTN [5]. Developing countries account for almost 80% of these deaths [5]. Among the list of noncommunicable diseases plaguing the general Ghanaian population, HTN is said to be the most prevalent [6, 7]. Efforts geared towards improving lifestyles, controlling lifestyle-related major cardiovascular risk factors, absolutely will contribute to the prevention of cardiovascular diseases [1, 5]. The Ghana Health Service (GHS) also estimated that the prevalence rate of HTN in Ghana among adults of 18 years and above was 29.9 per cent for males and 27.6 per cent for females (GHS, 2014). It has been reported that blood pressure (BP) control among hypertensives in Ghana is largely poor due to noncompliance to therapy [8]. Noncompliance to antihypertensive therapy (AHT) involves the interplay of the healthcare-provider/health system, therapy, condition, client, and socioeconomic factors [3, 8, 9].

The annual health report of the Kintampo Municipality continues to show HTN ranking among the top 10 diseases over the past 5 years (Municipal Health Year Report, 2015). Moreover, it was the fourth leading cause of death in the municipality. Failure to maintain a well-controlled blood pressure (BP) has been mainly attributed to noncompliance to AHT [2, 3]. To the best of our knowledge, no published study has been conducted to determine noncompliance among hypertensives in the municipality. The health belief model (HBM) is one of the most classical theories devised by social psychologists to describe social behaviour as well as public participation in medical programs [10]. The model was further extended to the study of range of health behaviours which included dietary behaviour, smoking, contraceptives, physical activities alcohol use and drinking, and obstetrics outcome [11–13]. The model contains several cognitive constructs that predict why people take actions to control their illness including perceived susceptibility, perceived severity, perceived benefits, perceived barriers, and cues to actions. HBM has strength to allow patient diagnosed with HTN to consider the benefits to be gained from compliance (behaviour), is worth the cost, and also assess his or her severity and vulnerability to HTN complications before making the decision [14]. There is limited research evidence on the implications of health behaviour from low income countries such as Ghana, although the applications of this model have been widely used in developed countries. Several studies have investigated the prevalence of antihypertensive compliance and its determinants in Ghana [15–18]; no study has focused on the applicability of HBM. It was against this background that the study sought to evaluate noncompliance to AHT among Ghanaian hypertensive patients using HBM.

2. Material and Methods

2.1. Study Design and Setting.
This study was a cross-sectional descriptive study among hypertensives attending the Hypertension Clinic at the Kintampo Municipal Hospital. The Kintampo Municipal Hospital is the major source of health care for the inhabitants of the Kintampo Municipality. The Hypertension Clinic was established in April 2015 under the auspices of the Kintampo Municipal Health Directorate and operates only on Wednesdays. The clinic is being run by a medical doctor, a physician assistant, a general nurse, an enrolled nurse, and two health extension workers.

2.2. Study Population and Subject Selection.
The targeted population was hypertensive patients who were on antihypertensive therapy and attending the Hypertension Clinic. Simple random sampling technique was used to recruit six hundred and seventy-eight (678) hypertensive patients who consented for the study at the Hypertension Clinic at the Kintampo Municipal Hospital. Each hypertensive patient was given a number and then a table of random numbers to decide which patient to include. Depending on the total number of patients per each clinic, a range of 20 to 24 patients were randomly sampled weekly until sample size was achieved. Hypertensive patients who had been diagnosed or were on medication for hypertension for one year or more were included in the study as well as hypertensive patients aged 30 years and above. Moreover, hypertensives with or without other existing comorbidities such as diabetes, cardiovascular diseases, and renal diseases were also included in the study. Hypertensive patients who did not consent and were seriously ill (too sick to be interviewed) were excluded from the study

2.3. Data Collection Tool.
For validity and reliability of the study, a pilot study was conducted using the research instrument. This was aimed at testing the strength of the research instrument to elicit the needed responses for the study. The pilot study was carefully evaluated by the researchers and an expert in the field of research. Necessary amendments were made and the resulting questionnaire was used for the main data collection process. Reliability coefficients ranging from 0.00 to 1.00, with higher coefficients indicating higher levels of reliability, were used to determine the validity and the reliability of the questionnaire. The reliability coefficients for all the questions were 0.903.

The questionnaire developed for this study was adopted from studies conducted by Joho [19]. It was made up of three sections. Section A collects the sociodemographic characteristics data of the participants. Section B was designed to collect information on treatment compliance, which comprised both medication regimen compliance and lifestyle modification. Medication regimen compliance was composed of 8 items, asking how often they forgot to take their medicine, did they stop taking their medicine because they felt better, because they felt worse, because they believed that medicine was ineffective, because they feared side effects, because they tried to avoid addiction, because of religious beliefs or they were using traditional medicine, and because of cost of medication. The responses were measured on a 4-point Likert scale (every day, frequently, rarely, or never). Lifestyle compliance composed of 5 items which included how often they did smoke, consumed alcohol, engaged in physical exercise, ate table salt, and ate meat with high animal fats. Participants were asked to respond to the single question based on a 4-point Likert scale: how often do desirable or undesirable behaviours related to control of hypertension. The responses were every day, frequently, rarely, or never. The responses were (1) every day, (2) frequently, (3) rarely, or (4) never. Some questions were set such that the highest score did not reflect the worst scenario of noncompliance. To resolve this, scores were reversed. For instance, how often do you engage in physical exercise: (4) every day, (3) frequently, (2) rarely, or (1) never. Section C constituted the HBM variables which include perceived severity of hypertension measured by six items which included whether BP was a serious problem, worried about their HTN condition, getting HTN was serious, getting HTN complications was very dangerous, and dying due HTN complication was dangerous; perceived susceptibility of being at risk of hypertension complications measured by six items, thus having stroke, developing visual impairment, heart problems, kidney problems, becoming burden for family, and career being negatively affected; perceived benefit treatments were each measured by six items which were keeping their BP under control, increasing their quality of life, increasing their sense of well-being, protecting them from complications, avoiding added financial burden to treat complications, and decreasing my chance of dying; and cues to action were measured by seven items. Participants were then asked to respond strongly agree (4), agree (3), disagree, (2) or strongly disagree (1). The remainder which is perception of barriers was also measured by five items, ineffective of the medicine to stabilize their BP, lack of motivation because they cannot be cured, not having enough time to exercise, lack of discipline to comply with dietary restriction, and lack of motivation to stop smoking. The responses were 'not at all' (1), 'to some extent' (2), 'to a larger extent' (3), or 'very much extent' (4). The 13 items measuring treatment compliance and life style compliance were added up to get sum index with a distribution ranging from 23 to 52 with mean 44.30 (SD =5.55), and the median split was used (46.0), which was dichotomized into two groups, i.e., 1 = those who are nontreatment compliant and 0 = treatment compliant which was 23-45 and 46-52. The variables comprising the number of items measuring compliance in the HBM were added up to get sum index with a distribution range, and the median split was used as a cut point. Dichotomization was done into two frequency groups, those who had low perceived severity, susceptibility, benefits, and vice versa. The entire questionnaire was available in English version but interviewed carefully with the proper translation of the official local language of the study population. The responses of the participants were translated back to English in the correct meaning as was interpreted.

2.4. Ethical Consideration. Approval for this study was obtained from Human Research, Publication and Ethics of the School of Medical Sciences (SMS), Kwame Nkrumah University of Science and Technology (KNUST) (CHRPE/AP/213/16). Participation was voluntary and written informed consent was obtained from each participant. Hypertensive clients were also given a short exposition on the essence of the study and their role to play to make it a success. The clients who were prospective subjects for the study were made to understand that the research was solely for academic purposes, and that no information would be handled with anything short of full privacy and confidentiality.

2.5. Statistical Analysis. Data was entered into excel worksheet and analysed using the statistical package for social sciences version (SPSS) 23.0. Continuous variables were

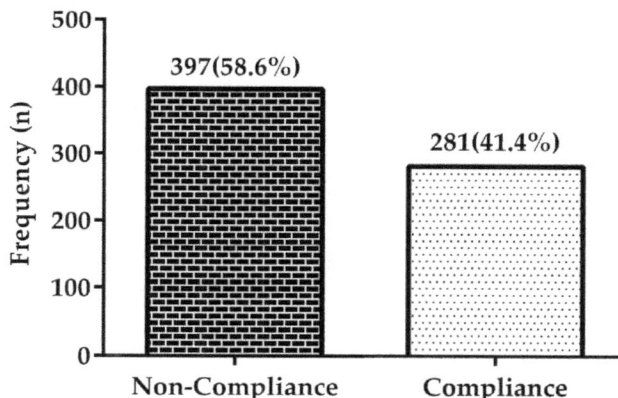

FIGURE 1: Frequency distribution of noncompliance and compliance among participants.

expressed as mean ± SD for normal distributed data and median (interquartile range) for not normally distributed data, respectively. Frequency distributions were done as sociodemographic data and then bivariate analysis using chisquire for association of sociodemographic characteristics and HBM with treatment noncompliance; and Pearson correlation between HBM variables was done. Logistic regressions were done with treatment noncompliance as the outcome variable and the rest of HBM variables as predictors. Statistical significance was assumed at $p < 0.05$.

3. Results

The mean age (SD) of the participants was 43.5(±5.2) years and median duration of the disease was 2 years. Majority of them were males (50.7%). Considerable proportions of the participants had no education (34.2%), were married (66.7%), and were private employees (50.8%). Most of the participants have had the condition for less than 5 years (72.0%). Moreover, more than half of the participants (60.8%) did not have regular income [**Table 1**].

Three hundred and ninety-seven (58.6%) participants were not compliant to AHT, while 41.4% complied [**Figure 1**].

Participants with high cues to actions and perceived benefits had reduced odds for noncompliance [aOR=0.59(0.38-0.90), p=0.0008); OR=0.55(0.36-0.82), p=0.0001)]. Moreover, participants with high perceptions of severity had significantly increased odds for noncompliance [aOR=4.20(2.93-6.00), p<0.0001)]. Participant with high perception of susceptibility [aOR=3.05, (2.20-4.25), p<0.0001)] and high perceived barriers [aOR=2.14(1.56-2.92), p<0.0001)] were more likely to be noncompliant to AHT [**Table 2**].

As shown in **Table 3**, treatment noncompliance showed significant and positive association with perceived severity (r=0.19, p<0.0001) and susceptibility (r=0.33, p<0.001). Furthermore, treatment noncompliance was significantly negatively associated benefits (r= -0.449, p<0.0001).

Participant who had completed tertiary education had significantly reduced odds for noncompliance to AHT [aOR=0.27(0.17-0.43), p<0.0001)]. However, being a

TABLE 1: Sociodemographic characteristics of study participants.

Variables	Frequency (n=678)	Percentages (%)
Age (years) (Mean ± SD)	43.5±6.2	
Age Groups		
31-40	301	44.4%
41-50	264	38.9%
51-60	113	16.7%
Gender		
Male	344	50.7%
Female	334	49.3%
Marital Status		
Single	90	13.3%
Married	452	66.7%
Divorced	51	7.5%
Separate	38	5.6%
Widowed	30	4.4%
Cohabiting	17	2.5%
Education Level		
Uneducated	232	34.2%
Basic	203	30.0%
SHS	115	16.9%
Tertiary	128	18.9%
Occupational Status		
Government employee	230	33.9%
Private employee	344	50.7%
Self-employed	65	9.6%
Student	5	0.7%
Unemployed	34	5.0%
Duration of Condition(years)		
<5	488	72.0%
5-10	179	26.4%
>10	12	1.6%
Regular Source Income		
No	412	60.8%
Yes	266	39.2%
Duration of Condition (years) (Median, IQR)	2.0(1.0-5.0)	
Duration of Treatment (years) (Median, IQR)	2.0(1.0-5.0)	

SD: standard deviation, IQR: interquartile range, JHS: junior high school, and SHS: senior high school.

government employee [aOR=4.16(1.93-8.96), p=0.0002)] was significantly associated with increased likelihood of being noncompliant to AHT. Participants who had regular source of income had lower odds for noncompliance to AHT [aOR=0.52(0.38-0.71), p<0.0001)]. Being male [aOR= 1.33(0.98-1.81), p=0.074)], being divorced [aOR=2.00(0.98-4.09, p=0.077)], and duration of HTN 5-10 years [OR=1.37(0.96-1.95), p=0.092) had significant association with noncompliance to AHT [**Table 4**].

Lifestyle-related factors such as number of medicine taken (p=0.002), history of smoking (p<0.0001), and history of alcohol consumption (p<0.0001) had statistically significant association with noncompliance to AHT. Moreover, considerable proportions of the participants who had health compliant other than HTN (73.0%) and those on two different drugs (56.9%) were noncompliant to AHT [**Table 5**].

Multiple logistic regression analysis showed significant model fit for the data (F=24.7, p< 0.0001). The amount of variance in noncompliance to AHT which is explained by the predictors is 31.7 % (R^2=0.317) with perceived barrier being the strongest predictor of noncompliance to AHT ($\beta = 0.780$, p< 0.0001). Positive beta coefficient indicates a positive

TABLE 2: Association of constructs of HBM with participant's treatment compliance.

Variables	Non-compliance	Compliance	p-value	aOR (95%CI)
Cues to Action			**0.0008**	
Low	226(56.9%)	123(43.8%)		1
High	171(43.1%)	158(56.2%)		0.59(0.38-0.90)
Perception of benefits			**0.0001**	
Low	233(58.7%)	123(43.8%)		1
High	164(41.3%)	158(56.2%)		0.55(0.36-0.82)
Perception of severity			**<0.0001**	
Low	201(50.6%)	228(81.1%)		1
High	196(49.4%)	53(18.9%)		4.20(2.93-6.00)
Perception of susceptibility			**<0.0001**	
Low	188(47.4%)	206(73.3%)		1
High	209(52.6%)	75(26.7%)		3.05(2.20-4.25)
Perception to barriers			**<0.0001**	
Low	179(45.1 %)	179(63.7%)		1
High	218(54.9%)	102(36.3%)		2.14(1.56-2.92)

aOR: adjusted odds ratio; CI: confidence interval; p<0.05 is statistically significant; and 1∗ reference category.

TABLE 3: Partial correlation between HBM constructs controlling for age, gender, and duration of disease.

Variables		1	2	3	4	5	6
1.Treatmen non-compliance	r	-	0.19	0.33	-0.21	-0.449	-0.012
	p-value		**<0.0001**	**<0.0001**	**<0.0001**	**<0.0001**	0.820
2.Perceived Severity	r		-	0.539	-0.013	-0.294	0.087
	p-value			**<0.0001**	0.808	**<0.0001**	0.099
3.Perceived Susceptibility	r			-	0.067	-0.538	0.339
	p-value				0.206	**<0.0001**	**<0.0001**
4.Perceived Benefits	r				-	0.018	0.464
	p-value					0.735	**<0.0001**
5.Perceived Barriers	r					-	0.111
	p-value						**0.036**
6.Cues to Action	r						-
	p-value						

r: correlation coefficient; p<0.05 is statistically significant.

association between perceived barriers and noncompliance to AHT [**Table 6**].

4. Discussion

This study determined noncompliance to AHT and its associated factors among hypertensive patients in the Kintampo Municipality using HBM questionnaire. The rate of noncompliance to AHT was 58.6% which indicates that more than half of the participants were not complaint to their medication. This observed prevalence rate is lower compared to other cross-sectional studies done in the Ghanaian setting by Kretchy et al. [15] and Buabeng et al. [16] but higher compared to a study by Jambedu among Ghanaian hypertensive patients [17]. The possible explanations for these disparities in findings could be due to the differences in sample size and the type of questionnaire used, as previous studies did not employ the HBM. Conversely, the observed noncompliance rate in

this current study is comparable to range of reports from previous cross-sectional studies done elsewhere in Africa [8, 20–22]. These results highlight the fact that noncompliance to AHT is very common in the Ghanaian setting. The high noncompliance rate reported in this study is also consistent with some cross-sectional studies in Pakistan [23, 24], China [25, 26], and Iran [27].

Several retrospective and prospective studies have provided extensive support for the HBM in evaluating a range of health-related behaviours, although some other studies do not fully support this theory [11, 28, 29]. The HBM performed fairly well in predicting noncompliance to AHT among Ghanaian hypertensive patients in this study. The amount of variance in treatment noncompliance which is explained by the five constructs was 31.7 % with an overall prediction accuracy of 77.5% after adjusting age, gender, and duration of condition. This indicates that HBM is generally reliable in predicting noncompliance to AHT and framing intervention

TABLE 4: Sociodemographics of study participants and relation to compliance.

Variables	Non-compliance	Compliance	X^2, df	P-value	aOR (95% CI)	p-value
Age Groups (years)			1.3,2	0.519		
31-40	167(42.1%)	134(47.7%)			1	
41-50	164(41.3%)	100(35.6%)			1.32(0.94-1.84)	0.124
51-60	66(16.6%)	47(16.7%)			1.13(0.73-1.75)	0.657
Gender						
Male	214(53.9%)	130(46.2%)			1.33(0.98-1.81)	0.074
Female	187(46.1%)	151(53.8%)			1	
Marital Status			3.6, 6	0.724		
Single	45(11.3%)	45(16.0%)			1	
Married	264(66.5%)	189(67.3%)			1.40(0.88-2.20)	0.163
Divorced	34(8.6%)	17(6.0%)			2.00(0.98-4.09)	0.077
Separate	23(5.8%)	15(5.4%)			1.53(0.71-3.31)	0.334
Widowed	20(5.0%)	9(3.2%)			2.22(0.91-5.41)	0.089
Cohabiting	11(2.8%)	6(2.1%)			1.83(0.62-5.39)	0.301
Educational Level			20.8, 4	**<0.0001**		
Unschooled	154(38.9%)	77(27.4%)			1	
Basic	132(33.2%)	72(25.6%)			0.92(0.61-1.36)	0.686
SHS	66(16.6%)	49(17.4%)			0.67(0.42-1.07)	0.098
Tertiary	45(11.3%)	83(29.6%)			0.27(0.17-0.43)	**<0.0001**
Occupational Status			13.1, 4	**0.011**		
Government employee	153(38.5%)	77(27.4%)			4.16(1.93-8.96)	**0.0002**
Private employee	201(50.6%)	143(50.9%)			2.94(1.39-6.22)	**0.006**
Self-employed	32(8.1%)	32(11.4%)			2.09(0.88-4.99)	0.134
Student	0(0.0%)	6(2.0%)			-	-
Unemployed	11(2.8%)	23(8.2%)			1	
Duration of Condition(years)			1.8,2	0.411		
<5	277(69.8%)	211(75.1%)			1	
5 -10	115(29.0%)	64(22.8%)			1.37(0.96-1.95)	0.092
>10	5(1.2%)	6(2.1%)			0.63(0.19-2.11)	0.544
Regular Source Income			10.0,1	**0.007**		
No	267(67.2%)	145(51.6%)			1	
Yes	130(32.8%)	136(48.4%)			0.52(0.38-0.71)	**<0.0001**

X^2: *Chi-square, df: degree of freedom, aOR: adjusted odds ratio, CI: confidence interval, JHS: junior high school, and SHS: senior high school; p<0.05 is statistically significant;*1 reference category.*

measures to reduce noncompliance to AHT among Ghanaian hypertensive patients.

Perceived barrier was observed to be the strongest predictor of treatment noncompliance which is consistent with finding observed by Day et al. [30]. It was also observed that higher levels of perceived barriers were associated with increased odds of noncompliance to AHT. This result corresponds closely to finding from previous study conducted by Haynes et al., who reported that perceived barrier was the strongest predictor of noncompliance to AHT [31]. Higher perceived benefit of using medicine and cue to actions significantly correlated with reduced odds of noncompliance to AHT. These findings concur with current literature on hypertensive medication adherence among Chinese [25, 32]. Thus, intervention measures suitable for Ghanaian hypertensive patients should mainly focus on reducing perceived

susceptibility, perceived severity, and perceived barriers but increase cues to action and perceived benefits.

In this study, the average age of all included hypertensive patients was 43.5 years indicating high prevalence of hypertension in younger adults compared to the elderly. This is inconsistent with studies by Almas et al. [33] and Okwuonu et al. [20], where mean age within the fifties were reported, depicting higher prevalence of hypertension among the elderly. However, current literature indicates that the prevalence rate of hypertension in the Ghanaians population is higher in the 40-55 years age groups [16, 34, 35]. Our current study confirms this change of trend, where now the prevalence is higher in those in their forties and fifties. The high prevalence in the young adults in our population could be due to change in lifestyle and adaptation of Westernized diets, full of salts and fats that could predispose them

TABLE 5: Association of lifestyle-related factors with treatment noncompliance.

Variables	Non-compliance	Compliance	P-value
Health complaint other than HTN			0.069
Yes	290(73.0%)	223(79.3%)	
No	107(27.0%)	58(20.7%)	
Number of Medicine taken			**0.002**
1	38(9.6%)	8(2.9%)	
2	226(56.9%)	177(63.0%)	
3	115(29.0%)	90(32.0%)	
≥4	18(4.5%)	6(2.1%)	
History of smoking			**<0.0001**
No	344(86.6%)	279(99.3%)	
Yes	53(13.4%)	2(0.7%)	
History of alcohol consumption			**<0.0001**
No	269(67.8%)	257(91.4%)	
Yes	128(32.2%)	24(8.6%)	

P<0.05 is statistically significant.

TABLE 6: Cross-sectional association and predictability of HBM variables for noncompliance.

Health belief model variables	Beta	SE	aOR (95%)	P-value
Perceived Severity	-0.007	0.078	0.99(0.25-1.78)	0.933
Perceived susceptibility	0.142	0.067	1.15(0.75-2.72	**0.034**
Perceived benefits	-0.414	0.099	0.66(0.09-1.62)	**<0.0001**
Perceived barriers	0.780	0.115	2.18(1.09-4.12)	**<0.0001**
Cues to actions	-0.006	0.062	0.98(0.22-1.64)	0.925

R^2=0.317, F=24.7(p<0.0001), SE: standard error, p<0.05 is statistically significant, and aOR: adjusted odd ratio.

to hypertension. Moreover, logistic regression models in this study showed that participants within 41-50 years had increased odds for noncompliance to AHT. The majority of the previous studies had shown that age is related to compliance, although a few researchers found age not to be a factor causing noncompliance [36–38]. Patients in this age ranges (middle-aged patients) always have other priorities in their daily life; due to their work and other commitments, they may not be able to attend for treatment or spend a long time waiting for clinic appointments

Participants who have had tertiary education had significant reduced odds for noncompliance to AHT in this study. This is consistent with studies by Okuno et al. [39], Ghods and Nasrollahzadeh [40], and Yaruz et al. [41] who found that patients with higher educational level have higher compliance to their medication. Intuitively, it may be expected that patients with higher educational level should have better knowledge about the disease and therapy and therefore be more compliant. Sufficient knowledge about hypertension in patients has been associated with greater medication adherence and better BP control in previous studies [33, 42]. Other studies have also reported contrasting results where high level of education was associated with low compliance [43, 44]

Findings from this study showed that government and private employees had significant increased odds for noncompliance to AHT. It is assumed that patients who are

employed can afford the cost of medication and treatment and hence more likely to be compliant to medication. However, high noncompliance was observed among employed participants and this could be attributed to the busy work schedules and patients having less time for self-care or management [45, 46]. Other studies have also reported contrasting results whereby prevalence of noncompliance to AHT was found to be higher among unemployed individuals with low socioeconomic status [24]. Furthermore, participants with regular source of income had lower odds for noncompliance to AHT. This result is supported by cross-sectional studies conducted in Egypt, by Awad et al. [47] and in Saudi Arabia and Sudan by EL-Zubier [48] who reported that the insufficient income will possibly affect compliance principally if patient is receiving numerous drugs or the drug is expensive. Distribution of participants by reasons of compliant to antihypertensive medication was determined. The main reason for noncompliance reported by participants was cost of medication, stopping medication when feeling well, fear of side effects, forgetfulness, and use of traditional medicine. These findings are supported by reports from previous cross-sectional studies conducted by Almas et al. [33] and Hashim et al. [49].

Although findings in this study concur with reports from other studies and highlight the burden of noncompliance to AHT in the Kintampo municipality and probable associated factors such as health beliefs and lifestyle, there were some limitations. This was a cross-sectional study conducted with small sample size which limited our ability to explain the causal correlations between variables and noncompliance. All participants came from one municipality, and thus, the findings may not represent all of Ghana. The current HBM only includes five cognitively based constructs. It does not consider the emotional, environmental, and social components of health behaviour, which should be added to the HBM in future studies.

5. Conclusion

The study showed that noncompliance to AHT was considerably high and HBM is generally reliable in assessing treatment noncompliance in the Ghanaian hypertensive patients. The study further identified sociodemographic characteristics such as educational level, occupational status, and regular source of income to be significantly associated with noncompliance in the hypertensive patients higher level of perceived barriers; susceptibility and severity were significant predictors of noncompliance: therefore, intervention programmes for noncompliance can be directed towards a greater involvement of increased perceived benefits, cues to action, and personality characteristics such as locus of control.

Acknowledgments

The authors express their gratitude to the clinical staff and patients of the Kintampo Municipal Hospital who actively participated in this study.

References

[1] G. Santulli, "Epidemiology of cardiovascular disease in the 21st century: updated numbers and updated facts," *Journal of Cardiovascular Disease Research*, vol. 1, no. 1, pp. 1-2, 2013.

[2] E. C. Yiannakopoulou, J. S. Papadopulos, D. V. Cokkinos, and T. D. Mountokalakis, "Adherence to antihypertensive treatment: a critical factor for blood pressure control," *European Journal of Cardiovascular Prevention and Rehabilitation*, vol. 12, no. 3, pp. 243–249, 2005.

[3] M. U. Khan, S. Shah, and T. Hameed, "Barriers to and determinants of medication adherence among hypertensive patients attended National Health Service Hospital, Sunderland," *Journal of Pharmacy and Bioallied Sciences*, vol. 6, no. 2, pp. 104–108, 2014.

[4] S. H. S. Lo, J. P. C. Chau, J. Woo, D. R. Thompson, and K. C. Choi, "Adherence to antihypertensive medication in older adults with hypertension," *Journal of Cardiovascular Nursing*, vol. 31, no. 4, pp. 296–303, 2016.

[5] J. Mathew, S. Krishnamoorthy, L. Chacko et al., "Non Compliance to Anti-Hypertensive Medications and Associated Factors-Community Based Cross Sectional Study from Kerala," *Scholars Journal of Applied Medical Sciences*, vol. 4, no. 6, pp. 1956–1959, 2016.

[6] J. Addo, C. Agyemang, L. Smeeth, A. de-Graft Aikins, A. K. Edusei, and O. Ogedegbe, "A review of population-based studies on hypertension in Ghana," *Ghana Medical Journal*, vol. 46, supplement, no. 2, pp. 4–11, 2012.

[7] W. K. Bosu, "Epidemic of hypertension in Ghana: a systematic review," *BMC Public Health*, vol. 10, article 418, 2010.

[8] V. Boima, A. D. Ademola, A. O. Odusola et al., "Factors Associated with Medication Nonadherence among Hypertensives in Ghana and Nigeria," *International Journal of Hypertension*, vol. 2015, Article ID 205716, 2015.

[9] S. A. Alghurair, C. A. Hughes, S. H. Simpson, and L. M. Guirguis, "A systematic review of patient self-reported barriers of adherence to antihypertensive medications using the world health organization multidimensional adherence model," *The Journal of Clinical Hypertension*, vol. 14, no. 12, pp. 877–886, 2012.

[10] N. K. Janz and M. H. Becker, "The health belief model: a decade later," *Health Education Journal*, vol. 11, no. 1, pp. 1–47, 1984.

[11] C. J. Carpenter, "A meta-analysis of the effectiveness of health belief model variables in predicting behavior," *Health Communication*, vol. 25, no. 8, pp. 661–669, 2010.

[12] S. Olsen, S. Smith, T. Oei, and J. Douglas, "Health belief model predicts adherence to CPAP before experience with CPAP," *European Respiratory Journal*, vol. 32, no. 3, pp. 710–717, 2008.

[13] J. N. Harvey and V. L. Lawson, "The importance of health belief models in determining self-care behaviour in diabetes," *Diabetic Medicine*, vol. 26, no. 1, pp. 5–13, 2009.

[14] K. Glanz, BK. Rimer, and K. Viswanath, *Health behavior and health education: theory, research, and practice*, John Wiley Sons, and practice, 2008.

[15] I. A. Kretchy, F. Owusu-Daaku, and S. Danquah, "Patterns and determinants of the use of complementary and alternative medicine: a cross-sectional study of hypertensive patients in Ghana," *BMC Complementary and Alternative Medicine*, vol. 14, article 44, 2014.

[16] K. O. Buabeng, L. Matowe, and J. Plange-Rhule, "Unaffordable drug prices: the major cause of non-compliance with hypertension medication in Ghana," *Journal of Pharmacy & Pharmaceutical Sciences*, vol. 7, no. 3, pp. 350–352, 2004.

[17] H. A. Jambedu, *Adherence to anti-hypertensive medication regimens among patients attending the GPHA Hospital in Takoradi-Ghana*, 2006.

[18] Y. Obirikorang, C. Obirikorang, E. Acheampong et al., "Adherence to Lifestyle Modification among Hypertensive Clients: A Descriptive Cross-Sectional Study," *OALib*, vol. 05, no. 02, pp. 1–13, 2018.

[19] A. A. Joho, *Factors affecting treatment compliance among hypertension patients in three DISTRICT hospitals-dar es salaam*, Muhimbili University of Health and Allied Sciences, Joho, 2012.

[20] C. G. Okwuonu, N. E. Ojimadu, E. I. Okaka, and F. M. Akemokwe, "Patient-related barriers to hypertension control in a Nigerian population," *Journal of General Internal Medicine*, vol. 7, pp. 345–353, 2014.

[21] K. Peltzer, "Health beliefs and prescription medication compliance among diagnosed hypertension clinic attenders in a rural South African Hospital," *Curationis*, vol. 27, no. 3, pp. 15–23, 2004.

[22] N. G. Nkosi and S. C. Wright, "Knowledge related to nutrition and hypertension management practices of adults in Ga-Rankuwa day clinics," *Curationis*, vol. 33, no. 2, pp. 33–40, 2010.

[23] N. Ahmed, M. Abdul Khaliq, S. H. Shah, and W. Anwar, "Compliance to antihypertensive drugs, salt restriction, exercise and control of systemic hypertension in hypertensive patients at Abbottabad.," *Journal of Ayub Medical College*, vol. 20, no. 2, pp. 66–69, 2008.

[24] A. Bilal, M. Riaz, N.-U. Shafiq, M. Ahmed, S. Sheikh, and S. Rasheed, "Non-Compliance to Anti-Hypertensive Medication And Its Associated Factors among Hypertensives," *Journal of Ayub Medical College*, vol. 27, no. 1, pp. 158–163, 2015.

[25] S. Yang, C. He, X. Zhang et al., "Determinants of antihypertensive adherence among patients in Beijing: Application of the health belief model," *Patient Education and Counseling*, vol. 99, no. 11, pp. 1894–1900, 2016.

[26] H. Guo, H. He, and J. Jiang, "Study on the compliance of anti-hypertensive drugs in patients with hypertension," *Zhonghua liu xing bing xue za zhi = Zhonghua liuxingbingxue zazhi*, vol. 22, no. 6, pp. 418–420, 2001.

[27] A. Kamran, S. S. Ahari, M. Biria, A. Malpour, and H. Heydari, "Determinants of patient's adherence to hypertension medications: application of health belief model among rural patients," *Annals of Medical and Health Sciences Research*, vol. 4, no. 6, pp. 922–927, 2014.

[28] S. S. Tavafian, L. Hasani, T. Aghamolaei, S. Zare, and D. Gregory, "Prediction of breast self-examination in a sample of Iranian women: An application of the Health Belief Model," *BMC Women's Health*, vol. 9, article no. 37, 2009.

[29] E. E. Tanner-Smith and T. N. Brown, "Evaluating the health belief model: A critical review of studies predicting mammographic and pap screening," *Social Theory & Health*, vol. 8, no. 1, pp. 95–125, 2010.

[30] D. SEA, P. T. Van Dort, and K. Tay-Teo, *Improving participation in cancer screening programs: A review of social cognitive models, factors affecting participation, and strategies to improve participation*, Victorian Cytology Service, 2010.

[31] R. B. Haynes, H. P. McDonald, and A. X. Garg, "Helping patients follow prescribed treatment: Clinical applications," *Journal of the American Medical Association*, vol. 288, no. 22, pp. 2880–2883, 2002.

[32] Z. Yue, C. Li, Q. Weilin, and W. Bin, "Application of the health belief model to improve the understanding of antihypertensive medication adherence among Chinese patients," *Patient Education and Counseling*, vol. 98, no. 5, pp. 669–673, 2015.

[33] A. Almas, S. S. Godil, S. Lalani, Z. A. Samani, and A. H. Khan, "Good knowledge about hypertension is linked to better control of hypertension; A multicentre cross sectional study in Karachi, Pakistan," *BMC Research Notes*, vol. 5, article no. 579, 2012.

[34] S. H. Nyarko, "Prevalence and Sociodemographic Determinants of Hypertension History among Women in Reproductive Age in Ghana," *International Journal of Hypertension*, vol. 2016, Article ID 3292938, 2016.

[35] R. Ofori-Asenso and D. Garcia, "Cardiovascular diseases in Ghana within the context of globalization," *Cardiovascular Diagnosis and Therapy*, vol. 6, no. 1, pp. 67–77, 2016.

[36] C.-T. Wai, M.-L. Wong, S. Ng et al., "Utility of the health belief model in predicting compliance of screening in patients with chronic hepatitis B," *Alimentary Pharmacology & Therapeutics*, vol. 21, no. 10, pp. 1255–1262, 2005.

[37] M. R. Wild, H. M. Engleman, N. J. Douglas, and C. A. Espie, "Can psychological factors help us to determine adherence to CPAP? A prospective study," *European Respiratory Journal*, vol. 24, no. 3, pp. 461–465, 2004.

[38] N. Iihara, T. Tsukamoto, S. Morita, C. Miyoshi, K. Takabatake, and Y. Kurosaki, "Beliefs of chronically ill Japanese patients that lead to intentional non-adherence to medication," *Journal of Clinical Pharmacy and Therapeutics*, vol. 29, no. 5, pp. 417–424, 2004.

[39] J. Okuno, H. Yanagi, and S. Tomura, "Is cognitive impairment a risk factor for poor compliance among Japanese elderly in the community?" *European Journal of Clinical Pharmacology*, vol. 57, no. 8, pp. 589–594, 2001.

[40] A. J. Ghods and D. Nasrollahzadeh, "Noncompliance with immunnosuppressive medications after renal transplantation.," *Exp Clin Transplant*, vol. 1, no. 1, pp. 39–47, 2003.

[41] A. Yavuz, M. Tuncer, O. Erdoğan et al., "Is there any effect of compliance on clinical parameters of renal transplant recipients?" *Transplantation Proceedings*, vol. 36, no. 1, pp. 120-121, 2004.

[42] R. W. Sanson-Fisher and K. Clover, "Compliance in the treatment of hypertension: A need for action," *American Journal of Hypertension*, vol. 8, no. 10, pp. 82–88, 1995.

[43] H. Kyngäs and T. Lahdenperä, "Compliance of patients with hypertension and associated factors," *Journal of Advanced Nursing*, vol. 29, no. 4, pp. 832–839, 1999.

[44] V. Senior, T. M. Marteau, and J. Weinman, "Self-reported adherence to cholesterol-lowering medication in patients with familial hypercholesterolaemia: The role of illness perceptions," *Cardiovascular Drugs and Therapy*, vol. 18, no. 6, pp. 475–481, 2004.

[45] F. Alsolami, X. Hou, and I. Correa-Velez, "Factors Affecting Antihypertensive Medications Adherence among Hypertensive Patients in Saudi Arabia," *Journal of Hypertension*, vol. 34, p. e132, 2016.

[46] E. P. Jolles, R. S. Padwal, A. M. Clark, and B. Braam, "A Qualitative Study of Patient Perspectives about Hypertension," *ISRN Hypertension*, vol. 2013, pp. 1–10, 2013.

[47] E. Y. Awad, B. E. Gwaied, and L. M. Fouda, "Compliance of hypertensive patients with treatment regimen and its effect on their quality of life," *Health*, vol. 13, p. 16, 2015.

[48] A. El Zubier, "Drug compliance among hypertensive patients in Kassala, eastern Sudan," 2000.

[49] S. K. Hashmi, M. B. Afridi, K. Abbas et al., "Factors associated with adherence to anti-hypertensive treatment in Pakistan," *PLoS ONE*, vol. 2, no. 3, article e280, 2007.

16

Sleep as a Mediator in the Pathway Linking Environmental Factors to Hypertension

Oluwaseun A. Akinseye,[1] **Stephen K. Williams,**[2]
Azizi Seixas,[2] **Seithikurippu R. Pandi-Perumal,**[2] **Julian Vallon,**[2]
Ferdinand Zizi,[2] **and Girardin Jean-Louis**[2]

[1]*Department of Medicine, Icahn School of Medicine at Mount Sinai, Queens Hospital Center, 82-68 164th Street,
Jamaica, NY 11432, USA*
[2]*Center for Healthful Behavior Change, Department of Population Health, NYU School of Medicine, 227 East 30th Street,
New York, NY 10016, USA*

Correspondence should be addressed to Girardin Jean-Louis; girardin.jean-louis@nyumc.org

Academic Editor: Tomohiro Katsuya

Environmental factors, such as noise exposure and air pollution, are associated with hypertension. These environmental factors also affect sleep quality. Given the growing evidence linking sleep quality with hypertension, the purpose of this review is to investigate the role of sleep as a key mediator in the association between hypertension and environmental factors. Through this narrative review of the extant literature, we highlight that poor sleep quality mediates the relationship between environmental factors and hypertension. The conceptual model proposed in this review offers opportunities to address healthcare disparities in hypertension among African Americans by highlighting the disparate impact that the predictors (environmental factors) and mediator (sleep) have on the African-American community. Understanding the impact of these factors is crucial since the main outcome variable (hypertension) severely burdens the African-American community.

1. Introduction

Chronic noise exposure and air pollution have become a significant public health issue given its ubiquity in urban environments [1, 2]. For the first time in history, more than 50% of the world's population lives in an urban environment, and it is estimated that it will likely rise to 70% by 2050 [1]. Urban environments teeming with subways, airplanes, road traffic, and emergency vehicle sirens are epicenters of chronic noise and pollutant exposure [3]. The health implications of chronic exposure to noise and pollutants are becoming more evident based on increased levels of related chronic disease, deaths, and impaired quality of life issues in urban populations. Noise complaints in New York City (NYC) were the primary insult to quality of life in the late 90s [4]. It is estimated that air pollution is responsible for 6% of annual deaths in NYC [5].

Although the association between hypertension and environmental factors, such as ambient noise exposure [6] and air pollutants [7, 8], is well documented primarily in laboratory-based studies [9–12], field-based studies accounting for chronic exposures will likely provide more clinically and ecologically relevant hypertension risk factors. Hypertension has a multifactorial etiology [13] and sleep quality has been identified as a factor associated with hypertension [14–17]. Hypertension and sleep disorders are common in the USA. It is estimated that 60–70 million Americans suffer from hypertension [18] and a similar number of Americans also suffer from chronic inadequate sleep, hindering daily functioning and adversely affecting health and longevity [19].

The theory that sleep could be a mediator in the role between environmental factors and cardiovascular health outcomes has been proposed in the past [20]. As per the Baron and Kenny model [21], to satisfy the conceptual model for mediating a predictor-outcome relationship, the following relationships must be present: (1) The proposed environmental factors (predictor variables) are significantly

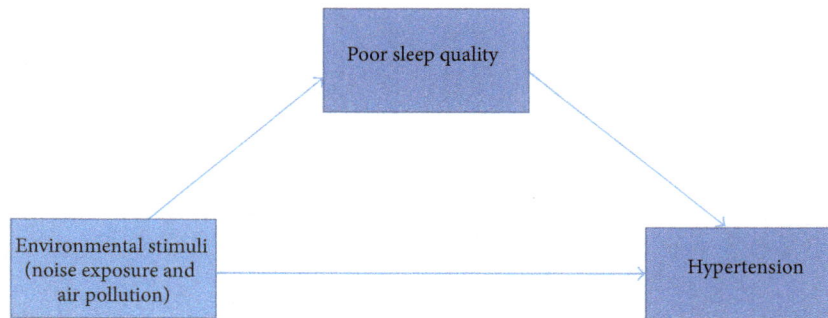

FIGURE 1: Conceptual model proposing sleep quality as a mediator in the pathway linking environmental stimuli to hypertension.

associated with hypertension (outcome variable); (2) the environmental factors must be significantly associated with sleep (mediating variable); and (3) sleep must be associated with hypertension (Figure 1). In a previous study, noise sensitivity and health complaints were noted to be associated and sleep was found to be a mediating variable [22]. Additionally, noisy neighborhoods were associated with lower self-rated physical health and the association was also mediated by sleep [23]. Conversely, in a study evaluating the adverse impact of night-time aircraft noise on endothelial function, sleep quality was not noted to be a mediating factor [24].

The purpose of this review is to summarize: (1) the relationship of hypertension to noise and air pollutants; (2) the relationship between sleep and the aforementioned environmental factors; and (3) the relationship between hypertension and sleep. We propose that relationships between these environmental factors and hypertension among Blacks would be especially relevant clinically because of the greater exposure to the aforementioned environmental factors as well as the greater prevalence of poor sleep quality in that population.

2. Sleep and Hypertension

Sleep has become of great interest in the field of hypertension because of the potential interventions that could be administered with resultant improvement in hypertension and its related adverse outcomes. The CARDIA Sleep Study, a longitudinal study examining the association between hypertension and sleep quality, showed an increase in the odds of hypertension among individuals with shorter sleep duration [25]. Data from a cross-sectional analysis of the 2009 National Health Interview Survey (NHIS) showed a higher likelihood of hypertension among individuals who reported daily sleep durations of 6 hours or less [26]. This is consistent with findings from the National Health and Nutrition Examination Survey (NHANES) I Epidemiologic Follow-Up Study that revealed a hazard ratio of 1.60 (95% CI: 1.19, 2.14) for developing hypertension over 8 to 10 years among individuals reporting sleep duration of 5 hours or less compared with those sleeping 7 to 8 hours [15].

3. Environmental Factors and Hypertension

Environmental factors are included under the social determinants of health and are emphasized in the Healthy People

2020 initiative [27]. The environmental factors that this review will emphasize are limited to chronic ambient noise exposure (nonoccupational) and chronic ambient air pollution (Table 1). The air pollutants that will be discussed are predominantly $PM_{2.5}$, which is defined as fine particulate matter <2.5 μm in diameter.

4. Noise and Hypertension

"Noise is generally defined as unwanted sound or set of sounds." [28] Noise disturbance is one of the most frequent complaints among urban-dwelling populations [28] and can be due to amplification of the noise levels by reflections off rigid urban area structures [29]. These areas are also more likely to have higher volume of vehicular traffic, train tracks, and airports [30]. Chronic exposure to subway traffic noise in New York City has been documented to have potential for significant adverse health effects with decibel levels exceeding 100 dB(A) [30, 31]. Decibel levels > 70 dB(A) are thought to be associated with harmful cardiovascular health effects [32].

The epidemiologic evidence associating noise with higher risk of developing hypertension continues to grow [33–35]. The Hypertension and Exposure to Noise near Airport (HYENA) study, comprising almost 5,000 participants living close to several European airports, showed a significant exposure-response relationship between night-time aircraft, average daily road traffic noise exposure, and risk of hypertension [36]. Evidence shows a 1.14 (95% CI: 1.01, 1.29) increase in the odds of developing hypertension with each 10 dB increase in exposure to night-time aircraft noise, and similar exposure-response relationships were seen for road traffic noise in the highest exposure category of >65 dB with a significant odds ratio (OR) of 1.54 (95% CI: 0.99, 2.40) [36]. Furthermore, an increase of 0.26 mmHg in systolic blood pressure (BP) per 10 dB increase in road traffic noise levels and a 8% higher risk of hypertension with exposure to railway noise > 60 dB were reported in another study [37]. A smaller study found that there were a 1.06 to 1.80 increased odds of hypertension for every 5 dB increase in noise exposure and the association was stronger among those who had lived at the same address for >10 years [38], suggesting additional impact among those with more chronic exposure. This finding was supported by another cross-sectional study that showed a stronger estimate of noise effect on the risk of hypertension in individuals with

TABLE 1: Highlighted studies on effect of long-term environmental factor exposure on population-level samples.

(a) Environmental noise and hypertension

First author, year (design)	Sample size (N)	Country	Exposure assessment method	Hypertension assessment	Main finding	Effect size: ES r (95% CI)
Jarup, 2008 [36] (cross-sectional)	4861	United Kingdom, Germany, Netherlands, Sweden, Italy, Greece	Country specific noise exposure models: both aircraft and road traffic noise	Home BP readings with hypertension defined as ≥140/90 mmHg OR self-reported physician diagnosis of hypertension OR use of antihypertensive medication	Significant exposure-response relationship between night-time aircraft noise, average daily road traffic noise exposure, and risk of hypertension	Night-time aircraft noise: OR 1.14 (95% CI: 1.01–1.29) of hypertension with 10 dB(A) increase in exposure; average road traffic noise: OR 1.097 (95% CI: 1.00–1.20) of hypertension with 10 dB(A) increase in exposure
Bluhm, 2007 [38] (cross-sectional)	667	Sweden	Nordic prediction model for road traffic noise	Self-report on survey	Significant relationship between exposure to residential road traffic noise and hypertension; association stronger among women and among those who have lived at the address for >10 years; exposure-response relationship suggested	The odds ratio for hypertension was 1.38 for every 5 dB(A) increase in noise exposure
Sorensen, 2011 [37] (cross-sectional)	44,083	Denmark	Nordic prediction model for road traffic noise and railway noise	Incident hypertension over 5 years identified by questionnaire; baseline association between measured blood pressure and residential exposure to road traffic noise	Exposure-response relationship between road traffic noise and systolic blood pressure levels; effect size statistically significant only in males; no association between road traffic noise levels and diastolic BP; there was a borderline statistically significant relationship between railway noise and incident hypertension cases	Cross section: increase of 0.59 mmHg in systolic BP (95% CI: 0.13–1.05) per 10 dB(A) increase in road traffic noise levels; prospective: 8% higher risk of hypertension with exposure to railway noise above 60 dB(A) (95% CI: −2%–19%)
Babisch, 2014 [39] (cross-sectional)	1770	Berlin, Germany	City noise map for road traffic noise	Self-reported physician diagnosis, use of antihypertensive medications, measured blood pressure ≥140/90	Stronger significant estimates of the noise effect were found in subjects with long residence time and with respect to the exposure of the living room during daytime, no association with respect to exposure of the bedroom during night-time	OR for developing hypertension while living at the residence was 1.11 interval (95% CI: 1.00–1.23) per noise level increment of 10 dB(A); effect size stronger with resident time >10 years (OR: 1.20; 95% CI: 1.05–1.37); OR for development of hypertension was 1.24 (95% CI: 1.08–1.41) in those living with exposure of the living room during daytime

(a) Continued.

First author, year (design)	Sample size (N)	Country	Exposure assessment method	Hypertension assessment	Main finding	Effect size: ES r (95% CI)
Eriksson, 2012 [40] (cross-sectional)	25,851	Sweden	Traffic load (millions of vehicle kilometers per year) within 500 m around residential address; subpopulation had additional assessment using Nordic prediction method	Self-reported physician diagnosis of hypertension	No significant association noted between traffic load and hypertension	OR for diagnosis of HTN with exposure to ≥65 dB(A) with <50 dB(A) as reference was 0.96 (95% CI 0.59–1.59)
de Kluizenaar, 2007 [45] (cross-sectional)	2 samples Sample 1: 40,856 Sample 2: 8592	2 samples (1) City of Groningen sample (2) Sample from observational study: Prevention of Renal and Vascular End-Stage Disease (PREVEND)	Road traffic noise exposure of the subjects was calculated at the most exposed facade of the dwelling with standard method	Groningen subjects were defined as having hypertension when they reported using medication for elevated blood pressure	Adjusted ORs summarizing noise exposure and hypertension were not significant; significant findings in subjects who were between 45 and 55 years old; associations seemed to be stronger at higher noise levels	In the Groningen sample, adjusted OR for having hypertension in subjects between 45 and 55 years old was 1.19 (95% CI: 1.02–1.40) per 10 dB increase in noise level (Lden) PREVEND cohort OR 1.39 (1.08–1.77)
Haralabidis, 2011 [42] (cross-sectional)	149	4 European airports with night-time flights permitted	Long-term noise exposure as per HYENA study protocol (aircraft and road traffic)	Ambulatory blood pressure measurement for 24 hr	Only road traffic noise, and not aircraft noise, was associated with decreased BP dipping	Pooled estimates: with a 5 dB(A) increase in measured road traffic noise, there is 0.8% less dipping (95% CI: −1.55 % to −0.05%)
Dratva, 2012 [41] (cross-sectional)	6,450	Switzerland	SONBASE national data repository on railway and traffic noise linked to residential addresses	Measured at rest by study staff	Positive association of railway noise with SBP and DBP; effect size stronger among subjects with reported physician-diagnosed hypertension, DM, or CVD; traffic noise was not impressive except for people with DM	For a 10 dB(A) increase in railway noise during the night 0.84 mmHg increase in SBP (95% CI: 0.22–1.46) and during the day 0.60 mmHg increase (0.07–1.13)

(a) Continued.

First author, year (design)	Sample size (N)	Country	Exposure assessment method	Hypertension assessment	Main finding	Effect size: ES r (95% CI)
Belojević, 2008 [43] (cross-sectional)	2,503	Belgrade	Grouped into noisy areas (equivalent noise level [Leq] > 45 dB(A)) and quiet areas (Leq ≤ 45 dB(A))	Use of antihypertensive medication OR measured BP with values ≥140/90 mmHg defined as hypertension	Night-time urban road traffic noise might be related to occurrence of hypertension; no significant findings in women	In men, OR for hypertension was 1.58 (95% CI: 1.03–2.42).
Barregard, 2009 [44] (cross-sectional)	1386	Sweden	GIS and validated model to assess road and railway traffic noise	Self-report of physician diagnosis or taking antihypertensive medications	Association between road traffic and hypertension noted along with an exposure-response relationship; there were no clear associations in women or for railway noise	OR for hypertension was 1.9 (95% CI: 1.1 to 3.5) in the highest noise category for road traffic noise; OR for hypertension was higher in men—3.8 (95% CI: 1.6 to 9.0)
Eriksson, 2007 [35] (prospective)	2,754 men	Stockholm airport	Geographical information systems techniques	Incidence cases of hypertension defined by self-report of physician diagnosis or use of medications or BP measured at ≥140/90 mmHg	Long-term aircraft noise exposure increases risk for hypertension	For subjects exposed to energy-averaged levels above 50 dB(A) the adjusted relative risk for hypertension was 1.19 (95% CI: 1.03–1.37); maximum aircraft noise levels presented similar results, with a relative risk of 1.20 (1.03–1.40) for those exposed above 70 dB(A)

(b) Ambient air pollution and hypertension

First author, year (design)	Sample size	Country	Air pollution assessment method	Hypertension assessment	Main finding	Effect size: ES r (95% CI)
Fuks, 2011 [61] (cross-sectional)	4,291	Urban West Germany	$PM_{2.5}$ using validated dispersion model system	Measured systolic BP ≥140 mmHg or diastolic BP ≥90 mmHg or current use of antihypertensive therapy	Long-term exposure to $PM_{2.5}$ is associated with increased blood pressure; more impressive findings with traffic noise proximity	An IQR increase in $PM_{2.5}$ (2.4 $\mu g/m^3$) was associated with estimated increases in mean systolic and diastolic BP of 1.4 mmHg [CI 95%: 0.5–2.3] and 0.9 mmHg (CI 95% CI: 0.4–1.4), respectively

(b) Continued.

First author, year (design)	Sample size	Country	Air pollution assessment method	Hypertension assessment	Main finding	Effect size: ES r (95% CI)
Auchincloss, 2008 [62] (cross-sectional)	5,112	North America: Multiethnic Study of Atherosclerosis (MESA)	$PM_{2.5}$ using 24-hour integrated samplers with 5 retrospective exposure phases recorded	Resting seated BP	Stronger effect sizes from longer exposures (1-2 months) of ambient $PM_{2.5}$ exposure compared with shorter (≤ 1 week) exposures; systolic blood pressure was only significantly affected (diastolic was not); effects stronger in the presence of higher traffic exposure	$10\,\mu g/m^3$ increase in $PM_{2.5}$ prior 30-day mean was associated with 2.8 mmHg SBP (95% CI: 1.38 to 4.22) **Note that this is a relatively short exposure study**
Chuang, 2011 [65] (cross-sectional)	1,023	Taiwan	1-year averaged criteria air pollutants measured by local monitoring stations ($PM_{2.5}$, PM_{10}, nitrogen dioxide (NO(2)), and ozone (O3))	Measured blood pressure	$PM_{2.5}$ retained the strongest association with blood pressure (both systolic and diastolic) among the four air pollutants	For an IQR increase in $PM_{2.5}$ ($20.42\,\mu g/m^3$), there were 32.4 mmHg (95% CI: 22.4–42.5) and 29.3 mmHg (95% CI: 19.2–39.3) increases in systolic and diastolic blood pressure, respectively, (controlling for ozone), and 31.1 mmHg (95% CI: 21.1 to 41.2) and 30.0 mmHg (95% CI 18.0 to 41.9) increases in systolic and diastolic blood pressure, respectively, (controlling for NO(2))
Dong, 2013 [58] (cross-sectional)	24,845	China	Local monitoring stations: three-year average concentration PM_{10}, sulfur dioxide (SO2), nitrogen dioxides (NO2), and ozone (O3)	Measured blood pressure	Note that these are findings for more coarse particles, comparing apples and oranges; it addresses exposures to a mixture including not only $PM_{2.5}$	Odds ratio for hypertension increased by 1.12 (CI 95%: 1.08–1.16) per $19\,\mu g/m^3$ increase in PM_{10}; the estimated increases in mean systolic and diastolic blood pressure were 0.87 mmHg (95% CI, 0.48–1.27) and 0.32 mmHg (95% CI, 0.08–0.56) per $19\,\mu g/m^3$ increase in PM_{10}

(b) Continued.

First author, year (design)	Sample size	Country	Air pollution assessment method	Hypertension assessment	Main finding	Effect size: ES r (95% CI)
Coogan, 2012 [56] (prospective)	4,204	USA	Participants' residential addresses with land use regression models (nitrogen oxides) and interpolation from monitoring station measurements ($PM_{2.5}$)	Incident case of hypertension as self-report of physician-diagnosed hypertension during follow-up and concurrent use of antihypertensive medications	Exposure to ambient fine particulate pollution increased risk; association did not quite reach statistical significance and got weaker when controlling for nitrogen containing air pollutants	Over 10-year follow-up incidence rate ratio for hypertension for a 10 $\mu g/m^3$ increase in $PM_{2.5}$ was 1.48 (95% CI, 0.95–2.31)
Johnson, 2009 [55] (cross-sectional)	132,224 National Health Interview Survey (NHIS)	USA	$PM_{2.5}$ data from the US Environmental Protection Agency	Self-reported physician diagnosis of hypertension or use of medications	Odds ratio for prevalent hypertension was higher with higher levels of $PM_{2.5}$ in Whites and not Blacks	Amongst Whites, a 10 $\mu g/m^3$ increase in $PM_{2.5}$ exposure was associated with a small elevated risk of hypertension (adjusted odds ratio (OR) 1.05, 95% confidence interval (CI) 1.04–1.17); OR in Blacks was 0.90 (95% CI: 0.79–1.03)
Sørensen, 2012 [64] (cross-sectional and prospective)	57,053	Denmark	Dispersion model to calculate residential long-term nitrogen oxide	Self-reported incident hypertension was assessed by questionnaire	Nitrogen oxide (a measure of traffic air pollution that correlates well with fine particles and is easier to measure) was inversely associated with systolic and diastolic BP and the prevalence of self-reported hypertension, and there was no association with the risk of incident self-reported hypertension during approximately 5 years of follow-up	There were 0.53 mmHg and 0.50 mmHg decrease in systolic BP with nitrogen oxide exposure during 1- and 5-year periods preceding enrollment, respectively; the OR of self-reported hypertension with long-term exposure was 0.96 (95% CI: 0.91, 1.00)
Chuang, 2010 [57] (cross-sectional)	26,685	Taiwan	Monitoring stations by Taiwan Environmental Protection Agency	Measured BP	PM_{10} was associated with elevated systolic BP, triglyceride, apolipoprotein B, hemoglobin A1c, and reduced high-density lipoprotein cholesterol; elevated ozone was associated with increased diastolic BP	Increase of 0.47 mmHg; (95% CI, −0.09 to 1.02) with each interquartile range (34 $\mu g/m^3$) PM_{10}

(b) Continued.

First author, year (design)	Sample size	Country	Air pollution assessment method	Hypertension assessment	Main finding	Effect size: ES r (95% CI)
Schwartz, 2012 [63] (longitudinal)	853 elderly VA patients	USA	Traffic black soot	Measured BP	Increase in black soot was associated with increase in systolic and diastolic BP	An IQR increase in 1-year average black soot exposure ($0.32\ \mu g/m^3$) was associated with a 2.64 mmHg increase in systolic blood pressure (95% CI 1.47 to 3.80) and a 2.41 mmHg increase in diastolic blood pressure (95% CI 1.77 to 3.05)

(c) Environmental noise and sleep quality

First author, year (design)	Sample size	Country	Noise assessment method	Sleep quality assessment method	Main finding	Effect size: ES r (95% CI)
Saremi, 2008 [67] (cross-sectional)	38	France	Recorded train noise at 40–50 dB(A)	Polysomnography	Arousal responsiveness increased with sound levels; awakenings (>10 s) were produced more frequently by freight train (compared to automotive/passenger)	Increase in noise level had main effect on the percentage of awakenings ($F_{(2,50)} = 26.94$, $P < 0.00001$), and microarousals ($F_{(2,50)} = 64.29$, $P < 0.00001$); there were increase in sleep fragmentation ($P < 0.001$) and a shorter arousal onset latency ($F_{(1,36)} = 16.18$, $P = 0.0002$), with increasing noise level
Basner, 2011 [68] (cross-sectional)	72	Germany	Traffic noise events were recorded with class 1 sound level meters in bedrooms of residents living close to a road, a railway track, or an airport	Polysomnography, actigraphs, self-report	Subjective sleep assessment and recuperation were affected; indicators for sleep continuity were pronounced significantly except for awakening frequency	There were difficulty falling asleep (+89, P = 0.013), increased sleep disturbance (+126, P < 0.001), lighter sleep (+121, P < 0.001), and less recuperative sleep (+111, P < 0.001) in triple compared to single night exposure to noise; slow-wave sleep latency was 5.2 min longer in triple than single exposure night; REM latency was 9.0 min longer with the same exposure; time spent in REM was shorter in the triple than single or double exposure nights

(c) Continued.

First author, year (design)	Sample size	Country	Noise assessment method	Sleep quality assessment method	Main finding	Effect size: ES r (95% CI)
Basner, 2005 [72] (cross-sectional)	128	Germany	Noise (45–80 dB(A)) was recorded with class 1 sound level meters (NC-10, Cortex Industries) in the vicinity of Dusseldorf Airport with closed or tilted windows	Polysomnography	Aircraft noise was associated with signs of sleep fragmentation (increased stage 1 and number of awakenings)	Slow-wave sleep was significantly reduced by 5.3 min, and total sleep time increased on average by 2.5 min
Agarwal, 2011 [71] (cross-sectional)	550	India	Self-report and objective assessment of noise indices (traffic volume and associated noise)	Self-report	Reported loss of sleep as a result of noise pollution	67% of respondents reported loss of sleep
Griefahn, 2006 [73] (experimental)	32	Germany	Noise range 32–74 dB(A) was applied	Polysomnography, self-report	Subjectively evaluated sleep quality decreased gradually with increasing noise levels; SWS latency prolongation, total sleep time reduction, and decrease of SWS during first sleep cycle were significant	The SWS latency and waketime after sleep onset were increased; total sleep time (TST) and sleep efficiency were decreased; In relation to sleep period time (SPT), the amount of time awake and in stage S1 (S0 and 1) was increased (+13 min), but REM-sleep and SWS were decreased (−11.7 min)
Horne, 1994 [82] (cross-sectional)	400	UK Airports	Aircraft noise event (ANE) was unit of measure	Wrist actigraphs and sleep logs	Minority of ANEs disrupted sleep; domestic idiosyncratic factors had greater impact on sleep	Effect size not available for qualitative-type study

(c) Continued.

First author, year (design)	Sample size	Country	Noise assessment method	Sleep quality assessment method	Main finding	Effect size: ES r (95% CI)
Öhrström, 2004 [80] (literature review)	—	Sweden	Nordic prediction method for road traffic	Sleep survey	Reduction in road traffic after improvement in road traffic pattern resulted in improved self-reported sleep quality	Noise reduction from range of 56–69 dB(A) to 44–57 dB(A) resulted in improvement in self-reported sleep quality

(d) Air pollution and sleep quality

First author, year (design)	Sample size	Country	Air pollution assessment	Sleep quality assessment	Main finding	Effect size: ES r (95% CI)
Zanobetti, 2010 [51] (cross-sectional)	6441	USA	PM_{10}	Polysomnography	Air pollution associated with increases in respiratory disturbance index and decrease in sleep efficiency	In the summer period, for every interquartile increase in short-term PM_{10} levels, there were 12.9% increase (95% CI: 2.77, 24.09) in RDI, 19.4% increase (95% CI: 3.67, 37.5) in percentage of sleep time at <90% oxygen saturation, and 1.20% decrease (95% CI: −2.40, −0.004) in sleep efficiency
Fang, 2014 [76] (cross-sectional)	3,821	USA	Black carbon (BC)	Self-report, Berlin Sleep Questionnaire	Increased sleep duration with annual BC in Blacks with no observation in Whites and Hispanics; sleep duration decreased in men and those with low socioeconomic status (SES) per IQR increase in BC but not in women and those with medium or high SES	OR for short sleep in men is 1.7 per IQR increase in BC (95% CI: 1.1, 2.6) and 1.6 (95% CI: 1.1, 2.3) for low socioeconomic status; OR for short sleep in Hispanics is 1.4 (95% CI: 1.1, 1.8); Blacks experienced increased sleep duration with increasing BC ($\beta = 0.34$ per IQR; 95% CI: 0.12, 0.57)
Abou-Khadra, 2013 [75] (cross-sectional)	276	Egypt	PM_{10}	Self-report	PM_{10} and disorder of initiation and maintaining sleep were significantly associated ($P = 0.012$) and sleep hyperhidrosis was 0.045; PM_{10} and global sleep disturbance were marginally associated ($P = 0.073$)	Effect size was not reported

chronic noise exposure [39]. More significant estimates of the noise effect were found in subjects with long residence time (OR: 1.20, 95% CI: 1.05–1.37) and with exposure of the living room during daytime (OR 1.24, 95% CI: 1.08–1.41) compared with the exposure of the bedroom during night-time [39].

In contrast, the ROADSIDE study found no statistically significant association between road traffic noise and traffic load and self-reported hypertension [40]. This finding was reproduced by Dratva et al. [41], who showed no significant association between traffic noise and hypertension except in diabetics. Analysis of the HYENA study also supported this differential effect of the source of noise on hypertension [42]. Other studies found the association between noise and hypertension to be gender [43, 44] and age [45] dependent.

5. Air Pollution and Hypertension

The urbanization of most American cities is likely to worsen the problem of air pollution. In addition to soot, smog, smoke, dust, ozone, sulfur, carbon monoxide, nitrogen dioxide, and lead which make up the particulates, suspended particulates in the air come from increased combustion of motor vehicle fuel in the urbanized environment, posing a serious health threat among urban dwellers. Recommended limits for $PM_{2.5}$ are 35 $\mu g/m^3$ daily and 15.0 $\mu g/m^3$ annually [46]. In 2000, the annual average in downtown NYC was 17.5 $\mu g/m^3$ [47]. Both indoor and outdoor pollution have been associated with adverse effects on human health [48–54]. Even though asthma is typically the disease associated with air pollution, accumulating evidence suggests that hypertension is associated with air pollution [55–58].

Data from a meta-analysis suggested that blood pressure (BP) was positively related to $PM_{2.5}$ exposure, resulting in an increase of 1.393 mmHg and 0.895 mmHg per 10 $\mu g/m^3$ increase in $PM_{2.5}$ exposure for systolic BP and diastolic BP, respectively [41]. Further supporting a causal mechanism was the finding that, with long-term exposure, there was a stronger association with BP increase [2]. This is consistent with findings in another study that found a 2.8 mmHg, 2.7 mmHg, and 2.7 mmHg increase in resting systolic, diastolic, and mean arterial BP, respectively, following exposure to mean $PM_{2.5}$ level of 10.5 $\mu g/m^3$ [59]. Dvonch et al. [60] also noted similar associations between $PM_{2.5}$ and BP, and larger effects were observed when urban location was controlled for in the analysis. An interquartile range (IQR) increase in $PM_{2.5}$ (2.4 $\mu g/m^3$) was found to be associated with estimated increases in mean systolic and diastolic BP of 1.4 mmHg and 0.9 mmHg, respectively [61], and stronger effect sizes from chronic exposure to ambient air pollution [62] and other air pollutants [63] have been reported. There are conflicting results with the finding that long-term exposure to traffic air pollution is inversely associated with systolic and diastolic BP and the prevalence of self-reported hypertension [64]; however it should be noted that there were differences in the method that traffic air pollution was assessed in this study. The fact that nitric oxide (NO), but not $PM_{2.5}$, was assessed makes direct comparison with the majority of the traffic air pollution studies difficult. It is also worthy of note that

$PM_{2.5}$ retained the strongest association with blood pressure (both systolic and diastolic) among four air pollutants (ozone (O(3)), nitrogen dioxide (NO(2)), sulfur dioxide, and carbon monoxide) in a recent study [65].

6. Environmental Factors and Sleep Quality

Urban communities are more likely than rural communities to have certain neighborhood characteristics (i.e., noise and air pollution) that affect sleep quality. The odds of having short sleep are highest for those who live in central city environments with over 1 million people compared with residents of more rural, nonmetropolitan environments even after adjusting for socioeconomic and health characteristics [66].

7. Noise and Sleep Quality

Noise is independently associated with reduced sleep quality [67, 68]. Data from a cross-sectional study showed that residing in noisy area is associated with difficulties falling asleep, falling back to sleep, waking up at night, and having poor sleep quality [69]. In a related study, chronic exposure to loud noise over a year was strongly associated with poor sleep efficiency resulting in a decrease in total rapid eye movement time, none rapid eye movement time, slow-wave sleep time, sleep onset latency, and total sleep time [70]. A Norwegian study also developed a model that presented sleep disturbance as a mediator of the noise and poor health relationship. It is interesting that a phenomenon of "noise annoyance" was found to be a mediator factor suggesting that a vulnerable subset of the population was more likely to suffer from the adverse health effects of noise [20]. Different populations have been noted to rate different sources of noise population as being noxious [68, 71]. Environmental noise elevates arousal levels and fragments sleep resulting in a redistribution of time spent in the different sleep stages [68], typically increasing wake and stage 1 sleep and decreasing slow-wave and REM sleep [72, 73]. The method by which sleep quality is assessed must be considered in examining the research literature since it has been reported that subjective assessment of sleep quality after exposure to noise does not correlate well with objective findings [68, 74].

8. Air Pollution and Sleep Quality

Decreases in sleep efficiency have been associated with increases in short-term variation of particulate air matter less than 10 μm in aerodynamic diameter [51]. An analysis of a cross-sectional study showed a statistically significant association between higher PM_{10} exposure and disorders of initiation and maintenance of sleep assessed by the Sleep Disturbance Scale for children questionnaire [75]. Exposure to black carbon (a marker of traffic-related air pollution) in urban Boston was associated with short sleep duration in men and in the lower socioeconomic (SES) population. However, the complexities in such analysis are highlighted by associations with longer sleep duration in Blacks, an association not found in Whites or Hispanics [76].

9. Discussion

Even though there is accumulating evidence on the association between hypertension and environmental factors such as air and noise pollution, there remains a significant gap in elucidating the mechanism of this association. In the USA, there is a paucity of published research that has examined the association between hypertension and environmental factors with most of the cited research originating from the Scandinavian countries. This finding is somewhat surprising given the urbanization of our nation's communities. Nonetheless, these environmental factors, in particular air pollution, have become a critical issue for the American Heart Association (AHA) [54]. Given the evidence that environment plays a significant role in determining blood pressure levels and hypertension prevalence, it is imperative that the United States derived data be gathered in the interest of the nation's public health [77, 78].

The proposed model presented in this review is simple by virtue of the paucity of data on the relationships. Field studies, as opposed to laboratory studies, are indicated to correlate long-term exposure to environmental factors to hypertension and sleep. There is evidence that sleep responses to noise in the field are different to laboratory exposure [79] likely because of physiological factors such as habituation [80] and behavioral factors such as subject self-selection for living in particular locations [81]. Idiosyncratic domestic stimuli, such as bed partner movement and children going to bathrooms, have been shown to be more influential on sleep patterns than road traffic or aircraft noise [82, 83]. Future models will need to clarify the relative contributions of genetics to the environment-hypertension association.

The premise of this paper is that there is a glaring gap in extant literature investigating the mediating effect of sleep on the noise-BP association, given the well-established associations of noise-BP and noise-sleep. The HYENA study demonstrated a relationship between exposure to aircraft noise and hypertension with a stronger relationship noted with night-time exposure to noise as opposed to daytime [36]. The implication of these findings is that night-time noise disturbance may be more significant by virtue of sleep disturbance. In a separate study of exposure to aircraft noise, while greater perception of noise disturbance was associated with poorer subjective sleep quality, higher objective measures of noise were associated with higher BP levels [84]. There is even more of a paucity of clinical research when exploring the air pollution-BP and the air pollution-sleep association. An intriguing area of exploration is the common denominator of electroencephalography (EEG) arousals in both the pathogenesis of BP physiology and sleep architecture. It is well established that EEG findings are instrumental in describing sleep architecture [85]. EEG changes have been observed when individuals are exposed to air pollutants [86], and similarly EEG findings have been shown to precede changes in BP homeostasis [87]. These findings suggest a gap in our understanding of the associations between environmental factors and BP, warranting further investigations.

In the United States, there is the opportunity to link data sets such as NHANES with validated spatiotemporal models or data such as the NYC community air survey (NYCCAS) to investigate cross-sectional associations of environmental factors and hypertension. Such endeavors are in the infancy of being funded by the National Institute of Health (NIH) [88]. This recently funded study uses a cohort from Black Women's Health Study to determine the incidence of hypertension and diabetes associated with $PM_{2.5}$ while controlling for noise confounded using innovative modelling.

Finally, the proposed model has the potential to address ethnic/racial disparities in the field of hypertension. Innovative research methods from Southern California have illustrated the excess exposure to road traffic and its pollutants that minority populations experience [89, 90]. The National Institute of Environmental Health Sciences is a branch of the NIH that has at its core mandate a stated mission to address environmental health disparities. There is a higher prevalence of hypertension in the African American population and African Americans disproportionately suffer from poor sleep quality, relative to other racial/ethnic groups [66, 91–94]. They also dwell predominantly in urban populations and are subjected to a unique array of intense and prolonged environmental stimuli. There should be opportunities for further funding from the NIH to address these relevant issues.

10. Conclusions

In summary, sleep as a mediator in the pathway of the relationship between environmental factors and hypertension is an intriguing model with promising avenues for therapeutic intervention. The factors comprising the conceptual model are especially common and small improvements in the proposed predictor and mediator variables could lead to significant improvements in the management of hypertension. In addition, the epidemiology of the discussed variables is such that they promise to address racial/ethnic disparities in hypertension.

Authors' Contribution

Oluwaseun A. Akinseye, Stephen K. Williams, Azizi Seixas, Ferdinand Zizi, and Girardin Jean-Louis conceived and designed the outline of review. Oluwaseun A. Akinseye, Stephen K. Williams, Seithikurippu R. Pandi-Perumal, Julian Vallon, and Girardin Jean-Louis performed the literature search. Oluwaseun A. Akinseye, Stephen K. Williams, Azizi Seixas, Seithikurippu R. Pandi-Perumal, and Girardin Jean-Louis wrote the paper. All authors approved the final version of the paper that was submitted for publication.

Acknowledgment

This research was supported by funding from the National Institute of Health (U54NS081765, R01HL095799, and R01MD007716). However, the funders had no role in the preparation or decision to publish the paper.

References

[1] B. L. City and E. Assessment, "Urbanization and health," *Bulletin of the World Health Organization*, vol. 88, no. 4, pp. 245–246, 2010.

[2] S. Luzzi, "Urban noise management and its practical implementation," in *Proceedings 20th International Congress on Sound and Vibration (ICSV20 '13)*, Bangkok, Thailand, July 2013.

[3] A. Skånberg and E. Öhrström, "Adverse health effects in relation to urban residential soundscapes," *Journal of Sound and Vibration*, vol. 250, no. 1, pp. 151–155, 2002.

[4] L. Goines and L. Hagler, "Noise pollution: a modern plague," *Southern Medical Journal*, vol. 100, no. 3, pp. 287–294, 2007.

[5] New York City Department of Environmental Protection, *Air Pollution*, New York City Environmental Protection Web site, 2014, http://www.nyc.gov/html/dep/html/air/index.shtml.

[6] E. van Kempen and W. Babisch, "The quantitative relationship between road traffic noise and hypertension: a meta-analysis," *Journal of Hypertension*, vol. 30, no. 6, pp. 1075–1086, 2012.

[7] R. Liang, B. Zhang, X. Zhao, Y. Ruan, H. Lian, and Z. Fan, "Effect of exposure to PM2.5 on blood pressure: a systematic review and meta-analysis," *Journal of Hypertension*, vol. 32, no. 11, pp. 2130–2141, 2014.

[8] R. D. Brook, "Why physicians who treat hypertension should know more about air pollution," *The Journal of Clinical Hypertension*, vol. 9, no. 8, pp. 629–635, 2007.

[9] L. Andren, "Cardiovascular effects of noise," *Acta medica Scandinavica. Supplementum*, vol. 657, pp. 1–45, 1982.

[10] L. Andren, L. Hansson, R. Eggertsen, T. Hedner, and B. E. Karlberg, "Circulatory effects of noise," *Acta Medica Scandinavica*, vol. 213, no. 1, pp. 31–35, 1983.

[11] L. Andrén, G. Lindstedt, M. Björkman, K. O. Borg, and L. Hansson, "Effect of noise on blood pressure and 'stress' hormones," *Clinical Science*, vol. 62, no. 2, pp. 137–141, 1982.

[12] B. Urch, F. Silverman, P. Corey et al., "Acute blood pressure responses in healthy adults during controlled air pollution exposures," *Environmental Health Perspectives*, vol. 113, no. 8, pp. 1052–1055, 2005.

[13] World Health Organization, *A Global Brief on Hypertension: Silent Killer, Global Public Health Crisis: World Health Day 2013*, 2013.

[14] J. Fang, A. G. Wheaton, N. L. Keenan, K. J. Greenlund, G. S. Perry, and J. B. Croft, "Association of sleep duration and hypertension among us adults varies by age and sex," *The American Journal of Hypertension*, vol. 25, no. 3, pp. 335–341, 2012.

[15] J. E. Gangwisch, S. B. Heymsfield, B. Boden-Albala et al., "Short sleep duration as a risk factor for hypertension: analyses of the first National Health and Nutrition Examination Survey," *Hypertension*, vol. 47, no. 5, pp. 833–839, 2006.

[16] L. Meng, Y. Zheng, and R. Hui, "The relationship of sleep duration and insomnia to risk of hypertension incidence: a meta-analysis of prospective cohort studies," *Hypertension Research*, vol. 36, no. 11, pp. 985–995, 2013.

[17] X. Guo, L. Zheng, J. Wang, X. Zhang, J. Li, and Y. Sun, "Epidemiological evidence for the link between sleep duration and high blood pressure: a systematic review and meta-analysis," *Sleep Medicine*, vol. 14, no. 4, pp. 324–332, 2013.

[18] Centers for Disease Control and Prevention (CDC), "Vital signs: awareness and treatment of uncontrolled hypertension among adults—United States, 2003–2010," *Morbidity and Mortality Weekly Report*, vol. 61, no. 35, pp. 703–709, 2012.

[19] H. Colten and B. Altevogt, *Sleep Disorders and Sleep Deprivation*, The National Academies Press, 2006.

[20] A. Fyhri and G. M. Aasvang, "Noise, sleep and poor health: modeling the relationship between road traffic noise and cardiovascular problems," *Science of the Total Environment*, vol. 408, no. 21, pp. 4935–4942, 2010.

[21] R. M. Baron and D. A. Kenny, "The moderator-mediator variable distinction in social psychological research: conceptual, strategic, and statistical considerations," *Journal of Personality and Social Psychology*, vol. 51, no. 6, pp. 1173–1182, 1986.

[22] E. M. Hill, R. Billington, and C. Krägeloh, "Noise sensitivity and diminished health: testing moderators and mediators of the relationship," *Noise and Health*, vol. 16, no. 68, pp. 47–56, 2014.

[23] L. Hale, T. D. Hill, and A. M. Burdette, "Does sleep quality mediate the association between neighborhood disorder and self-rated physical health?" *Preventive Medicine*, vol. 51, no. 3-4, pp. 275–278, 2010.

[24] F. Schmidt, K. Kolle, K. Kreuder et al., "Nighttime aircraft noise impairs endothelial function and increases blood pressure in patients with or at high risk for coronary artery disease," *Clinical Research in Cardiology*, vol. 104, no. 1, pp. 23–30, 2015.

[25] K. L. Knutson, E. van Cauter, P. J. Rathouz et al., "Association between sleep and blood pressure in midlife: the CARDIA sleep study," *Archives of Internal Medicine*, vol. 169, no. 11, pp. 1055–1061, 2009.

[26] A. Pandey, N. Williams, M. Donat et al., "Linking sleep to hypertension: greater risk for blacks," *International Journal of Hypertension*, vol. 2013, Article ID 436502, 7 pages, 2013.

[27] U.S. Department of Health and Human Services, Determinants of health, 2014, https://www.healthypeople.gov/2020/about/foundation-health-measures/Determinants-of-Health.

[28] A. Muzet, "Environmental noise, sleep and health," *Sleep Medicine Reviews*, vol. 11, no. 2, pp. 135–142, 2007.

[29] T. van Renterghem and D. Botteldooren, "Focused study on the quiet side effect in dwellings highly exposed to road traffic noise," *International Journal of Environmental Research and Public Health*, vol. 9, no. 12, pp. 4292–4310, 2012.

[30] R. R. M. Gershon, R. Neitzel, M. A. Barrera, and M. Akram, "Pilot survey of subway and bus stop noise levels," *Journal of Urban Health*, vol. 83, no. 5, pp. 802–812, 2006.

[31] New York City Department of Environmental Protection, "Transit operations strategies, new york city noise code," Local law 113 of 2005, 2010, http://www.nyc.gov/, http://www.nyc.gov/html/dep/pdf/noise/transit-noise-study.pdf.

[32] W. Passchier-Vermeer and W. F. Passchier, "Noise exposure and public health," *Environmental Health Perspectives*, vol. 108, supplement 1, pp. 123–131, 2000.

[33] T.-Y. Chang, R. Beelen, S.-F. Li et al., "Road traffic noise frequency and prevalent hypertension in Taichung, Taiwan: a cross-sectional study," *Environmental Health*, vol. 13, article 37, 2014.

[34] T.-Y. Chang, Y.-A. Lai, H.-H. Hsieh, J.-S. Lai, and C.-S. Liu, "Effects of environmental noise exposure on ambulatory blood pressure in young adults," *Environmental Research*, vol. 109, no. 7, pp. 900–905, 2009.

[35] C. Eriksson, M. Rosenlund, G. Pershagen, A. Hilding, C.-G. Östenson, and G. Bluhm, "Aircraft noise and incidence of hypertension," *Epidemiology*, vol. 18, no. 6, pp. 716–721, 2007.

[36] L. Jarup, W. Babisch, D. Houthuijs et al., "Hypertension and exposure to noise near airports: the HYENA study," *Environmental Health Perspectives*, vol. 116, no. 3, pp. 329–333, 2008.

[37] M. Sørensen, M. Hvidberg, B. Hoffmann et al., "Exposure to road traffic and railway noise and associations with blood pressure and self-reported hypertension: a cohort study," *Environmental Health*, vol. 10, no. 1, article 92, 2011.

[38] G. L. Bluhm, N. Berglind, E. Nordling, and M. Rosenlund, "Road traffic noise and hypertension," *Occupational and Environmental Medicine*, vol. 64, no. 2, pp. 122–126, 2007.

[39] W. Babisch, G. Wölke, J. Heinrich, and W. Straff, "Road traffic noise and hypertension—accounting for the location of rooms," *Environmental Research*, vol. 133, pp. 380–387, 2014.

[40] C. Eriksson, M. E. Nilsson, S. M. Willers, L. Gidhagen, T. Bellander, and G. Pershagen, "Traffic noise and cardiovascular health in Sweden: the roadside study," *Noise and Health*, vol. 14, no. 59, pp. 140–147, 2012.

[41] J. Dratva, H. C. Phuleria, M. Foraster et al., "Transportation noise and blood pressure in a population-based sample of adults," *Environmental Health Perspectives*, vol. 120, no. 1, pp. 50–55, 2012.

[42] A. S. Haralabidis, K. Dimakopoulou, V. Velonaki et al., "Can exposure to noise affect the 24 h blood pressure profile? Results from the HYENA study," *Journal of Epidemiology and Community Health*, vol. 65, no. 6, pp. 535–541, 2011.

[43] G. A. Belojević, B. D. Jakovljević, V. J. Stojanov, V. Ž. Slep and K. Ž. Paunović, "Nighttime road-traffic noise and arterial hypertension in an urban population," *Hypertension Research* vol. 31, no. 4, pp. 775–781, 2008.

[44] L. Barregard, E. Bonde, and E. Öhrström, "Risk of hypertension from exposure to road traffic noise in a population-based sample," *Occupational and Environmental Medicine*, vol. 66, no. 6, pp. 410–415, 2009.

[45] Y. de Kluizenaar, R. T. Gansevoort, H. M. E. Miedema, and P. E. de Jong, "Hypertension and road traffic noise exposure," of Occupational & Environmental Medicine, vol. 49, no. 5, pp. 484–492, 2007.

[46] U.S. Environmental Protection Agency, *National Ambient Air Quality Standards (NAAQS)*, 2011, http://www.epa.gov/ www.epa.gov/air/criteria.html.

[47] New York State Department of Environmental Conservation, PM2.5 / PM10 monitoring data, 2011, http://www.dec.ny.gov/ chemical/8888.html.

[48] N. Canha, S. M. Almeida, M. C. Freitas, and H. T. Wolterbeek, "Indoor and outdoor biomonitoring using lichens at urban and rural primary schools," *Journal of Toxicology and Environmental Health A*, vol. 77, no. 14–16, pp. 900–915, 2014.

[49] A. Hajat, A. V. Diez-Roux, N. Jenny, A. Szpiro, and J. Kaufman, "Long-term exposure to air pollution and markers of inflammation, coagulation and endothelial activation: a repeat measures analysis in the multi-ethnic study of atherosclerosis," *Circulation*, vol. 129, supplement 1, p. AP243, 2014.

[50] D. L. DeMeo, A. Zanobetti, A. A. Litonjua, B. A. Coull, J. Schwartz, and D. R. Gold, "Ambient air pollution and oxygen saturation," *The American Journal of Respiratory and Critical Care Medicine*, vol. 170, no. 4, pp. 383–387, 2004.

[51] A. Zanobetti, S. Redline, J. Schwartz et al., "Associations of PM10 with sleep and sleep-disordered breathing in adults from seven U.S. urban areas," *The American Journal of Respiratory and Critical Care Medicine*, vol. 182, no. 6, pp. 819–825, 2010.

[52] H. Luttmann-Gibson, S. E. Sarnat, H. H. Suh et al., "Short-term effects of air pollution on oxygen saturation in a cohort of senior adults in steubenville, Ohio," *Journal of Occupational and Environmental Medicine*, vol. 56, no. 2, pp. 149–154, 2014.

[53] P. L. Ljungman and M. A. Mittleman, "Ambient air pollution and stroke," *Stroke*, vol. 45, no. 12, pp. 3734–3741, 2014.

[54] R. D. Brook, S. Rajagopalan, C. A. Pope III et al., "Particulate matter air pollution and cardiovascular disease: an update to the scientific statement from the American Heart Association," *Circulation*, vol. 121, no. 21, pp. 2331–2378, 2010.

[55] D. Johnson and J. D. Parker, "Air pollution exposure and self-reported cardiovascular disease," *Environmental Research*, vol. 109, no. 5, pp. 582–589, 2009.

[56] P. F. Coogan, L. F. White, M. Jerrett et al., "Air pollution and incidence of hypertension and diabetes mellitus in black women living in Los Angeles," *Circulation*, vol. 125, no. 6, pp. 767–772, 2012.

[57] K. J. Chuang, Y. H. Yan, and T. J. Cheng, "Effect of air pollution on blood pressure, blood lipids, and blood sugar: a population-based approach," *Journal of Occupational and Environmental Medicine*, vol. 52, no. 3, pp. 258–262, 2010.

[58] F. M. Dong, Y. Z. Mo, G. X. Li, M. M. Xu, and X. C. Pan, "Association between ambient $PM_{10}/PM_{2.5}$ levels and population mortality of circulatory diseases: a case-crossover study in Beijing," *Beijing Da Xue Xue Bao*, vol. 45, no. 3, pp. 398–404, 2013.

[59] A. Zanobetti, M. J. Canner, P. H. Stone et al., "Ambient pollution and blood pressure in cardiac rehabilitation patients," *Circulation*, vol. 110, no. 15, pp. 2184–2189, 2004.

[60] J. T. Dvonch, S. Kannan, A. J. Schulz et al., "Acute effects of ambient particulate matter on blood pressure: differential effects across urban communities," *Hypertension*, vol. 53, no. 5, pp. 853–859, 2009.

[61] K. Fuks, S. Moebus, S. Hertel et al., "Long-term urban particulate air pollution, traffic noise, and arterial blood pressure," *Environmental Health Perspectives*, vol. 119, no. 12, pp. 1706–1711, 2011.

[62] A. H. Auchincloss, A. V. Diez Roux, J. T. Dvonch et al., "Associations between recent exposure to ambient fine particulate matter and blood pressure in the multi-ethnic study of atherosclerosis (MESA)," *Environmental Health Perspectives*, vol. 116, no. 4, pp. 486–491, 2008.

[63] J. Schwartz, S. E. Alexeeff, I. Mordukhovich et al., "Association between long-term exposure to traffic particles and blood pressure in the veterans administration normative aging study," *Occupational & Environmental Medicine*, vol. 69, no. 6, pp. 422–427, 2012.

[64] M. Sørensen, B. Hoffmann, M. Hvidberg et al., "Long-term exposure to traffic-related air pollution associated with blood pressure and self-reported hypertension in a Danish Cohort," *Environmental Health Perspectives*, vol. 120, no. 3, pp. 418–424, 2012.

[65] K. J. Chuang, Y. H. Yan, S. Y. Chiu, and T. J. Cheng, "Long-term air pollution exposure and risk factors for cardiovascular diseases among the elderly in Taiwan," *Occupational and Environmental Medicine*

[66] L. Hale and D. P. Do, "Racial differences in self-reports of sleep duration in a population-based study," *Sleep*, vol. 30, no. 9, pp. 1096–1103, 2007.

[67] M. Saremi, J. Grenèche, A. Bonnefond, O. Rohmer, A. Eschenlauer, and P. Tassi, "Effects of nocturnal railway noise on sleep fragmentation in young and middle-aged subjects as a function of type of train and sound level," *International Journal of Psy-*

chophysiology, vol. 70, no. 3, pp. 184–191, 2008.

[68] M. Basner, U. Müller, and E.-M. Elmenhorst, "Single and combined effects of air, road, and rail traffic noise on sleep and recuperation," *Sleep*, vol. 34, no. 1, pp. 11–23, 2011.

[69] B. Jakovljević, G. Belojević, K. Paunović, and V. Stojanov, "Road traffic noise and sleep disturbances in an urban population: cross-sectional study," *Croatian Medical Journal*, vol. 47, no. 1, pp. 125–133, 2006.

[70] B. Gitanjali and R. Dhamotharan, "Effect of occupational noise on the nocturnal sleep architecture of healthy subjects," *Journal of Physiology and Pharmacology*, vol. 47, no. 4, pp. 415–422, 2003.

[71] S. Agarwal and B. L. Swami, "Road traffic noise, annoyance and community health survey—a case study for an Indian city," *Noise and Health*, vol. 13, no. 53, pp. 272–276, 2011.

[72] M. Basner and A. Samel, "Effects of nocturnal aircraft noise on sleep structure," *Somnologie*, vol. 9, no. 2, pp. 84–95, 2005.

[73] B. Griefahn, A. Marks, and S. Robens, "Noise emitted from road, rail and air traffic and their effects on sleep," *Journal of Sound and Vibration*, vol. 295, no. 1-2, pp. 129–140, 2006.

[74] S. Pirrera, E. de Valck, and R. Cluydts, "Field study on the impact of nocturnal road traffic noise on sleep: the importance of in- and outdoor noise assessment, the bedroom location and nighttime noise disturbances," *Science of the Total Environment* vol. 500-501, pp. 84–90, 2014.

[75] M. K. Abou-Khadra, "Association between PM10 exposure and sleep of Egyptian school children," *Sleep and Breathing*, vol. 17, no. 2, pp. 653–657, 2013.

[76] S. C. Fang, J. Schwartz, M. Yang, H. K. Yaggi, D. L. Bliwise, and A. B. Araujo, "Traffic-related air pollution and sleep in the Boston area community health survey," *Journal of Exposure Science and Environmental Epidemiology*, 2014.

[77] K. Wolf-Maier, R. S. Cooper, J. R. Banegas et al., "Hypertension prevalence and blood pressure levels in 6 European countries, Canada, and the United States," *The Journal of the American Medical Association*, vol. 289, no. 18, pp. 2363–2369, 2003.

[78] T. A. Kotchen and J. M. Kotchen, "Regional variations of blood pressure: environment or genes?" *Circulation*, vol. 96, no. 4, pp. 1071–1073, 1997.

[79] S. Fidell, K. Pearsons, B. Tabachnick, R. Howe, L. Silvati, and D. S. Barber, "Field study of noise-induced sleep disturbance," *Journal of the Acoustical Society of America*, vol. 98, no. 2, pp. 1025–1033, 1995.

[80] E. Öhrström, "Longitudinal surveys on effects of changes in road traffic noise—annoyance, activity disturbances, and psycho-social well-being," *The Journal of the Acoustical Society of America*, vol. 115, no. 2, pp. 719–729, 2004.

[81] S. Fidell, K. Pearsons, B. G. Tabachnick, and R. Howe, "Effects on sleep disturbance of changes in aircraft noise near three airports," *Journal of the Acoustical Society of America*, vol. 107, no. 5, pp. 2535–2547, 2000.

[82] J. A. Horne, F. L. Pankhurst, L. A. Reyner, K. Hume, and I. D. Diamond, "A field study of sleep disturbance: effects of aircraft noise and other factors on 5,742 nights of actimetrically monitored sleep in a large subject sample," *Sleep*, vol. 17, no. 2, pp. 146–159, 1994.

[83] D. S. Michaud, S. Fidell, K. Pearsons, K. C. Campbell, and S. E. Keith, "Review of field studies of aircraft noise-induced sleep disturbance," *Journal of the Acoustical Society of America*, vol. 121, no. 1, pp. 32–41, 2007.

[84] Y. Aydin and M. Kaltenbach, "Noise perception, heart rate and blood pressure in relation to aircraft noise in the vicinity of the Frankfurt airport," *Clinical Research in Cardiology*, vol. 96, no. 6, pp. 347–358, 2007.

[85] W. Dement and N. Kleitman, "Cyclic variations in EEG during sleep and their relation to eye movements, body motility, and dreaming," *Electroencephalography and Clinical Neurophysiology*, vol. 9, no. 4, pp. 673–690, 1957.

[86] B. Crüts, L. van Etten, H. Törnqvist et al., "Exposure to diesel exhaust induces changes in EEG in human volunteers," *Particle and Fibre Toxicology*, vol. 5, article no. 11, 2008.

[87] R. J. O. Davies, P. J. Belt, S. J. Roberts, N. J. Ali, and J. R. Stradling, "Arterial blood pressure responses to graded transient arousal from sleep in normal humans," *Journal of Applied Physiology*, vol. 74, no. 3, pp. 1123–1130, 1993.

[88] National Institute of Health, Air pollution and risk of incident hypertension and diabetes in U.S. black women, 2014, http://projectreporter.nih.gov/project_info_description.cfm?aid=8650890&icde=22795915&ddparam=&ddvalue=&ddsub=&cr=2&csb=default&cs=ASC.

[89] W. Choi, S. Hu, M. He et al., "Neighborhood-scale air quality impacts of emissions from motor vehicles and aircraft," *Atmospheric Environment*, vol. 80, pp. 310–321, 2013.

[90] D. Houston, J. Wu, P. Ong, and A. Winer, "Structural disparities of urban traffic in Southern California: implications for vehicle-related air pollution exposure in minority and high-poverty neighborhoods," *Journal of Urban Affairs*, vol. 26, no. 5, pp. 565–592, 2004.

[91] N. P. Patel, M. A. Grandner, D. Xie, C. C. Branas, and N. Gooneratne, "'Sleep disparity' in the population: poor sleep quality is strongly associated with poverty and ethnicity," *BMC Public Health*, vol. 10, article 475, 2010.

[92] J. Whinnery, N. Jackson, P. Rattanaumpawan, and M. A. Grandner, "Short and long sleep duration associated with race/ethnicity, sociodemographics, and Socioeconomic position," *Sleep*, vol. 37, no. 3, pp. 601–611, 2014.

[93] Y. Song, S. Ancoli-Israel, C. E. Lewis, S. Redline, S. L. Harrison, and K. L. Stone, "The association of race/ethnicity with objectively measured sleep characteristics in older men," *Behavioral Sleep Medicine*, vol. 10, no. 1, pp. 54–69, 2011.

[94] D. S. Lauderdale, K. L. Knutson, L. L. Yan et al., "Objectively measured sleep characteristics among early-middle-aged adults: the CARDIA study," *The American Journal of Epidemiology*, vol. 164, no. 1, pp. 5–16, 2006.

17

Beneficial Effects of Dietary Nitrate on Endothelial Function and Blood Pressure Levels

Jenifer d'El-Rei, Ana Rosa Cunha, Michelle Trindade, and Mario Fritsch Neves

Department of Clinical Medicine, State University of Rio de Janeiro, 20551-030 Rio de Janeiro, RJ, Brazil

Correspondence should be addressed to Jenifer d'El-Rei; jeniferdelrei@gmail.com

Academic Editor: Claudio Borghi

Poor eating habits may represent cardiovascular risk factors since high intake of fat and saturated fatty acids contributes to dyslipidemia, obesity, diabetes mellitus, and hypertension. Thus, nutritional interventions are recognized as important strategies for primary prevention of hypertension and as adjuvants to pharmacological therapies to reduce cardiovascular risk. The DASH (Dietary Approach to Stop Hypertension) plan is one of the most effective strategies for the prevention and nonpharmacological management of hypertension. The beneficial effects of DASH diet on blood pressure might be related to the high inorganic nitrate content of some food products included in this meal plan. The beetroot and other food plants considered as nitrate sources account for approximately 60–80% of the daily nitrate exposure in the western population. The increased levels of nitrite by nitrate intake seem to have beneficial effects in many of the physiological and clinical settings. Several clinical trials are being conducted to determine the broad therapeutic potential of increasing the bioavailability of nitrite in human health and disease, including studies related to vascular aging. In conclusion, the dietary inorganic nitrate seems to represent a promising complementary therapy to support hypertension treatment with benefits for cardiovascular health.

1. Introduction

Hypertension is a multifactorial condition characterized by high and sustained levels of blood pressure (BP). It is the most common condition in primary care and often associated with functional and/or structural changes in target organs and metabolic disorders, increasing the risk of fatal and nonfatal cardiovascular events [1, 2]. Among the risk factors for mortality from cardiovascular disease (CVD), hypertension explains 40% and 25% of deaths from stroke and coronary artery disease (CAD), respectively [3].

BP is a biological and dynamic variable, dependent on many factors. Endothelial cells of the vascular system are responsible for many biochemical reactions that maintain vascular homeostasis and consequently the BP levels [4]. Endothelium modulates vascular tone, not only by producing vasodilator substances but also by releasing vasoconstrictive substances through prostanoid of endothelin generation, as well as through conversion of angiotensin I (AI) in angiotensin II (AII) on the endothelial surface. These vasoconstrictor agents not only act mainly locally but also present some systemic effects, playing an important role in regulating the vascular function and remodeling the arterial wall. In healthy individuals, there is a balance among these substances, tending to vasodilatation when endothelial function is normal [5].

2. Nitric Oxide (NO), Endothelial Dysfunction, and Metabolic Syndrome

Changes in endothelial function precede morphological changes of blood vessels and contribute to the development of clinical complications of cardiovascular diseases. Thus, the beginning and the clinical course of adverse cardiovascular events depend directly on changes in vascular biology. Lately, it became clear that the endothelium is responsible for promoting vascular homeostasis [5].

The limited NO bioavailability is the main mechanism involved in endothelial dysfunction, which is crucial for the development of CVD [6]. In fact, endothelial dysfunction in peripheral and coronary vessels is an independent predictor of cardiovascular events and represents an early stage of

CAD [7]. As endothelial dysfunction is reversible, early detection and intervention could have critical therapeutic and prognostic implications for patients with risk for, or even with established, CVD [7, 8]. Therefore, an improvement in the NO bioavailability can have a major effect on endothelial function and, consequently, on CVD prevention and treatment [9, 10].

Metabolic syndrome can be considered a clinical and biochemical expression of insulin resistance, representing a clustering of central obesity, hypertension, hyperglycemia, and dyslipidemia [19, 20]. Recently, experimental models and clinical studies demonstrated that reductions in the NO bioavailability play a central role in the pathophysiology of metabolic dysfunction. Endothelial nitric oxide synthase- (eNOS-) deficient mice were able to develop high BP and metabolic dysfunction, and both might be the result of insulin resistance [21, 22]. In the same experimental model, several features of metabolic syndrome could be reversed by dietary supplementation with sodium nitrate. The amount of dietary nitrate used for this effect was comparable to those derived from eNOS under normal conditions, which corresponds to a rich intake of vegetables for humans. Besides, dietary nitrate was able to increase tissue and plasma levels of bioactive nitrogen oxides. Lastly, chronic nitrate supplementation prevented the prediabetic phenotype in these animals by reducing visceral fat accumulation and circulating levels of triglycerides [23]. In humans, eNOS polymorphisms have been associated with insulin resistance, type 2 diabetes mellitus, and metabolic syndrome [21]. Furthermore, recent evidences have shown that obese subjects present a reduced ability to produce NO [10, 24]. Therefore, the dietary nitrate has been widely studied in clinical trials as an alternative form of the classical pathway of L-arginine to NO production.

3. Sources and Beneficial Effects of Dietary Nitrate

Poor eating habits may be considered as risk factors for CVD. In fact, high intake of foods rich in cholesterol, lipids, and saturated fatty acids and low consumption of fiber sources are related to dyslipidemia, obesity, diabetes mellitus, and hypertension [25]. Thus, nutritional interventions associated with changes in lifestyle are recognized as important strategies for primary prevention of hypertension and are auxiliary to pharmacological therapies to reduce cardiovascular risk [26].

Epidemiological evidences suggest that vegetable consumption reduces BP and risk of CVD [27–29]. DASH (Dietary Approach to Stop Hypertension) eating plan is one of the major effective strategies for prevention and nonpharmacological management of hypertension [30]. This eating proposal highlights the importance of increasing fruit and vegetables intake [31], and recent research suggests that the beneficial effects of DASH plan on BP are related to high inorganic nitrate content of food included in this eating plan (e.g., green leaves and root vegetables) [32, 33].

Beetroots, lettuce, chard, arugula, and spinach are the vegetables containing the highest amount of nitrate, >250 mg nitrate/100 g [32]. Table 1 shows the vegetables

TABLE 1: Vegetables grouping according to the nitrate concentration [11].

Nitrate content (mg/100 g of fresh food)	Vegetables
Very low, <20 mg	Asparagus, garlic, onion, green bean, pepper, potato, sweet potato, tomato, and watermelon
Low, 20–<50 mg	Broccoli, carrot, cauliflower, and chicory
Regular, 50–<100 mg	Cabbage, turnip, and dill
High, 100–<250 mg	Endive, sweet leaf, parsley, and leek
Very high, >250 mg	Celery, chard, lettuce, beetroot, spinach, arugula, and watercress

classification according to the nitrate content. Beetroot is a vegetable, particularly rich in inorganic nitrate, which contains an average of 2056 mg of nitrate in a traditional cultivation. There are some studies using beetroot to test the effects of inorganic nitrate intake on BP [18].

Nitrate (NO_3^-) and nitrite (NO_2^-), present in beetroot and in other food sources, were recently related to cardiovascular benefits. However, they were previously considered as toxic compounds due to the development of malignancies such as gastric cancer. Therefore, strict rules regarding these inorganic anions are regulated in food and in drinking water [34].

Beetroot and other vegetables sources of nitrate contain approximately 60–80% of the daily nitrate intake in the western population [32]. Nitrate content in vegetables may be influenced by factors related to the plant itself, such as variety, species, and maturity, and to the environment, such as temperature, light intensity, lack of some nutrients, and fertilizer use [11].

International organizations indicate that the consumption of dietary nitrate is about 31 to 185 mg/day in Europe and 40 to 100 mg/day in USA [35], and the oral bioavailability of dietary nitrate is 100% [36]. In 1962, World Health Organization (WHO) set an upper limit of nitrate consumption in food. An acceptable daily intake is 3.7 mg NO_3^-/body weight (kg), which is the same value adopted by the European Authority for Food Safety. This amount is equivalent to 300 mg/day for an adult weighing 80 kg [37]. However, there is no evidence that nitrate intake is carcinogenic in humans. Instead, epidemiological evidence indicates that consumption of vegetables reduces risk of cancer [38].

After intake, dietary nitrate quickly increases in plasma, in about 30 minutes, reaching its peak in 90 minutes. In contrast, nitrite levels are considerably slower in circulation, reaching their peak in 2.5 to 3 hours. Most of inorganic nitrate, about 75% of absorbed nitrate, is excreted in urine and 25% of plasma nitrate is excreted in saliva [18, 39]. The exact mechanism of salivary concentration is unknown. As a result, there is supply of substrate for nitrate reductase expressed by bacteria that colonize the dorsal surface of the tongue, resulting in reduction of nitrate to nitrite. After nitrite is then swallowed, the stomach and the acid environment reduce it to NO. The remaining nitrite is reabsorbed again by the vascular flow [40]. NO and nitrite continue through the systemic circulation, and the remaining nitrite is reduced to NO in high resistance vessels, promoting vasodilatation and consequently lowering BP [18] (Figure 1). Both NO_3^- and NO_2^- from diet and via L-arginine participate in the NO synthesis [41]. Lately, there is a growing body of interest on the role of these two anions in biological function. The improvement in vascular dysfunction and in BP levels after dietary nitrate seems to be mediated by effects on oxidative stress and inflammation [42, 43].

4. Effects of Dietary Nitrate on Blood Pressure

After an acute intake of beetroot juice (500 mL), it is possible to observe reduction of 10 mmHg in systolic BP (after 2.5 h) and reduction of 8 mmHg in diastolic BP (after 3 h) in healthy individuals. The decrease in BP was sustained after 24 h of juice intake. The highest reduction in BP is correlated to the peak in plasma nitrite [18].

Liu et al. evaluated the effects of a meal rich in nitrate (based on spinach consumption) on BP and arterial stiffness in healthy individuals. Two hours after a nitrate-rich meal consumption (220 mg nitrate), there was a larger artery elasticity index, lower pulse pressure, and lower systolic BP compared to the values after a standard meal, low in nitrate [44].

Recent experimental studies [23, 45, 46] and clinical trials have shown that nitrate dietary intakes from beetroot juice [18, 47], beet-enriched bread [48], or inorganic nitrate supplements [49] have a protective effect against CVD because of reducing BP, platelet aggregation inhibition, and prevention of endothelial dysfunction.

Recently, Bondonno et al. have shown that chronic ingestion of beetroot juice (one week, 420 mg nitrate/day) did not improve the BP control in treated hypertensive patients [13]. In another study with overweight elderly subjects, Jajja et al. showed reduction of 7 mmHg in systolic BP, after three weeks of beetroot juice intake (350 mg nitrate/day). However, when BP was evaluated for 24 hours by ambulatory blood pressure monitoring (ABPM), no significant changes were shown in BP levels [14]. Table 2 shows some clinical trials that evaluated the effects of nitrate intake on BP and vascular function. In fact, there is no consensus about the effects of dietary inorganic nitrates on BP and endothelial function, and their effects on cardiovascular health, despite studies with positive results.

Since the initial investigations in healthy volunteers, studies using inorganic nitrate and formulations with nitrate salt showed promising results reducing BP, with nitrate doses ranging from 155 to 1484 mg/day, between 1 and 15 days, with reductions of 4 mmHg in systolic BP and of 1 mmHg in diastolic BP [33, 50]. In hypertensive patients, systolic BP remained significantly reduced in approximately 8 mmHg over 24 hours after the intervention, which is similar to the reduction provided by drug therapy (9 mmHg). This is important because the ingestion of dietary nitrate in a single

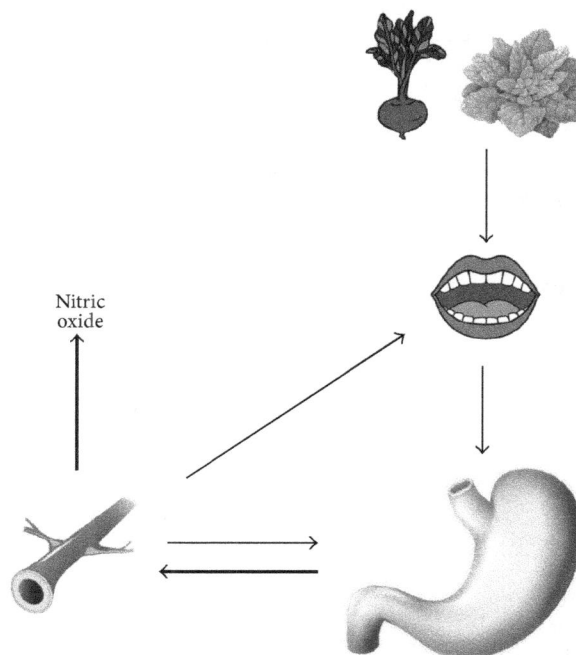

FIGURE 1: Nitrate (thin arrows) intake from the diet is swallowed and completely absorbed in the upper gastrointestinal tract. About 25% of this amount is concentrated in the salivary glands and still inside the mouth is reduced to nitrite by anaerobic bacteria present on the tongue and is swallowed again. In the stomach, nitrite acid undergoes reduction and is converted to NO (thick arrows) that has vasodilatory action on blood vessels.

dose per day may be sufficient to achieve benefits in lowering BP [50, 51].

5. Conclusion

Increasing nitrite levels by nitrate intake appears to have beneficial effects in many physiologic and clinical settings. Several clinical trials are being conducted to determine the great therapeutic potential of increasing the bioavailability of nitrite in human health and disease, including studies related to vascular aging. Nevertheless, there are many limitations in nitrate studies, such as the type of population enrolled in each trial and the dependent effect of the baseline BP. Therefore, the effects are unlikely to be the same among healthy and hypertensive individuals. In addition, when evaluating treated hypertensive patients, use of medications, such as calcium channel antagonists, may affect endothelial function and hence can interfere in some vascular parameters. Sample size is also a limiting factor considering the fact that it is small in most of nitrate studies. Indeed, large clinical trials are necessary to confirm the potential beneficial effects of inorganic nitrate in patients with CVD. Even with these considerations, dietary nitrate seems to represent an inexpensive and a promising complementary therapy to support hypertension treatment with benefits for cardiovascular health.

TABLE 2: Clinical trials evaluating the effects of dietary inorganic nitrate on cardiovascular health.

Population	Study design and duration	Nitrate dose	Control	Vascular parameter	Result	Reference
Hypertensive $n = 68$ 57 years 144/88 mmHg	Chronic 4 weeks	450 mg (250 mL beetroot juice)	Beetroot juice poor in nitrate	PWV FMD SBP DBP	↓ PWV, ↑ FMD ↓ SBP, ↓ DBP ↓ SBP$_{24h}$ ↓ DBP$_{24h}$	Kapil et al., 2015 [12]
Hypertensive $n = 27$ 63 years 133/77 mmHg	Chronic 1 week	420 mg (140 mL beetroot juice)	Beetroot juice poor in nitrate	SBP DBP	No effect	Bondonno et al., 2015 [13]
Overweight elderly $n = 24$ 63 years	Chronic 3 weeks	±350 mg (70 mL beetroot juice)	Blackcurrant juice	SBP DBP	↓ SBP No effect on DBP	Jajja et al., 2014 [14]
T2DM $n = 27$ 67 years 143/81 mmHg	Chronic 2 weeks	500 mg (250 mL beetroot juice)	Beetroot juice poor in nitrate	FMD	No effect	Gilchrist et al., 2013 [15]
Healthy $n = 30$ 47 years 112/68 mmHg	Acute 0–2 h	190 mg (200 g spinach)	Rice milk	FMD	2% ↑ after 2 h	Bondonno et al., 2012 [16]
Healthy $n = 9$ 25 years 121/71 mmHg	Acute 0–3 h	375 mg (250 mL beetroot juice)	Mineral water	SBP DBP	↓ SBP after 3 h No effect on DBP	Kapil et al., 2010 [17]
Healthy $n = 14$ 26 years 106/70 mmHg	Acute 0–6 h–24 h	1437 mg (500 mL beetroot juice)	Mineral water	SBP DBP MAP	↓ SBP ↓ DBP ↓ MAP	Webb et al., 2008 [18]
Healthy $n = 10$ 27 years	Acute 0–2 h	1437 mg (500 mL beetroot juice)	Mineral water	FMD	Protection against reperfusion ischemia after 2 h	Webb et al., 2008 [18]

T2DM, type 2 diabetes mellitus; PWV, pulse wave velocity; FMD, flow mediated dilation; SBP, systolic blood pressure; DBP, diastolic blood pressure; MAP, mean arterial pressure.

Competing Interests

The authors declare that they have no competing interests.

References

[1] P. A. James, S. Oparil, B. L. Carter et al., "2014 Evidence-based guideline for the management of high blood pressure in adults: report from the panel members appointed to the Eighth Joint National Committee (JNC 8)," *The Journal of the American Medical Association*, vol. 311, no. 5, pp. 507–520, 2014.

[2] M. Pereira, N. Lunet, A. Azevedo, and H. Barros, "Differences in prevalence, awareness, treatment and control of hypertension between developing and developed countries," *Journal of Hypertension*, vol. 27, no. 5, pp. 963–975, 2009.

[3] C. Lenfant, A. V. Chobanian, D. W. Jones, and E. J. Roccella, "Seventh report of the Joint National Committee on the Prevention, Detection, Evaluation, and Treatment of High Blood Pressure (JNC 7): resetting the hypertension sails," *Hypertension*, vol. 41, no. 6, pp. 1178–1179, 2003.

[4] F. Contreras, M. Rivera, J. Vásquez, M. A. De La Parte, and M. Velasco, "Endothelial dysfunction in arterial hypertension," *Journal of Human Hypertension*, vol. 14, supplement 1, pp. S20–S25, 2000.

[5] J. E. Deanfield, J. P. Halcox, and T. J. Rabelink, "Endothelial function and dysfunction: testing and clinical relevance," *Circulation*, vol. 115, no. 10, pp. 1285–1295, 2007.

[6] H. Cai and D. G. Harrison, "Endothelial dysfunction in cardiovascular diseases: the role of oxidant stress," *Circulation Research*, vol. 87, no. 10, pp. 840–844, 2000.

[7] J. D. Rossen, Y. Agmon, R. Gorlin, E. C. Abbott, K. Egashira, and A. Takeshita, "Endothelial dysfunction in microvascular angina," *The New England Journal of Medicine*, vol. 329, no. 23, pp. 1739–1740, 1993.

[8] P. O. Bonetti, G. M. Pumper, S. T. Higano, D. R. Holmes Jr., J. T. Kuvin, and A. Lerman, "Noninvasive identification of patients with early coronary atherosclerosis by assessment of digital reactive hyperemia," *Journal of the American College of Cardiology*, vol. 44, no. 11, pp. 2137–2141, 2004.

[9] D. A. Hobbs, T. W. George, and J. A. Lovegrove, "The effects of dietary nitrate on blood pressure and endothelial function: a review of human intervention studies," *Nutrition Research Reviews*, vol. 26, no. 2, pp. 210–222, 2013.

[10] B. McNally, J. L. Griffin, and L. D. Roberts, "Dietary inorganic nitrate: from villain to hero in metabolic disease?" *Molecular Nutrition & Food Research*, vol. 60, no. 1, pp. 67–78, 2016.

[11] A. H. Gorenjak and A. Cencič, "Nitrate in vegetables and their impact on human health. A review," *Acta Alimentaria*, vol. 42, no. 2, pp. 158–172, 2013.

[12] V. Kapil, R. S. Khambata, A. Robertson, M. J. Caulfield, and A. Ahluwalia, "Dietary nitrate provides sustained blood pressure lowering in hypertensive patients: a randomized, phase 2, double-blind, placebo-controlled study," *Hypertension*, vol. 65, no. 2, pp. 320–327, 2015.

[13] C. P. Bondonno, A. H. Liu, K. D. Croft et al., "Absence of an effect of high nitrate intake from beetroot juice on blood pressure in treated hypertensive individuals: a randomized controlled trial," *The American Journal of Clinical Nutrition*, vol. 102, no. 2, pp. 368–375, 2015.

[14] A. Jajja, A. Sutyarjoko, J. Lara et al., "Beetroot supplementation lowers daily systolic blood pressure in older, overweight subjects," *Nutrition Research*, vol. 34, no. 10, pp. 868–875, 2014.

[15] M. Gilchrist, P. G. Winyard, K. Aizawa, C. Anning, A. Shore, and N. Benjamin, "Effect of dietary nitrate on blood pressure, endothelial function, and insulin sensitivity in type 2 diabetes," *Free Radical Biology and Medicine*, vol. 60, pp. 89–97, 2013.

[16] C. P. Bondonno, K. D. Croft, I. B. Puddey et al., "Nitrate causes a dose-dependent augmentation of nitric oxide status in healthy women," *Food and Function*, vol. 3, no. 5, pp. 522–527, 2012.

[17] V. Kapil, A. J. Webb, and A. Ahluwalia, "Inorganic nitrate and the cardiovascular system," *Heart*, vol. 96, no. 21, pp. 1703–1709, 2010.

[18] A. J. Webb, N. Patel, S. Loukogeorgakis et al., "Acute blood pressure lowering, vasoprotective, and antiplatelet properties of dietary nitrate via bioconversion to nitrite," *Hypertension*, vol. 51, no. 3, pp. 784–790, 2008.

[19] P. L. Huang, "A comprehensive definition for metabolic syndrome," *Disease Models and Mechanisms*, vol. 2, no. 5-6, pp. 231–237, 2009.

[20] R. H. Eckel, S. M. Grundy, and P. Z. Zimmet, "The metabolic syndrome," *The Lancet*, vol. 365, no. 9468, pp. 1415–1428, 2005.

[21] L. D. Monti, C. Barlassina, L. Citterio et al., "Endothelial nitric oxide synthase polymorphisms are associated with type 2 diabetes and the insulin resistance syndrome," *Diabetes*, vol. 52, no. 5, pp. 1270–1275, 2003.

[22] P. L. Huang, "eNOS, metabolic syndrome and cardiovascular disease," *Trends in Endocrinology and Metabolism*, vol. 20, no. 6, pp. 295–302, 2009.

[23] M. Carlström, F. J. Larsen, T. Nyström et al., "Dietary inorganic nitrate reverses features of metabolic syndrome in endothelial nitric oxide synthase-deficient mice," *Proceedings of the National Academy of Sciences of the United States of America*, vol. 107, no. 41, pp. 17716–17720, 2010.

[24] M. Siervo, S. J. Jackson, and L. J. C. Bluck, "In-vivo nitric oxide synthesis is reduced in obese patients with metabolic syndrome: application of a novel stable isotopic method," *Journal of Hypertension*, vol. 29, no. 8, pp. 1515–1527, 2011.

[25] L. Van Horn, M. McCoin, P. M. Kris-Etherton et al., "The evidence for dietary prevention and treatment of cardiovascular disease," *Journal of the American Dietetic Association*, vol. 108, no. 2, pp. 287–331, 2008.

[26] V. Savica, G. Bellinghieri, and J. D. Kopple, "The effect of nutrition on blood pressure," *Annual Review of Nutrition*, vol. 30, pp. 365–401, 2010.

[27] L. A. Bazzano, J. He, L. G. Ogden et al., "Fruit and vegetable intake and risk of cardiovascular disease in US adults: the first National Health and Nutrition Examination Survey Epidemiologic Follow-up study," *American Journal of Clinical Nutrition*, vol. 76, no. 1, pp. 93–99, 2002.

[28] K. J. Joshipura, F. B. Hu, J. E. Manson et al., "The effect of fruit and vegetable intake on risk for coronary heart disease," *Annals of Internal Medicine*, vol. 134, no. 12, pp. 1106–1114, 2001.

[29] E. R. Miller III, T. P. Erlinger, and L. J. Appel, "The effects of macronutrients on blood pressure and lipids: an overview of the DASH and OmniHeart trials," *Current Atherosclerosis Reports*, vol. 8, no. 6, pp. 460–465, 2006.

[30] L. J. Appel, M. W. Brands, S. R. Daniels, N. Karanja, P. J. Elmer, and F. M. Sacks, "Dietary approaches to prevent and treat hypertension: a scientific statement from the American Heart Association," *Hypertension*, vol. 47, no. 2, pp. 296–308, 2006.

[31] T. J. Moore, P. R. Conlin, J. Ard, and L. P. Svetkey, "DASH (Dietary Approaches to Stop Hypertension) diet is effective treatment for stage 1 isolated systolic hypertension," *Hypertension*, vol. 38, no. 2, pp. 155–158, 2001.

[32] N. G. Hord, Y. Tang, and N. S. Bryan, "Food sources of nitrates and nitrites: the physiologic context for potential health benefits," *The American Journal of Clinical Nutrition*, vol. 90, no. 1, pp. 1–10, 2009.

[33] M. Siervo, J. Lara, I. Ogbonmwan, and J. C. Mathers, "Inorganic nitrate and beetroot juice supplementation reduces blood pressure in adults: a systematic review and meta-analysis," *Journal of Nutrition*, vol. 143, no. 6, pp. 818–826, 2013.

[34] S. S. Mirvish, "Role of N-nitroso compounds (NOC) and N-nitrosation in etiology of gastric, esophageal, nasopharyngeal and bladder cancer and contribution to cancer of known exposures to NOC," *Cancer Letters*, vol. 93, no. 1, pp. 17–48, 1995.

[35] T. T. Mensinga, G. J. A. Speijers, and J. Meulenbelt, "Health implications of exposure to environmental nitrogenous compounds," *Toxicological Reviews*, vol. 22, no. 1, pp. 41–51, 2003.

[36] A. G. van Velzen, A. J. A. M. Sips, R. C. Schothorst, A. C. Lambers, and J. Meulenbelt, "The oral bioavailability of nitrate from nitrate-rich vegetables in humans," *Toxicology Letters*, vol. 181, no. 3, pp. 177–181, 2008.

[37] M. B. Katan, "Nitrate in foods: harmful or healthy?" *American Journal of Clinical Nutrition*, vol. 90, no. 1, pp. 11–12, 2009.

[38] P. Terry, J. B. Terry, and A. Wolk, "Fruit and vegetable consumption in the prevention of cancer: an update," *Journal of Internal Medicine*, vol. 250, no. 4, pp. 280–290, 2001.

[39] S. R. Tannenbaum, M. Weisman, and D. Fett, "The effect of nitrate intake on nitrite formation in human saliva," *Food and Cosmetics Toxicology*, vol. 14, no. 6, pp. 549–552, 1976.

[40] J. O. Lundberg, E. Weitzberg, J. A. Cole, and N. Benjamin, "Nitrate, bacteria and human health," *Nature Reviews Microbiology*, vol. 2, no. 7, pp. 593–602, 2004.

[41] D. A. Hobbs, M. G. Goulding, A. Nguyen et al., "Acute ingestion of beetroot bread increases endothelium-independent vasodilation and lowers diastolic blood pressure in healthymen: a randomized controlled trial," *Journal of Nutrition*, vol. 143, no. 9, pp. 1399–1405, 2013.

[42] X. Gao, T. Yang, M. Liu et al., "NADPH oxidase in the renal microvasculature is a primary target for blood pressure-lowering effects by inorganic nitrate and nitrite," *Hypertension*, vol. 65, no. 1, pp. 161–170, 2015.

[43] M. P. Hezel, M. Liu, T. A. Schiffer et al., "Effects of long-term dietary nitrate supplementation in mice," *Redox Biology*, vol. 5, pp. 234–242, 2015.

[44] A. H. Liu, C. P. Bondonno, K. D. Croft et al., "Effects of a nitrate-rich meal on arterial stiffness and blood pressure in healthy volunteers," *Nitric Oxide*, vol. 35, pp. 123–130, 2013.

[45] M. Govoni, E. Å. Jansson, E. Weitzberg, and J. O. Lundberg, "The increase in plasma nitrite after a dietary nitrate load is markedly attenuated by an antibacterial mouthwash," *Nitric Oxide*, vol. 19, no. 4, pp. 333–337, 2008.

[46] E. Å. Jansson, L. Huang, R. Malkey et al., "A mammalian functional nitrate reductase that regulates nitrite and nitric oxide homeostasis," *Nature Chemical Biology*, vol. 4, no. 7, pp. 411–417, 2008.

[47] V. Kapil, A. B. Milsom, M. Okorie et al., "Inorganic nitrate supplementation lowers blood pressure in humans: role for nitrite-derived no," *Hypertension*, vol. 56, no. 2, pp. 274–281, 2010.

[48] D. A. Hobbs, N. Kaffa, T. W. George, L. Methven, and J. A. Lovegrove, "Blood pressure-lowering effects of beetroot juice and novel beetroot-enriched bread products in normotensive male subjects," *British Journal of Nutrition*, vol. 108, no. 11, pp. 2066–2074, 2012.

[49] F. J. Larsen, B. Ekblom, K. Sahlin, J. O. Lundberg, and E. Weitzberg, "Effects of dietary nitrate on blood pressure in healthy volunteers," *The New England Journal of Medicine*, vol. 355, no. 26, pp. 2792–2793, 2006.

[50] V. Kapil, E. Weitzberg, J. O. Lundberg, and A. Ahluwalia, "Clinical evidence demonstrating the utility of inorganic nitrate in cardiovascular health," *Nitric Oxide—Biology and Chemistry*, vol. 38, no. 1, pp. 45–57, 2014.

[51] M. R. Law, J. K. Morris, and N. J. Wald, "Use of blood pressure lowering drugs in the prevention of cardiovascular disease: meta-analysis of 147 randomised trials in the context of expectations from prospective epidemiological studies," *The British Medical Journal*, vol. 338, no. 7705, p. 1245, 2009.

18

Doctors' Knowledge of Hypertension Guidelines Recommendations Reflected in Their Practice

Nafees Ahmad [ID],[1] Amer Hayat Khan [ID],[2] Irfanullah Khan,[2]
Amjad Khan [ID],[3] and Muhammad Atif[4]

[1]Faculty of Pharmacy and Health Sciences, University of Balochistan, Balochistan, Pakistan
[2]Discipline of Clinical Pharmacy, School of Pharmaceutical Sciences, Universiti Sains Malaysia, Pulau Pinang, Malaysia
[3]Department of Pharmacy, Quaid-e-Azam University, Islamabad, Pakistan
[4]Department of Pharmacy, The Islamia University, Bahawalpur, Pakistan

Correspondence should be addressed to Nafees Ahmad; nafeesuob@gmail.com

Academic Editor: Franco Veglio

Aim. To evaluate doctors' knowledge, attitude, and practices and predictors of adherence to Malaysian hypertension guidelines (CPG 2008). *Methods.* Twenty-six doctors involved in hypertension management at Penang General Hospital were enrolled in a cross-sectional study. Doctors' knowledge and attitudes towards guidelines were evaluated through a self-administered questionnaire. Their practices were evaluated by noting their prescriptions written to 520 established hypertensive outpatients (20 prescriptions/doctor). SPSS 17 was used for data analysis. *Results.* Nineteen doctors (73.07%) had adequate knowledge of guidelines. Specialists and consultants had significantly better knowledge about guidelines' recommendations. Doctors were positive towards guidelines with mean attitude score of 23.15 ± 1.34 points on a 30-point scale. The median number of guidelines compliant prescriptions was 13 (range 5–20). Statistically significant correlation (r_s = 0.635, P < 0.001) was observed between doctors' knowledge and practice scores. A total of 349 (67.1%) prescriptions written were guidelines compliant. In multivariate analysis hypertension clinic (OR = 0.398, P = 0.008), left ventricular hypertrophy (OR = 0.091, P = 0.001) and heart failure (OR = 1.923, P = 0.039) were significantly associated with guidelines adherence. *Conclusion.* Doctors' knowledge of guidelines is reflected in their practice. The gap between guidelines recommendations and practice was seen in the pharmacotherapy of uncomplicated hypertension and hypertension with left ventricular hypertrophy, renal disease, and diabetes mellitus.

1. Introduction

High prevalence and poor control of hypertension have challenged the public health around the world. Malaysia has an effective and widespread system of healthcare working mainly under Ministry of Health. Infant mortality rate, a yard stick in determining the overall efficiency of healthcare, in 2005 was 10, comparing favorably with the United States and Western Europe. Malaysian healthcare consists of a dual-tiered system: government led and funded public sector and a coexisting private healthcare system. The public sector which provides healthcare services to >65% of the population has the country's best healthcare facilities and equipment but the shortage of doctors in government hospitals is the main drawback [1]. Despite the effective healthcare system,

the latest National Health and Morbidity Survey (2015) revealed that situation regarding prevalence (30.3%) and control of hypertension (26.8% to 48.5%) in Malaysia is not different than the global picture [2, 3]. Factors contributing to suboptimal control of hypertension are arbitrarily classified into patients, healthcare providers, and system related factors [4]. In order to improve hypertension control, a large number of hypertension management guidelines have been developed and disseminated worldwide. Despite guidelines' availability, dissemination, and potential to improve hypertension control [5–8], published literature from US [6, 9], Zimbabwe [10], Malaysia [3, 11–13], India [14], South Africa [15], Cyprus [16], Sweden [17], Kuwait [18], Jordan [19], Pakistan [20], and Italy [21] suggests the presence of a wide gap between guidelines recommended and actual clinical practices. According to

Cabana et al., barriers limiting adherence to guidelines are classified into three categories: *knowledge related factors*, such as lack of awareness and familiarity, *attitude related factors* such as lack of agreement, lack of outcome expectancy, self-efficacy, and motivation, and *behavior related factors*, such as characteristics of patients, guidelines, and practice [22].

Literature review revealed several weaknesses in previous research regarding evaluation of doctors' adherence to hypertension guidelines. As hypertension occurs in isolation in less than 20% cases and is almost always accompanied by other risk factors [23], addressing comorbidities is an important consideration while measuring doctors' adherence with hypertension guidelines. Some of the studies which had evaluated doctors prescribing practices against the guidelines failed to address comorbidities [24], excluded comorbidities [11, 25], or included only one comorbidity [13, 26], while some failed to define explicit criteria for defining guidelines adherence [24]. The majority of these studies had not conducted the review of patient's medical record to find whether divergence from guidelines was justifiable or not [13, 24, 26, 27]. The studies which had used survey data as a tool for measuring adherence with guidelines had the major limitation of reliance on self-reported practices [17, 19, 21], which are always subject to bias [28]. Doctors' attitudes towards guidelines play a significant role in their implementation in clinical practice. Doctors' intentions to use guidelines can be predicted from their attitudes towards guidelines, which are influenced by many factors, such as their knowledge, past clinical experience, beliefs about guidelines, outcome expectations, peers' opinions, and guidelines characteristics [22]. In order to overcome limitations associated with the above-mentioned studies, we evaluated doctors' subjective (knowledge of guidelines recommendations) as well as objective (actual) prescribing practices, addressed multiple comorbidities, developed explicit criteria for measuring guidelines adherence, conducted detailed review of patients' medical records, and evaluated doctors' attitude towards hypertension guidelines. In addition, we also examined relationship between doctors' knowledge, attitudes, and practices on Malaysian Clinical Practice Guidelines on Management of Hypertension (CPG 2008).

2. Methods

This was a cross-sectional study conducted at cardiology, nephrology, diabetic, and hypertension clinics of Penang General Hospital (PGH) Malaysia from October 2010 to April 2011. All the doctors practicing at the four clinics ($n = 26$: 13 at cardiology, 5 at nephrology, and 4 at diabetic and hypertension clinics each) were enrolled in the study. Written consent was taken prior to the beginning of the study. CPG 2008 available at http://www.acadmed.org.my/view_file.cfm?fileid=245 was used as reference.

3. Evaluation of Doctors' Knowledge and Attitude on CPG 2008

3.1. Tool Development. A self-developed, validated, and reliable questionnaire (in Appendix) was used as a tool for evaluating doctors' knowledge and attitudes on CPG 2008. Content validity of the questionnaire was assessed by a panel of experts composed of a cardiologist, a nephrologist, an endocrinologist, a general physician, and a clinical pharmacist. Construct validity of the tool was established by using key check and item response analysis [29]. Face validity of the questionnaire was established by giving it to a group of 10 participants other than those enrolled in the study [29]. Questionnaire was finalized after a series of discussions with the group. Internal consistency of the knowledge evaluating portion of the tool assessed by using Kuder-Richardson formula 20 (K-R 20) [23] yielded good internal consistency of K-R 20 coefficient = 0.733, while internal consistency of attitude evaluating portion was Cronbach's alpha = 0.808 [29]. To assess the stability of the tool, test-retest correlation was used. Pearson's r product moment correlation of 0.885 ($P < 0.001$) and 0.890 ($P < 0.001$) yielded an excellent stability of the knowledge and attitude evaluating portion of the tool, respectively [29].

3.2. Tool Administration and Scoring. Questionnaire was administered by the principal investigator (NA). In order to avoid the bias of respondents referring to CPG (2008) for answering the questions, they were requested to fill the questionnaire on spot. The knowledge evaluating portion of the questionnaire consisted of 11 multiple-choice questions. A score of "1" point was credited to each correct answer and "0" to each wrong answer and unanswered question. Adequate knowledge of CPG (2008) was defined as "correctly answering 7 out of 11 questions (>60%). As hypertension cannot be treated properly without correctly diagnosing it, therefore a correct answer regarding hypertension definition according to CPG (2008) was included in these 7 answers" [30]. Questions and correct answers included in the knowledge portion of the questionnaire were derived from recommendations included in CPG 2008.

Attitude evaluation portion, consisting of 6 items, was developed on the basis of extensive literature review. These items were based on a 5-point Likert scale ranging from "Strongly Disagree" to "Strongly Agree" and scored as strongly disagree = 1, disagree = 2, undecided = 3, agree = 4, and strongly agree = 5. Negative items were scored reversely, so that the high score reflects more positive attitude.

4. Evaluation of Doctors' Practices

In order to evaluate objective prescribing practices, a total of 520 (20 prescriptions per enrolled doctor) prescriptions written to established hypertensive patients were noted. The inclusion criteria were prescription written to hypertensive outpatients with and without comorbidities and aged > 18 and <80 years. A purpose-developed validated data collection form was used to collect patients' demographic and clinical data. Diagnosis of hypertension and other comorbidities was based on documentation from patients' medical record. Multiple comorbidities were noted and reported as different disease entity; diabetes mellitus, renal disease, stroke, and so on were reported individually. Drugs prescribed to the patients were noted by their generic names. Detailed review

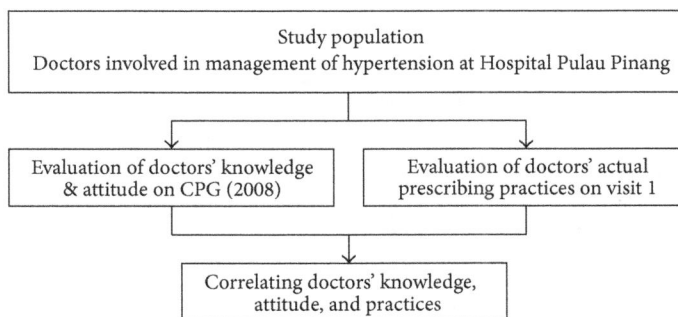

FIGURE 1: Flowchart of study methodology.

of the patients' medical record was conducted. Adverse drug reactions, contraindications, and statement about the inefficacy of a drug, due to which the drug is changed or not prescribed, were noted to find acceptable rationales for nonadherence with guidelines.

Prescription written was considered in compliance with guidelines when

(1) CPG 2008 recommended first-line agent for the particular condition was prescribed,

(2) CPG 2008 recommended first-line agents having no contraindications to their use were prescribed to patients with multiple comorbidities,

(3) CPG 2008 recommended first-line agent for a particular condition was not prescribed because of adverse effects caused by the recommended drug, contraindication to its use, or the drug was changed because of inefficacy.

A score of point "1" was credited to each guidelines compliant and "0" to noncompliant prescription. Doctors' knowledge and attitude were correlated to their prescribing practices scores. Flowchart of the study methodology is given in Figure 1.

5. Statistical Analysis

Data were analyzed by using SPSS 17. Percentages and frequencies were used for categorical variables, and means, medians, and standard deviations were calculated for continuous variables. Chi-squared and Fisher exact tests were used to observe significance between categorical variables. Mann–Whitney U test was performed to observe difference between doctors' demographics and their knowledge, attitude, and practice scores. Univariate logistic regression analysis was conducted to find association between independent variables and CPG adherence. Multivariate analysis was used to obtain a final model describing the significant independent predictors of guidelines adherence. All those variables which had statistically significant association with CPG adherence in univariate analysis were included in multivariate model. The fit of the model was assessed by Hosmer and Lemeshow test and overall classification percentage. Spearman rank order correlation was used to note correlation between doctors' knowledge, attitude, and practice scores. Significance of the statistical tests was taken at a P value of <0.05.

TABLE 1: Doctors' demographics.

Variables	Mean ± SD	Number (%)
Gender		
Male		10 (38.5)
Female		16 (61.5)
Age (years)	35 ± 6.45	
Years in practice	8.23 ± 5.11	
Ethnicity		
Malay		4 (15.4)
Chinese		17 (65.4)
Indian		4 (15.4)
Others		1 (3.8)
Designation		
Medical officers		12 (46.2)
Specialists		6 (23.1)
Consultants		8 (30.8)
Place of graduation		
Malaysia		19 (73.1)
Abroad		7 (26.9)

This study was approved by the Ministry of Health Medical Research Ethics Committee (MREC), Malaysia (ref: KKM/NIHSEC/08/0804/P-10-453).

6. Results

Demographics of the enrolled doctors are given in Table 1. Of the 520 established hypertensive patients included in the final analysis, 304 (58.8%) were males. Mean age of the patients was 61.28 ± 10.98 years. The patients sample was ethnically diverse and consisted of Chinese (259) (49.8%), Malay (168) (32.3%), Indian (81) (15.6%), and other ethnicities (12) (2.3%). A total of 1060 comorbidities were recorded. The most common comorbidity was dyslipidemia (24.62%) ($n = 261$) followed by diabetes mellitus (22.45%) ($n = 238$), IHD (22.45%) ($n = 238$), chronic kidney disease without proteinuria (11.50%) ($n = 122$), HF (8.30%) ($n = 88$), cerebrovascular disease (3.20%) ($n = 34$), asthma (2.35%) ($n = 25$), left ventricular hypertrophy (1.22%) ($n = 13$), gout (1.22%) ($n = 13$), chronic kidney disease with proteinuria

TABLE 2: Percentages of answers conforming to the recommendations of CPG (2008).

Question number	Number and percentage of answers conforming to the guidelines
(1)	24 (92.3)
(2)	22 (84.6)
(3)	22 (84.6)
(4)	16 (61.5)
(5)	10 (48.5)
(6)	22 (84.6)
(7)	24 (92.3)
(8)	17 (64.5)
(9)	6 (23.1)
(10)	9 (34.6)
(11)	20 (76.9)

(1.13%) ($n = 12$), diabetic nephropathy (1.03%) ($n = 11$), and peripheral vascular disease (PVD) (0.47%) ($n = 5$).

7. Doctors' Knowledge and Attitude on CPG (2008)

The percentages of correct answers to the 11 questions are shown in Table 2. The mean number of correct answers was 7.96 ± 1.82 (range 5–11). On the basis of criterion used for adequate awareness, 19 (73.07%) doctors had adequate knowledge of CPG 2008 recommendations. Only three doctors correctly answered all 11 questions. On the basis of designation, we divided doctors into two groups, medical officers and others (specialists and consultants). The results of Mann–Whitney U test showed a significant difference ($U = 17.5$, P value < 0.001) between knowledge possessed by two groups. Group composed of specialists and consultants was identified to be more knowledgeable (mean rank = 18.25) as compared to medical officers group (mean rank = 7.96).

Doctors in the present study were highly positive towards the CPG (2008), with mean attitude score of 23.15 ± 1.34, ranging from 19 to 24 on a 30-point scale. Doctors' responses to attitude statements are given in Table 3.

8. Prescribing Practices

A total of 349 (67.1%) prescriptions were written in compliance with guidelines. The mean number of guidelines compliant prescriptions was 13.42 ± 3.42 ranging from 5 to 20. The results of Mann–Whitney U test showed a significant difference ($U = 31.5$, $P = 0.007$) of CPG 2008 adherence score between two groups of doctors. Group composed of specialists and consultants had more guideline adherent practice score (mean rank = 17.25) as compared to medical officers group (mean rank = 9.12).

In univariate analysis, we evaluated association between CPG adherence and patients' age, gender, presence of any comorbidity, HF, LVH, CKD, DM, dyslipidemia, cerebrovascular disease, receiving treatment at cardiology, hypertension, and nephrology clinics. The results of univariate analysis

showed that CPG adherence had significant association with comorbidity status, HF, LVH, and treatment at cardiology and hypertension clinics (Table 4). In multivariate analysis, LVH (OR = 0.091, $P = 0.001$) and hypertension clinic (OR = 0.400, $P = 0.008$) had significant negative association, whereas HF had significant positive association (OR = 1.923, $P = 0.039$) with CPG adherence (Table 5). This model fit was based on a nonsignificant Hosmer-Lemeshow test ($P = 0.975$) and overall percentage of 71.1% from the classification table.

Spearman rank correlation yielded a statistically significant strong positive correlation ($r_s = 0.635$, $P < 0.001$) between doctors' knowledge and practice scores.

9. Discussion

Familiarity with guidelines is considered the first step in their implementation in clinical practice [22]. The doctors in the present study possessed comparatively better knowledge than reported by some studies conducted elsewhere. Mean score of correct answers in the present study was 7.96 ± 1.82 points as compared to 5.3 points in a study conducted in Italy [21] and 4.5 in a study conducted in Germany [30]. In comparison to 73.07% of the doctors in the present study, only 23.7% of the German physicians had adequate knowledge about German Society of Hypertension guidelines [30]. However in the present study doctors' knowledge was poor in selecting guidelines recommended antihypertensive agents in LVH, renal disease, and uncomplicated hypertension.

Unfortunately, a very low percentage (23.1%) of doctors in the present study correctly identified the CPG (2008) recommended ARB as preferred antihypertensive therapy for patients with LVH. If we assume that the possible reason for this poor performance could be the nature of the disease, LVH, an advanced and complicated form of cardiovascular disease (CVD), supposed to be treated by cardiologists, still would not justify the doctors' poor performance, because, firstly, all the doctors are supposed to be familiar with guidelines recommendation for treating LVH and secondly half of our respondents ($n = 13$) were practicing in cardiology clinic.

CPG 2008 recommended ACE inhibitors as drug of choice in hypertension with renal disease. Unfortunately, a very low percentage (36.4%) of doctors ($n = 9$) in the present study selected ACE inhibitors as drug of choice in hypertension accompanied by renal disease. A similar low percentage (40.7%) of doctors had correctly answered the same question in a study conducted in Jordan [19].

Because of its association with higher incidence of new onset diabetes mellitus [31] and comparatively lower effectiveness in reducing BP and prevention of stroke [32], use of beta blockers (BB) in uncomplicated hypertension is discouraged by CPG 2008. In the present study, a low proportion (38.5%) of doctors correctly selected BB as antihypertensive agents discouraged in uncomplicated hypertension by CPG 2008. Similar low percentage of doctors had correctly answered the question regarding preferred antihypertensive agents in uncomplicated hypertension in a study conducted in Jordan [19].

TABLE 3: Frequencies of doctors' responses of attitude statements towards CPG (2008).

Statement	SA	A	UD	DA	SA
I have trust in the recommendations and developing committee of CPG (2008)	2	24	-	-	-
CPG (2008) on the management of hypertension is helpful for doctors	1	24	1	-	-
Adherence to CPG (2008) would produce desired outcome	1	25	-	-	-
CPG (2008) is motivated by desire to cut cost	-	3	6	17	-
CPG (2008) decreases doctors' autonomy	-	3	1	22	-
CPG (2008) is too rigid to apply to individual patients	-	2	3	21	-

CPG, clinical practice guidelines; SA, strongly agree; A, agree; UD, undecided; DA, disagree; SD, strongly disagree.

TABLE 4: Univariate analysis of predictors of CPG adherence.

Variables	CPG adherence (n, %)		Odds ratio	95% CI	P value
	Yes	No			
Gender					
Male	214 (70.4)	90 (29.6)	Reference		
Female	135 (62.5)	81 (36.5)	0.701	0.484–1.014	0.059
Age					
Elderly (≥65 years)	127 (65.5)	67 (34.5)	Reference		
Nonelderly	222 (68.1)	104 (31.9)	1.126	0.773–1.641	0.536
Comorbidity					
No	11 (30.6)	25 (69.4)	Reference		
Yes	338 (69.8)	146 (30.2)	5.26	2.52–10.97	0.000
Heart failure					
No	277 (64.12)	155 (35.88)	Reference		
Yes	72 (81.81)	16 (18.19)	2.209	1.271–3.841	0.005
LVH					
No	346 (68.2)	161 (31.6)	Reference		
Yes	3 (23.1)	10 (76.9)	0.140	0.038–0.514	0.003
Chronic kidney disease					
No	256 (66.3)	130 (33.7)	Reference		
Yes	93 (69.4)	41 (30.6)	1.124	0.745–1.698	0.577
Diabetes mellitus					
No	188 (66.7)	94 (33.3)	Reference		
Yes	161 (67.6)	77 (32.4)	1.068	0.740–1.541	0.725
Dyslipidemia					
No	164 (63.3)	95 (36.7)	Reference		
Yes	185 (70.9)	76 (29.1)	1.410	0.976–2.037	0.067
Cerebrovascular disease					
No	323 (66.5)	163 (33.5)	Reference		
Yes	26 (76.5)	8 (23.5)	1.640	0.726–3.703	0.234
Cardiology clinic					
No	158 (60.8)	102 (39.8)	Reference		
Yes	191 (73.5)	69 (26.5)	1.79	1.23–2.60	0.002
Hypertension clinic					
No	317 (72.0)	123 (28.0)	Reference		
Yes	32 (40.0)	48 (60.0)	0.26	0.16–0.42	0.004
Nephrology clinic					
No	279 (66.4)	141 (33.6)	Reference		
Yes	70 (70.0)	30 (30.0)	1.179	0.735–1.893	0.495
Diabetic clinic					
No	293 (66.7)	147 (33.3)	Reference		
Yes	56 (70.0)	24 (30.0)	1.171	0.698–1.964	0.551

CI, confidence interval; CPG, clinical practice guidelines; LVH, left ventricular hypertrophy. *Note.* Only statistically significant results are given in the table.

TABLE 5: Multivariate analysis of predictors of CPG adherence.

Variable	B	SE	P value	Odds ratio	95% CI
Left ventricular hypertrophy	−2.394	0.688	0.001	0.091	0.024–0.352
Heart failure	0.654	0.318	0.039	1.923	1.032–3.583
Hypertension clinic	−0.915	0.346	0.008	0.400	0.203–0.788

CI, confidence interval; B, beta; SE, standard error. *Note.* Only statistically significant results are given in the table.

All doctors in the present study had welcoming attitudes towards guidelines. They showed trust in both, CPG 2008 and its developers. They believed that CPG 2008 is useful for doctors and adherence to it would produce best patients' outcomes. The reason for doctors welcoming attitudes towards CPG 2008 might be the reputation of the bodies involved in its developing and dissemination. CPG 2008 is developed and disseminated by the Ministry of Health Malaysia in collaboration with Academy of Medicine, Malaysia, and Malaysian Society of Hypertension, the national bodies, which are often perceived to be credible [33]. Beside this, the inclusion of local data and publications in CPG 2008 to ensure local relevance and asking about a specific guideline, that is, CPG 2008, might have played an additional role in doctors' positive attitude towards it. Doctors are found to remain more positive when they are asked about a specific guideline as compared to guidelines in general [34].

Overall, a fair-to-good level of adherence to medication recommendations of CPG 2008 was observed at PGH. More than two-thirds of the patients (67.1%) received guidelines compliant prescriptions. Almost similar findings were reported by a cross-sectional study conducted at a family medicine clinic in Edmonton, where 64% of diabetic or renal disease patients were receiving Canadian Hypertension Education Program (CHEP) recommended therapy [35]. In our study, 67.9% of diabetic and 69% of renal disease patients were receiving CPG 2008 compliant therapy. Adherence to hypertension guidelines in the present study was comparatively better than other studies conducted in Malaysia. A study conducted in two primary clinics has reported that prescribing practices were not in accordance with CPG 2008, as the guidelines discouraged beta blockers were most commonly prescribed drugs in uncomplicated hypertension [11]. Similarly, in another study conducted at 11 primary healthcare clinics in Melaka, state of Malaysia, only 18.3% of diabetic hypertensive patients received guidelines recommended ACE inhibitors as compared to 67.9% in our study [13].

In the present study, doctors' knowledge of CPG 2008 was reflected in their prescribing practices. Doctors remained poorly adhered to those recommendations about which they had poor knowledge. Only 23.1% of the doctors selected guidelines recommended ARB as preferred agents in treating hypertension with LVH. Upon evaluation of the actual prescribing practices, we found only 23.1% of hypertensive patients with LVH were on guidelines compliant therapy. The majority (61.5%) of doctors were unable to correctly identify the guidelines discouraged BB in uncomplicated hypertension. As a consequence, a high percentage (69.4%) of uncomplicated hypertensive patients were on BB. Guidelines recommended BB were selected by almost 77% of the doctors as drug of choice in hypertension with CHD and were prescribed to 77% of patients. However, this relationship between doctors' knowledge and adherence to CPG 2008 medication recommendations did not follow the same sequence in case of diabetes mellitus. More than 86% of doctors selected guidelines recommended ACE inhibitors as drug of first choice in hypertension with diabetes mellitus, but only 64.3% of diabetic hypertensive patients received ACE inhibitors, despite the fact that only 3.6% of patients had contraindications to the use of ACE inhibitors. Similar finding of not implementing the knowledge in clinical practice was observed in studies conducted elsewhere [36, 37].

Hypertension clinic and LVH were the strong predictors of poor adherence to CPG (2008) in both univariate and multivariate analyses. In hypertension clinic, all the four enrolled doctors were medical officers, and in the present study it is observed that medical officers had significantly lower knowledge of CPG 2008 and guideline adherent practice scores as compared to specialists and consultants. Medical officers' inadequate familiarity with CPG 2008 seems to be the reason of poor adherence to guidelines at hypertension clinic. Beside this, all uncomplicated hypertensive patients in the present study were treated in hypertension clinic only. While evaluating doctors' knowledge, we found that the majority of doctors failed in correctly identifying CPG 2008 discouraged BB in uncomplicated hypertension. Prescription of BB to uncomplicated hypertensive patients was the major cause of poor adherence to CPG 2008 in hypertension clinic. Similar guidelines divergent antihypertensive prescriptions in uncomplicated hypertension have also been reported by studies conducted elsewhere. For example, only 18% of the uncomplicated hypertensive patients were on guidelines recommended diuretics in a study conducted elsewhere [25].

As per expectations, specialists and consultants who were more qualified and in practice for longer time performed better than medical officers both in knowledge on CPG 2008 and in practice. This finding is in line with the guidelines adherence models proposed by Cabana et al. [22]. Similarly in studies conducted in Hong Kong and Italy, doctors with higher qualifications and longer duration of practice performed better as compared to doctors with lower qualifications [21, 38]. The other reason for negative association between guidelines adherence and hypertension clinic was comparatively better practices at other clinics, where hypertensive patients with comorbidities were treated. Comparatively better adherence to guidelines at other clinics might be explained by the model proposed by Piette and Kerr [39]. According to the model, patients with concurrent comorbidities of overlapping pathophysiological pathways and management such as hypertension, CVD, and renal disease are likely to receive guidelines adherent management.

In the present study, medical officers at clinics other than hypertension clinic were used to discuss cases with specialists and consultants present at the clinics. In addition to writing guideline adherent prescriptions themselves, the presence of specialists and consultants in these clinics would have definitely helped medical officers in writing guidelines adherent prescriptions. In addition to the medical officers' lower familiarity of CPG (2008), the unavailability of specialists and consultants at hypertension clinic might have an additional effect on poor adherence to guidelines. The reason for poor guidelines adherence in LVH seems to be doctors' lower familiarity of guidelines recommendation as observed while evaluating their knowledge.

Heart failure was the strong predictor of better guidelines adherence in both univariate and multivariate analyses. The possible reason for doctors' good adherence to guidelines while treating patients with heart failure seems to be the wide range of antihypertensive classes (diuretics, ACE inhibitors, BB, ARB, and aldosterone antagonists) recommended by guidelines. The other possible reason for better guidelines adherence might be explained by model proposed by Piette and Kerr [39] which is explained above.

A strong positive relationship was observed between doctors' knowledge score on CPG 2008 and guidelines compliant practice scores. Doctors with higher knowledge of CPG 2008 wrote statistically significant higher numbers of guidelines compliant prescriptions. This finding was in line with the model proposed by Piette and Kerr [39] and studies conducted elsewhere [40, 41]. No significant association was observed among doctors' knowledge and attitude scores and attitude and practice scores. The reason for this lack of relationship seems be the doctors' very positive attitudes towards CPG (2008) irrespective of their knowledge and adherence to it, which made this variable somewhat constant.

10. Limitations

Relatively small number of doctors and being an older data set were the major limitations associated with the current study. The reason for doctors limited sample size was the co-relational design of the study. In order to avoid the bias associated with self-reported practices, we evaluated both subjective and objective practices of the doctors, due to which the study was conducted in a single hospital among the small number of doctors who were involved in the management of hypertension. Beside this, both knowledge and practice evaluation sections of the current study focused on hypertension pharmacotherapy, while hypertension management consists of several components including screening, life style interventions, pharmacotherapy, and continued follow-up.

11. Conclusion

To the best of our knowledge, this was the first study in Malaysian clinical setup which evaluated both the subjective and objective practices of hypertension management as well as their attitudes towards hypertension management guidelines. More than 73% of doctors were adequately familiar with guidelines recommendations. Lack of knowledge about the particular recommendations was reflected in their practice. Guidelines recommended ARB and ACE inhibitors were underutilized in treating hypertension with LVH and renal disease, while guidelines discouraged BB were prescribed to the patients with uncomplicated hypertension. Medical officers involved in the management of hypertension had significantly lower familiarity of CPG (2008) as compared to specialists and consultants. As lack of knowledge about particular recommendations was the major reason of guidelines divergent practices, multifaceted interventions including education interventions, using reminder tools that indicate appropriate pharmacotherapy, and the availability of clinical pharmacists to participate in collaborative practices which have shown effectiveness in enhancing doctors' adherence to clinical practice guidelines [42, 43] can be used to bridge the gap between evidence based medicines and hypertension management practices at the study site. Medical officers involved in the management of hypertension at (PGH) should be the preferred target population of such interventions. Findings of this study can be used as baseline data and guide for devising suitable interventions to improve doctors' adherence to hypertension guidelines, reduce practice variation, and optimize hypertension control. A large multicenter study including the primary care doctors and using the updated Malaysian CPG (2013) for the management of hypertension as a reference document is recommended to validate the findings of the current study.

Appendix

Questionnaire

Please answer the following questions about yourself:

(1) Gender

□ Male

□ Female

(2) Age (in years)_____

(3) Ethnicity

□ Malay

□ Chinese

□ Indian

□ Others, please specify_____

(4) Place of graduation

□ Malaysia

□ Other, please specify_____

(5) Designation

□ House medical officer

□ Medical officer

□ Consultant

□ Senior Consultant

□ Other, please specify_____

(6) I am in practice for last_____years.

Pick the single answer for each question that best matches your response.

(1) Which of the following blood pressure (BP) values defines hypertension in an adult subject without comorbidities?

☐ ≥150/90 mm Hg

☐ *≥140/90 mm Hg*

☐ ≥135/85 mm Hg

☐ ≥160/95 mm Hg

☐ Other please specify_____

(2) What is the target BP you would like to achieve in hypertensive patients with *diabetes mellitus and/or chronic kidney disease without proteinuria*?

☐ <150/95 mm Hg

☐ <140/90 mm Hg

☐ *<130/80 mm Hg*

☐ <135/85 mm Hg

☐ Other please specify_____

(3) The maximum observational period for a patient recently diagnosed with *Stage 1 Hypertension* having *no evident target organ involvement* and any *additional risk factor* is

☐ 1 week

☐ 1 month

☐ 9 months

☐ *6 months*

☐ Other please specify_____

(4) The absolute risk of cardiovascular events over *10 years* in *high risk* patients is

☐ <10%

☐ 10–20%

☐ *20–30%*

☐ >30%

☐ Other please specify_____

(5) In newly diagnosed, *uncomplicated hypertension* and no *compelling indications*, all of the following antihypertensive drug classes are agents of *choice of first line* monotherapy except,

☐ *Beta blockers*

☐ Angiotensin Receptor Blockers

☐ Diuretics

☐ Calcium Channel Blockers

☐ Angiotensin Converting Enzymes Inhibitors

(6) Which one of the following antihypertensive drug classes you would like to *prescribe* as first choice for hypertensive patients with *diabetes mellitus* having *no proteinuria*?

☐ Beta blockers

☐ Calcium Channel Blockers

☐ Diuretics

☐ Alpha blockers

☐ *Angiotensin Converting Enzymes Inhibitors*

(7) Which one of the following antihypertensive drugs you would like to prescribe as first choice for *pregnant hypertensive women*?

☐ *Methyldopa*

☐ Angiotensin Receptor Blocker

☐ Diuretics

☐ Angiotensin Converting Enzyme inhibitor

(8) Which one of the following antihypertensive drug classes you would *prefer* for *primary prevention* of stroke?

☐ Beta Blockers

☐ Angiotensin Receptor Blockers

☐ *Calcium Channel Blockers*

☐ Diuretics

(9) Which one of the following antihypertensive drug classes you would like to prescribe as *first choice* for hypertensive patient with *left ventricular hypertrophy*?

☐ Beta Blockers

☐ *Angiotensin Receptor Blockers*

☐ Calcium Channel Blockers

☐ Angiotensin Converting Enzyme Inhibitors

(10) Which one of the following antihypertensive drug classes you would like to prescribe as *first choice* for hypertensive patients with *non diabetic renal disease*?

☐ Beta Blockers

☐ Calcium Channel Blockers

☐ Alpha Blockers

☐ *Angiotensin Converting Enzyme Inhibitors*

(11) Which one of the following antihypertensive drug classes you would like to *prescribe* as *first choice* for hypertensive patients with *coronary heart diseases*?

☐ Angiotensin Receptor Blockers

☐ *Beta Blockers*

☐ Alpha Blockers

☐ Short acting Calcium Channel Blockers

Please circle the response that best describes your beliefs about CPG (2008) on the management of hypertension

(1) I have trust in the recommendations and developing committee of CPG (2008)

Strongly Disagree

Disagree

Undecided

Agree

Strongly Agree

(2) CPG (2008) on the management of hypertension is helpful for doctors

Strongly Disagree

Disagree

Undecided

Agree

Strongly Agree

(3) Adherence with CPG (2008) would produce desired outcome

Strongly Disagree

Disagree

Undecided

Agree

Strongly Agree

(4) CPG (2008) is motivated by desire to cut cost

Strongly Disagree

Disagree

Undecided

Agree

Strongly Agree

(5) CPG (2008) decreases doctors' autonomy

Strongly Disagree

Disagree

Undecided

Agree

Strongly Agree

(6) CPG (2008) is too rigid to apply to individual patients

Strongly Disagree

Disagree

Undecided

Agree

Strongly Agree

Conflicts of Interest

The authors declare no conflicts of interest, in part or whole.

Authors' Contributions

Nafees Ahmad and Amer Hayat Khan participated in conception and design of the study. Nafees Ahmad collected, analyzed, and interpreted the data. Nafees Ahmad and Muhammad Atif drafted the manuscript. All authors were involved in data interpretation. Amer Hayat Khan, Irfanullah Khan, Amjad Khan, and Muhammad Atif revised the manuscript critically. All the authors have read and approved the final manuscript.

Acknowledgments

The authors thank all the doctors and patients who participated in this study. Thanks are also due to the nursing and record-keeping staff of (PGH), Malaysia.

References

[1] D. Quek, "The Malaysian Health Care System: A Review," 1-11, 2014, https://www.researchgate.net/publication/237409933_The_Malaysian_Health_Care_System_A_Review.

[2] Institute for Public Health, "National health and morbidity survey 2015," in *Non-Communicable Diseases, Risk Factors and Other Health Problems*, vol. 2, p. 291, Ministry of Health, Kuala Lumpur, Malaysia, 2015.

[3] S. Teoh, A. Razlina, D. Norwati, and M. S. Siti, "Patients' blood pressure control and doctors' adherence to hypertension clinical practice guideline in managing patients at health clinics in Kuala Muda district, Kedah," *Medical Journal of Malaysia*, vol. 72, no. 1, pp. 18–25, 2017.

[4] N. Ahmad, Y. Hassan, B. Tangiisuran et al., "Guidelines adherence and hypertension control at a tertiary hospital in Malaysia," *Journal of Evaluation in Clinical Practice*, vol. 19, no. 5, pp. 798–804, 2013.

[5] R. Asmar, A. Achouba, P. Brunel, R. El Feghali, T. Denolle, and B. Vaisse, "A specific training on hypertension guidelines improves blood pressure control by more than 10% in hypertensive patients: the VALNORM study," *Journal of the American Society of Hypertension*, vol. 1, no. 4, pp. 278–285, 2007.

[6] C. G. Rowan, J. R. Turner, A. Shah, and J. A. Spaeder, "Antihypertensive treatment and blood pressure control relative to hypertension treatment guidelines," *Pharmacoepidemiology and Drug Safety*, vol. 23, no. 12, pp. 1294–1302, 2014.

[7] G. Li, A.-P. Cai, Y.-J. Mo et al., "Effects of guideline-based hypertension management in rural areas of Guangdong Province," *Chinese Medical Journal*, vol. 128, no. 6, pp. 799–803, 2015.

[8] J. H. Jackson, J. Sobolski, R. Krienke, K. S. Wong, F. Frech-Tamas, and B. Nightengale, "Blood pressure control and pharmacotherapy patterns in the United States before and after the release of the Joint National Committee on the Prevention, Detection, Evaluation, and Treatment of High Blood Pressure (JNC 7) guidelines," *Journal of the American Board of Family Medicine*, vol. 21, no. 6, pp. 512–521, 2008.

[9] J. Levy, L. M. Gerber, X. Wu, and S. J. Mann, "Nonadherence to recommended guidelines for blood pressure measurement," *The Journal of Clinical Hypertension*, vol. 18, no. 11, pp. 1157–1161, 2016.

[10] V. Basopo and P. N. Mujasi, "To what extent do prescribing practices for hypertension in the private sector in Zimbabwe follow the national treatment guidelines? An analysis of insurance medical claims," *Journal of Pharmaceutical Policy and Practice*, vol. 10, no. 1, p. 37, 2017.

[11] A. S. Ramli, M. Miskan, K. K. Ng et al., "Prescribing of antihypertensive agents in public primary care clinics - is it in accordance with current evidence," *Malaysian Family Physician*, vol. 5, no. 1, pp. 36–40, 2010.

[12] N. Ahmad, Y. Hassan, B. Tangiisuran, O. L. Meng, N. A. Aziz, and A. H. Khan, "Guidelines adherence and hypertension control in an outpatient cardiology clinic in Malaysia," *Tropical Journal of Pharmaceutical Research*, vol. 11, no. 4, pp. 665–672, 2012.

[13] G.-C. Chan, "Type 2 diabetes mellitus with hypertension at primary healthcare level in Malaysia: are they managed according to guidelines?" *Singapore Medical Journal*, vol. 46, no. 3, pp. 127–131, 2005.

[14] S. Raju, S. Solomon, N. Karthik, A. C. Joseph, and Venkatanarayanan, "Assessment of prescribing pattern for hypertension and comparison with jnc-8 guidelines-proposed intervention by clinical pharmacist," *Journal of Young Pharmacists*, vol. 8, no. 2, pp. 133–135, 2016.

[15] A. R. Adedeji, J. Tumbo, and I. Govender, "Adherence of doctors to a clinical guideline for hypertension in Bojanala district, North-West Province, South Africa," *African Journal of Primary Health Care and Family Medicine*, vol. 7, no. 1, pp. 1–6, 2015.

[16] M. Theodorou, P. Stafylas, G. Kourlaba, D. Kaitelidou, N. Maniadakis, and V. Papademetriou, "Physicians' perceptions and adherence to guidelines for the management of hypertension: a national, multicentre, prospective study," *International Journal of Hypertension*, vol. 2012, Article ID 503821, 11 pages, 2012.

[17] P. Midlöv, R. Ekesbo, L. Johansson et al., "Barriers to adherence to hypertension guidelines among GPs in southern Sweden: a survey," *Scandinavian Journal of Primary Health Care*, vol. 26, no. 3, pp. 154–159, 2008.

[18] K. A. Al-Ali, F. A. Al-Ghanim, A. M. Al-Furaih, N. Al-Otaibi, G. Makboul, and M. K. El-Shazly, "Awareness of hypertension guidelines among family physicians in primary health care," *Alexandria Journal of Medicine*, vol. 49, no. 1, pp. 81–87, 2013.

[19] S. I. Al-Azzam, R. B. Najjar, and Y. S. Khader, "Awareness of physicians in Jordan about the treatment of high blood pressure according to the seventh report of the Joint National Committee (JNC VII)," *European Journal of Cardiovascular Nursing*, vol. 6, no. 3, pp. 223–232, 2007.

[20] T. H. Jafar, S. Jessani, F. H. Jafary et al., "General practitioners' approach to hypertension in urban Pakistan: disturbing trends in practice," *Circulation*, vol. 111, no. 10, pp. 1278–1283, 2005.

[21] C. Cuspidi, I. Michev, S. Mean et al., "Awareness of hypertension guidelines in primary care: results of a regionwide survey in Italy," *Journal of Human Hypertension*, vol. 17, no. 8, pp. 541–547, 2003.

[22] M. D. Cabana, C. S. Rand, N. R. Powe et al., "Why don't physicians follow clinical practice guidelines? A framework for improvement," *Journal of the American Medical Association*, vol. 282, no. 15, pp. 1458–1465, 1999.

[23] A. N. Long and S. Dagogo-Jack, "Comorbidities of diabetes and hypertension: mechanisms and approach to target organ protection," *The Journal of Clinical Hypertension*, vol. 13, no. 4, pp. 244–251, 2011.

[24] D. Siegel and J. Lopez, "Trends in antihypertensive drug use in the United States: do the JNC V recommendations affect prescribing?" *Journal of the American Medical Association*, vol. 278, no. 21, pp. 1745–1748, 1997.

[25] P. E. Drawz, C. Bocirnea, K. B. Greer, J. Kim, F. Rader, and P. Murray, "Hypertension guideline adherence among nursing home patients," *Journal of General Internal Medicine*, vol. 24, no. 4, pp. 499–503, 2009.

[26] C. Russell, P. Dunbar, S. Salisbury, I. Sketris, and G. Kephart, "Hypertension control: Results from the Diabetes Care Program of Nova Scotia registry and impact of changing clinical practice guidelines," *Cardiovascular Diabetology*, vol. 4, article no. 11, 2005.

[27] D. J. Hyman and V. N. Pavlik, "Self-reported hypertension treatment practices among primary care physicians: blood pressure thresholds, drug choices, and the role of guidelines and evidence-based medicine," *JAMA Internal Medicine*, vol. 160, no. 15, pp. 2281–2286, 2000.

[28] A. S. Adams, S. B. Soumerai, J. Lomas, and D. Ross-Degnan, "Evidence of self-report bias in assessing adherence to guidelines," *International Journal for Quality in Health Care*, vol. 11, no. 3, pp. 187–192, 1999.

[29] J. Considine, M. Botti, and S. Thomas, "Design, format, validity and reliability of multiple choice questions for use in nursing research and education," *Journal of the Royal College of Nursing Australia*, vol. 12, no. 1, pp. 19–24, 2005.

[30] J. Hagemeister, C. A. Schneider, S. Barabas et al., "Hypertension guidelines and their limitations - The impact of physicians' compliance as evaluated by guideline awareness," *Journal of Hypertension*, vol. 19, no. 11, pp. 2079–2086, 2001.

[31] W. J. Elliott and P. M. Meyer, "Incident diabetes in clinical trials of antihypertensive drugs: a network meta-analysis," *The Lancet*, vol. 369, no. 9557, pp. 201–207, 2007.

[32] L. H. Lindholm, B. Carlberg, and O. Samuelsson, "Should β blockers remain first choice in the treatment of primary hypertension? A meta-analysis," *The Lancet*, vol. 366, no. 9496, pp. 1545–1553, 2005.

[33] A. Rashidian, M. P. Eccles, and I. Russell, "Falling on stony ground? A qualitative study of implementation of clinical guidelines' prescribing recommendations in primary care," *Health Policy*, vol. 85, no. 2, pp. 148–161, 2008.

[34] F. Olesen and T. Lauritzen, "Do general practitioners want guidelines?: attitudes toward a county- based and a national college-based approach," *Scandinavian Journal of Primary Health Care*, vol. 15, no. 3, pp. 141–145, 1997.

[35] S. J. Houlihan, S. H. Simpson, A. J. Cave et al., "Hypertension treatment and control rates: chart review in an academic family medicine clinic," *Canadian Family Physician*, vol. 55, no. 7, pp. 735–741, 2009.

[36] S. A. Oliveria, P. Lapuerta, B. D. McCarthy, G. J. L'Italien, D. R. Berlowitz, and S. M. Asch, "Physician-related barriers to the effective management of uncontrolled hypertension," *JAMA Internal Medicine*, vol. 162, no. 4, pp. 413–420, 2002.

[37] N. Holland, D. Segraves, V. O. Nnadi, D. A. Belletti, J. Wogen, and S. Arcona, "Identifying barriers to hypertension care: implications for quality improvement initiatives," *Population Health Management*, vol. 11, no. 2, pp. 71–77, 2008.

[38] T. Wae, C. Man, L. Tong, C. Wan, C. Yuk, and Y. Street, "Are we evidence-based in prescribing for hypertension?" *Asia Pacific Journal of Family Medicine*, vol. 5, no. 3, 2006.

[39] J. D. Piette and E. A. Kerr, "The impact of comorbid chronic conditions on diabetes care," *Diabetes Care*, vol. 29, no. 3, pp. 725–731, 2006.

[40] A. A. El-Solh, A. Alhajhusain, R. G. Saliba, and P. Drinka, "Physicians' attitudes toward guidelines for the treatment of hospitalized nursing home-acquired pneumonia," *Journal of the American Medical Directors Association*, vol. 12, no. 4, pp. 270–276, 2010.

[41] N. Ikeda, T. Hasegawa, T. Hasegawa, I. Saito, and T. Saruta, "Awareness of the Japanese Society of Hypertension Guidelines for the Management of Hypertension (JSH 2000) and compliance to its recommendations: surveys in 2000 and 2004," *Journal of Human Hypertension*, vol. 20, no. 4, pp. 263–266, 2006.

[42] O. Berwanger, H. P. Guimarães, L. N. Laranjeira et al., "Effect of a multifaceted intervention on use of evidence-based therapies in patients with acute coronary syndromes in Brazil:

19

Brain Oscillations Elicited by the Cold Pressor Test: A Putative Index of Untreated Essential Hypertension

Christos Papageorgiou,[1] Efstathios Manios,[1]
Eleftheria Tsaltas,[2] Eleni Koroboki,[1] Maria Alevizaki,[1]
Elias Angelopoulos,[2,3] Meletios-Athanasios Dimopoulos,[1]
Charalabos Papageorgiou,[2,3] and Nikolaos Zakopoulos[1]

[1]Department of Clinical Therapeutics, National and Kapodistrian University of Athens, Medical School, Athens, Greece
[2]1st Department of Psychiatry, National and Kapodistrian University of Athens, Medical School, "Eginition" Hospital, 115 28 Athens, Greece
[3]University Mental Health Research Institute (UMHRI), Athens, Greece

Correspondence should be addressed to Christos Papageorgiou; chrispapageorgio@gmail.com

Academic Editor: Tomohiro Katsuya

Objective. Essential hypertension is associated with reduced pain sensitivity of unclear aetiology. This study explores this issue using the Cold Pressor Test (CPT), a reliable pain/stress model, comparing CPT-related EEG activity in first episode hypertensives and controls. *Method.* 22 untreated hypertensives and 18 matched normotensives underwent 24-hour ambulatory blood pressure monitoring (ABPM). EEG recordings were taken before, during, and after CPT exposure. *Results.* Significant group differences in CPT-induced EEG oscillations were covaried with the most robust cardiovascular differentiators by means of a Canonical Analysis. Positive correlations were noted between ABPM variables and Delta (1–4 Hz) oscillations during the tolerance phase; in high-alpha (10–12 Hz) oscillations during the stress unit and posttest phase; and in low-alpha (8–10 Hz) oscillations during CPT phases overall. Negative correlations were found between ABPM variables and Beta2 oscillations (16.5–20 Hz) during the posttest phase and Gamma (28.5–45 Hz) oscillations during the CPT phases overall. These relationships were localised at several sites across the cerebral hemispheres with predominance in the right hemisphere and left frontal lobe. *Conclusions.* These findings provide a starting point for increasing our understanding of the complex relationships between cerebral activation and cardiovascular functioning involved in regulating blood pressure changes.

1. Introduction

Hypertension is a leading risk factor for cardiovascular disease and a major contributor to healthcare costs worldwide [1]. Given that autonomic nervous system (ANS) activity modulates transient changes in cardiovascular function, autonomic dysfunction has been implicated in the pathogenesis of essential hypertension (EH) [2]. Increased sympathetic activity [3] combined with parasympathetic inhibition may contribute to increased cardiac activity and/or peripheral vascular resistance and thereby to the early development of hypertension [4], although patients with borderline to mild hypertension often show normal vascular resistance at rest.

The central nervous system (CNS) has also been implicated in the aetiology and maintenance of some forms of EH. The CNS is a target of the disease which, if untreated, progresses to blood pressure (BP) levels threatening the integrity of cerebral vessels, potentially inducing stroke [5].

Considerable evidence supports the connection between pain perception and BP regulation. It has been proposed that acute BP increases may reduce pain, thus establishing hypertension through instrumental learning [6]. Hypoalgesia has been noted in animals and humans with high BP [7], but the issue of whether it precedes or follows hypertension remains equivocal.

TABLE 1: Outline of experimental measurements.

	Task	Measurements	Duration
Day 1	Habituation to laboratory environment and CPT conditions		1 hour approximately
	Onset of 24 hr ABPM procedure (Section 2.2.1)		24 hours
Day 2	Cold pressor test rest baseline	EEG recording period 1	3 min
	Hand immersion in 2°C water bath	EEG recording period 2 (unit of stress)	1 min
	Continuation of immersion (2°C) until spontaneous withdrawal	EEG recording period 3 (pain tolerance)	x min
	Cold pressor test recovery (Section 2.2.2)	EEG recording period 4	3 min

The layman concept that stress can cause hypertension still lacks strong empirical support. A review of studies examining the relationship of stress and hypertension [8] concluded that environmental measures of stress, such as natural disasters, unsafe neighborhood conditions, and work stress, were related to increased BP. In contrast, minimal association was noted between self-rated stress and BP.

Pain sensations, consisting of sensory, affective, and cognitive experiences, modulate EEG oscillations across a wide range of frequency bands, presumably reflecting the mechanisms involved in cortical activation and inhibition [9, 10]. Several studies have investigated the impact of experimental pain on human EEG. Most of these were based on the cold pressure test (CPT). There is consensus that the CPT produces decreased alpha EEG activity. Similarly, Beta and Theta bands activity has previously been reported to increase during CPT [11, 12].

Taking into consideration the issues presented above, the current study attempted an integrative approach to the factors interacting in the setting of hypertension. The objective was to compare well-characterised, untreated hypertensives and matched normotensive controls in terms of (i) arterial blood pressure variables (24-hour ambulatory blood pressure monitoring (ABPM)), (ii) CNS electrophysiological responsiveness (EEG), and (iii) behavioural responsiveness (pain perception and tolerance) under exposure to sympathoexcitatory stress and pain induced by the CPT.

Although the impact of experimental pain on EEG has attracted experimental interest, the existing available data do not warrant the formulation of specific hypotheses regarding the relationship between brain oscillations and newly diagnosed, untreated hypertension. Therefore this axis of our design has an exploratory character.

2. Methods

2.1. Study Population.
The hypertensive (HT) group consisted of 22 newly diagnosed untreated hypertensives (11 men, 11 women; mean age = 50.59 ± 11.45 years) referred to the hypertensive centre of the Department of Clinical Therapeutics (Athens University, Greece). The normotensive control (NT) group included 18 healthy volunteers (8 men and 10 women, mean age = 51.72 ± 8.33 years). All 40 participants were ambulatory and the two groups were matched for sex, age, and body mass index. They all fulfilled the following inclusion criteria: (1) no previous antihypertensive treatment; (2) absence of clinical signs or laboratory evidence of hypertension-related complications (coronary artery disease, heart failure, cerebrovascular disease, renal insufficiency, or peripheral artery disease) or of secondary causes of arterial hypertension; (3) absence of any other systematic disease; (4) absence of psychiatric disorders or psychiatric medication; (5) at least three valid BP measurements per hour over 24 hr ambulatory blood pressure monitoring (ABPM: 75% successful measurements). The cohort was initially evaluated by 24-hour ABPM and subjects were divided into 2 groups in terms of their ABPM measurements objectively on the basis of this measurement. Individuals with 24-hour ambulatory BP <130/80 mmHg were placed in the NT group; individuals with 24-hour ambulatory BP ≥130/80 mmHg were placed in the HT group. All subjects gave their informed consent for participation in the study, and the study protocol was approved by the hospital ethics review committee to ensure that the procedures followed were in accordance with the institutional guidelines.

2.2. Procedure.
Participants were instructed to abstain from alcohol, cigarette smoking, coffee/tea, and exercise for at least 30 minutes prior to testing. The study flow diagram can be seen in Table 1.

2.2.1. The 24-Hour ABPM Measurement [13, 14].
24-hour ABPM was conducted on all subjects on a usual working day by means of the Spacelabs 90217 ambulatory blood pressure monitor (Spacelabs Inc., Redmond, Wash). The appropriate sized cuff was placed around the nondominant arm and 3 consecutive blood pressure determinations were recorded along with sphygmomanometric measurements to verify that there was no difference greater than 5 mmHg on the average of the 2 sets of values. Throughout the 24-hour monitoring readings were obtained automatically at 15-minute intervals and all subjects had at least 3 valid readings per hour. The resulting 80 to 96 pairs of systolic and diastolic BP readings per recording with the corresponding recording time were used to calculate blood pressure derivatives. All subjects were instructed to maintain their usual daytime activities between

6:00 AM and 10:00 PM and rest-sleep between 10:00 PM and 6:00 AM [13]. In this context it is useful to outline the time rate (TR) of BP variation. The TR of BP variation was defined as the first derivative of the BP values against time and was calculated as the mean of the absolute ratios of the differences between successive BPs and the minutes between them. Details concerning the TR estimation have been described elsewhere [14]. This parameter focuses on the subsequent changes between consecutive BP recordings, how fast or how slow and in which direction BP values change, and is more sensitive to the sequential order of BP readings than the standard deviation index, which merely reflects the upward and downward BP excursions around the mean.

2.2.2. Cold Pressor Test (CPT). The CPT is a method commonly used to evoke a sympathoexcitatory stress response [15, 16]. Testing was conducted by trained experimenters in a quiet room. The cap for wireless EEG recording was attached, and the following EEG recording phases were carried out: (i) 3 min resting baseline period; (ii) immersion of the left hand to just above the wrist in a 2°C water bath with eyes closed for 1 min (unit of stress); (iii) continued immersion in the 2°C water bath until the participant, as previously directed, spontaneously withdrew the hand due to intolerability of the cold (pain tolerance assessment); (iv) 3 min resting/recovery phase. Time of immersion, time of 1 min exposure to the cold ("unit" of stress), and time of withdrawal of the hand (tolerance) were recorded. The CPT was well tolerated by all subjects, with no adverse effects noted. EEG monitoring during the CPT: EEG recording was continuous through the 3 min resting phase preceding the CPT, the 1st CPT minute (stress unit), the pain tolerance assessment phase, and the concluding 3 min post-CPT phase.

EEG data collection and analysis: for acquiring the EEG data, the EMOTIV Epoc EEG system was used (EMOTIV, 20141). This device has a wireless amplifier, and 14 wet saline electrodes, corresponding at the positions AF3, F7, F3, FC5, T7, P7, O1, O2, P8, T8, FC6, F4, F8, and AF4 according to the international 10–20 system (see Figure 7).

The device has also an embedded 16-bit ADC which was used to digitize the data with 128 Hz sampling frequency per channel. The data were sent via Bluetooth to a computer with the EMOTIV Control Panel software installed, allowing the visual monitoring of the impedance of the electrode contact to the scalp. The EMOTIV Epoc EEG device is part of a number of low-cost EEG systems, which have been recently applied for research aims. However, recent research assessing their reliability provides converging evidence indicating their capacity to measure consistently EEG signals [17–20].

Two electrodes located just above the subject's ears (P3, P4) were used as reference. Electrode resistance was kept constantly below 5 kΩ. The EEG signals were band-passed filtered with Butterworth 0.5–8 Hz, 8–12 Hz, 12–28 Hz, and 28–45.5 Hz filters.

In order to analyse the data from the experimental setup, a wavelet-based analysis was performed using EEGLAB 13.5.4b [21], an open-source toolbox for MATLAB (Mathworks, Inc., Natick, MA, USA). The data processing in our work is based on the wavelet transform, $W_x(t, f)$, that permits the accurate

decomposition of EEG waveforms into a set of component waveforms allowing the isolation of all scales of waveform structure [22]. According to this method, the complex Morlet wavelet is chosen as a mother wavelet, $\Psi(t)$, to be convolved with the original signal, $x(t)$. This convolution leads to a new signal, $W_x^{\Psi}(b, a)$, with b denoting the translation parameter and a the wavelet's scaling parameter. This signal consisted of coefficients which denote the correlation between the EEG signal and the wavelet function. In order to approximate the continuous wavelet transform, the convolution with the signal has to be done N times for each scale, where N is the number of points in the signal time series. Although the choice of N could be arbitrary, given the fact that the exact number of time segment data points of all CPT phases was known beforehand, the appropriate choice of repeated convolutions was made resulting in comparable wavelet coefficients for all time segments. Nevertheless, the wavelet transforms at each scale a have to be directly comparable to each other and to the transforms of other time series, so the wavelet function was normalized to have unit energy at all times. The wavelet power spectrum was then computed as $|W_x(t, f)^2|$ or as $|W_x(b, a)^2|$ in terms of translation and shifting parameters.

Furthermore, certain coefficients will be generated corresponding to the noise affected zones and some other coefficients will be generated in the areas corresponding to the actual EEG. Although these coefficients are associated with frequency components, they are modified in the time domain, where each coefficient corresponds to a time range. An appropriate choice of wavelet coefficients would result in removing the noisy part of the EEG signal to some extent, while retaining the useful part of the signal [23]. Noise filtering is therefore implemented simply by zeroing out any coefficients associated primarily with noise.

For each electrode the total measurements were divided into four time segments based on the previous described experimental procedure. The wavelet coefficients were split into the following eight standardized bands: Delta (1–4 Hz), Theta1 (4–6 Hz), Theta2 (6–8 Hz), Alpha1 (8–10 Hz), Alpha2 (10–12 Hz), Beta1 (12.5–16 Hz), Beta2 (16.5–20 Hz), Beta3 (20.5–28 Hz), and Gamma (28.5–45 Hz). The wavelet cycles of the transform were dynamically increased so that the time width of the wavelet corresponding to the highest frequency of the Gamma band is to be half the time width of that related to the lowest frequency of the Delta band, thus, allowing a higher frequency resolution (resulting from 3 cycles at 1 Hz to above 67 cycles at 45 Hz). The wavelet coefficients were averaged over time and then scales contained within each frequency band were summed together to yield the absolute activity within each band [12, 24]. For each time segment and frequency band, the Power Spectral Density was calculated by integrating the corresponding wavelet scalogram over time.

3. Statistical Analysis

Statistical analysis was performed with the STATISTICA 12.0 software for Windows. A first analysis involved a between-group, Repeated Measures design. Power spectrum density of EEG recordings from 14 electrodes was expressed as Delta,

TABLE 2

	Hypertensives N = 22		Controls N = 18		p
	Mean	SD	Mean	SD	
Mean MBP24	106.19	7.28	91.09	5.95	0.000
Max DBP day	118.59	11.15	98.22	25.97	0.002
Min HR day	62.18	8.87	52.27	16.33	0.019
Min MBP day	85.50	9.92	68.00	19.00	0.001

Theta1, Theta2, Alpha1, Alpha2, Beta1, Beta2, Beta3, and Gamma values. Each frequency was analysed as a dependent variable in separate, 1-way Repeated Measures ANOVAs. In each ANOVA, the independent variable was Group Membership ((1) normotensive controls versus (2) hypertensives); the Repeated Measures factor was phase, which included four levels corresponding to the stages of the Cold Pressor Test ((1) pretest resting phase, (2) stress unit phase, (3) tolerance phase, and (4) posttest resting phase). Special attention was given to interactions as those would provide the strongest evidence as to differential response profiles of hypertensives versus controls. The overall relationship among the clinical and the EEG variables was further investigated by Canonical Analysis; in order to ascertain the relative significance of the variables they showed the highest individual association with the two states of the subjects (i.e., healthy controls and hypertensives). On the left side of the equation we chose those EEG variables that clearly and statistically significant showed an interaction effect via the standard Repeated Measures ANOVA paradigm. Each subgroup of these variables was analysed separately so four Canonical Analyses were carried out, one for each group, that is, Gamma, Alpha1, Alpha2, Delta, and Theta1. On the right side of the equation we chose Maximum Diastolic Blood Pressure of the day (Max DBP day), Minimum Heart Rate of the day (Min HR day), Mean Blood Pressure 24 hours (Mean MBP24), and Minimum Diastolic Blood Pressure of the day (Min DBP day) by performing Discriminant Function Analysis that included all clinical variables and controls/hypertensives as the dependent variable.

We also performed the standard Student's t-test to check for differences between the groups regarding the behavioural performance in the pain tolerance of the subjects.

4. Results

4.1. Behavioural Variables. There was no significant difference between normotensives and hypertensives although a tendency was revealed towards greater pain tolerance in hypertensives measured as self-determined duration (min) of exposure to the cold bath (mean tolerance, controls = 4.62 ± 1.32 min; hypertensives 6.02 ± 2.79 min; $p = 0.059$).

4.2. Arterial Blood Pressure Variables. Overall the ABPM variables differed significantly between the two compared groups; however a Discriminant Function Analysis revealed the four most differentiators variables; see Table 2.

4.3. EEG Data. A significant main effect of phase was noted in several electrodes (Delta: O2 and F8; Theta1: F3; Alpha1: O2 and P8; Alpha2: F3 and AF4; Beta2: F3 and F4; and, finally, in Gamma electrodes AF3 and F7). Overall, signals tended to rise during the tolerance phase and drop during the posttest resting phase.

However, the central finding was the interactions observed between Group Membership and phase. Analyses revealed interactions in Delta, Theta1, Alpha1, Alpha2, Beta2, and Gamma values. In examining this relationship we encountered four distinct response patterns which support our hypothesis that hypertensives have a differential electrophysiological response profile to environmental stimuli as those are simulated by the phases of the Cold Pressor Test.

4.3.1. Delta Brain Activity (DBA). DBA at F3 and P8 leads had higher values for hypertensives than controls overall and particularly in the tolerance and posttest phases. A similar finding was noted for electrode O2 but with a greater difference between the two groups, with controls showing a continuous value decline from pretest to posttest. In the control group, lead F4 showed a sharp value drop at the posttest phase, whereas hypertensives demonstrated a slight increase at the same phase. In the control group the AF4 lead revealed a steady drop from the beginning of the procedure to the end, similarly to the O2 lead; in contrast, the hypertensives group sustained the same level of activity in all four experimental phases (Table 3, Figures 1 and 7). All five interactions were statistically significant (Table 3).

TBA 1 at F3 and AF4 leads produced a statistically significant interaction (Table 6), with hypertensives showing overall higher values peaking in the tolerance phase. In the same phase controls demonstrated a considerable value drop during the tolerance phase (Table 4, Figures 2 and 7).

Overall, ABA 1 values at O2 and P8 leads were higher in hypertensives than controls throughout the experiment, whereas controls showed a significant drop in the posttest resting phase (Table 5, Figures 3 and 7). This was a statistically significant interaction (Table 5).

In the case of Alpha1 electrode P8 the statistically significant interaction was due to the within the control group drop in the Power Spectral Density value at the posttest phase compared to the pretest ($p = 0.001$) rather than between the groups as noted in most measurements.

4.3.2. Alpha2 Brain Activity (A2BA). A2BA values showed significant interactions at leads AF3, F3, and AF4. The results followed a different pattern from that noted with A1BA. Both groups had similar values during the pretest, with the control group subsequently showing a marked drop during the stress unit phase. In contrast, in that phase hypertensives actually showed a small rise, which levelled off during the tolerance and the posttest phases (Table 6, Figures 4 and 7). These differences were statistically significant (Table 6).

B2BA showed a statistically significant interaction for lead T8 (Table 7). Hypertensives had lower values at the pretest resting phase and also at the tolerance and posttest resting

TABLE 3

	N	Pretest		Stress unit		Tolerance		Posttest		Interaction
		Mean	SD	Mean	SD	Mean	SD	Mean	SD	
Delta F3										
Controls	18	42.21	4.18	42.32	3.88	40.76	3.49	42.13	3.89	$F_3 = 6.65, p = 0.000$
Hypertensives	22	44.14	7.32	43.88	7.27	45.46	6.39	44.67	6.76	
Delta O2										
Controls	18	38.74	6.83	37.73	7.29	36.94	6.55	36.77	7.34	$F_3 = 4.37, p = 0.006$
Hypertensives	22	42.59	8.31	41.90	8.86	44.13	7.04	41.89	7.73	
Delta P8										
Controls	18	42.05	8.11	41.95	8.12	40.58	6.98	41.58	7.46	$F_3 = 5.64, p = 0.001$
Hypertensives	22	44.48	9.63	44.24	8.93	46.54	7.16	44.14	8.44	
Delta F8										
Controls	18	47.09	3.87	47.15	3.76	47.10	3.64	44.78	3.18	$F_3 = 13.85, p = 0.000$
Hypertensives	22	47.62	7.40	47.77	7.24	47.97	7.09	48.57	6.98	
Delta AF4										
Controls	18	44.71	5.63	44.64	6.03	43.66	5.63	43.05	4.71	$F_3 = 7.34, p = 0.004$
Hypertensives	22	47.19	8.40	47.11	8.30	48.24	7.19	47.78	8.19	

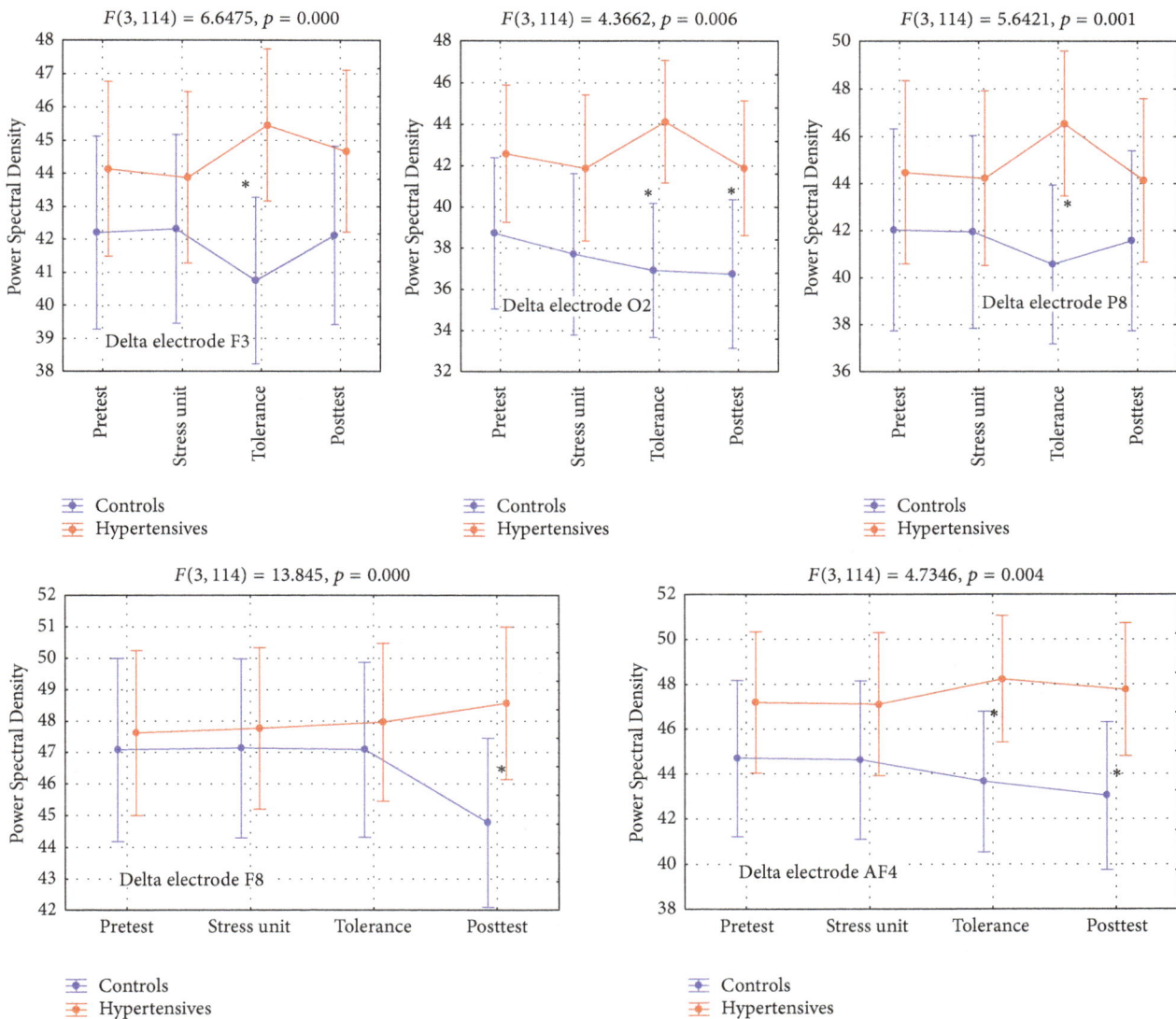

FIGURE 1: Delta brain activity (DBA). ∗ refers to statistically significant differences.

TABLE 4

	N	Pretest		Stress unit		Tolerance		Posttest		Interaction
		Mean	SD	Mean	SD	Mean	SD	Mean	SD	
Theta1 F3										
Controls	18	41.33	3.40	41.52	3.49	39.88	2.90	41.25	3.34	$F_3 = 8.43$, $p = 0.000$
Hypertensives	22	42.56	5.54	42.77	5.42	43.02	5.25	42.60	4.95	
Theta1 AF4										
Controls	18	43.65	5.10	43.80	5.79	42.04	4.79	43.43	5.43	$F_3 = 7.52$, $p = 0.000$
Hypertensives	22	45.55	7.01	45.80	6.68	46.11	6.60	45.29	6.51	

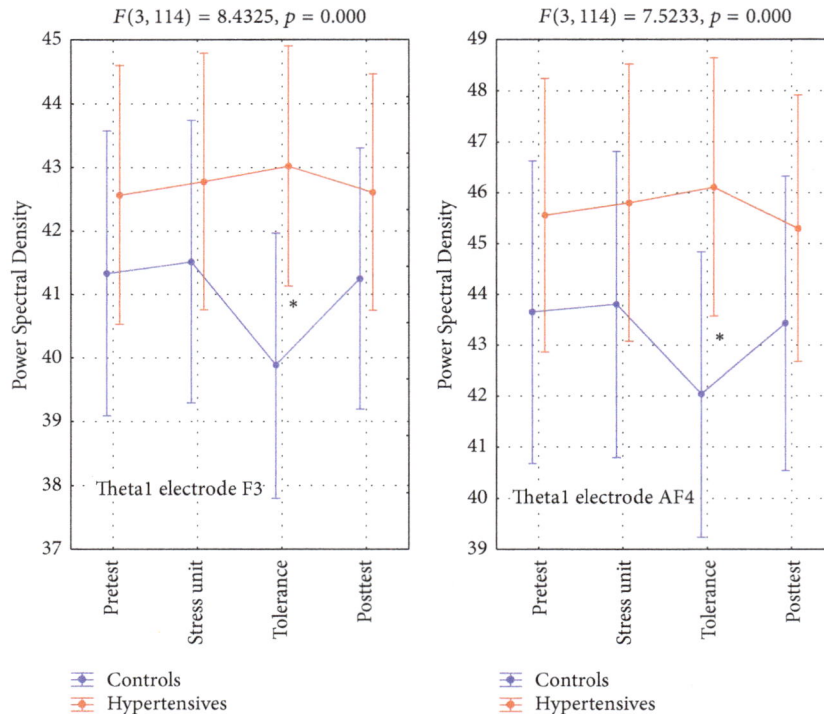

FIGURE 2: Theta1 brain activity (T1BA). ∗ refers to statistically significant differences.

phase, compared to healthy controls (Table 7, Figures 5 and 7).

As in the case of Alpha1 electrode P8 the statistically significant interaction in Beta2 electrode T8 was due to the within the control group rise in the Power Spectral Density value at the posttest phase compared to the stress unit phase ($p = 0.02$) rather than between the groups as noted in most measurements.

4.3.3. Gamma Brain Activity (GBA).
GBA values for leads T8, AF3, AF4, and FC6 revealed statistically significant Group X Phase interactions (Table 8). Multiple comparisons indicated AF3 values were lower in hypertensives at the pretest phase and again lower at the posttest phase whereas they were similar to controls during the stress unit and the tolerance phase.

T8 values showed the greatest difference between the two groups during the tolerance phase with hypertensives having higher values than controls.

The electrode FC6 recordings showed a general higher value range for controls especially during the tolerance and the posttest phases (Table 8, Figures 6 and 7).

Once more, the statistically significant interaction for Gamma electrode AF3 was due to statistically significant differences in the Power Spectral Density values what were noted in the hypertensives group who had a sharp rise from the pretest to the stress unit phase ($p = 0.001$) and the tolerance phase ($p = 0.000$) whereas no such changes were observed in the controls group whose values remained similar throughout the entire experiment.

On the left side of the equation we chose those EEG variables that clearly and statistically significantly showed an interaction effect via the standard Repeated Measures ANOVA paradigm. Each subgroup of these variables was analysed separately so four Canonical Analyses were carried out, one for each group, that is, Gamma, Alpha1, Alpha2, Delta, and Theta1. On the right side of the equation we chose Max DBP day, Min HR day, Min MBP24, and Min

TABLE 5

	N	Pretest		Stress unit		Tolerance		Posttest		Interaction
		Mean	SD	Mean	SD	Mean	SD	Mean	SD	
Alpha1 O2										
Controls	18	36.38	6.28	35.58	7.26	35.84	7.46	34.13	6.46	$F_3 = 3.18, p = 0.027$
Hypertensives	22	39.34	6.39	39.07	7.39	39.56	7.19	39.20	6.18	
Alpha1 P8										
Controls	18	39.39	7.02	39.08	7.28	39.63	7.11	36.84	5.46	$F_3 = 5.92, p = 0.00$
Hypertensives	22	41.41	8.01	41.09	7.24	41.70	7.81	41.27	7.35	

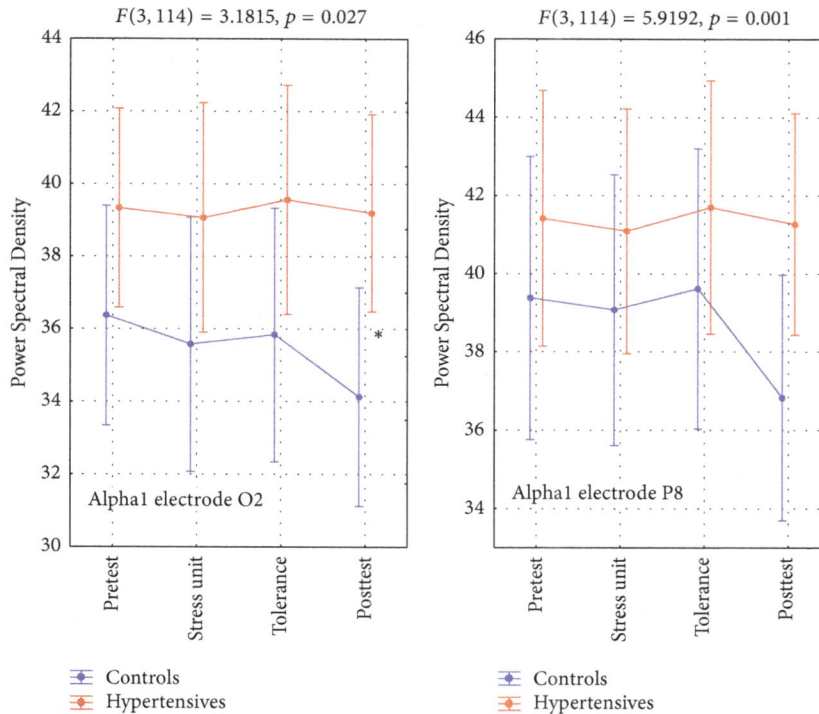

FIGURE 3: Alpha1 brain activity (A1BA). ∗ refers to statistically significant differences.

DBP day by performing Discriminant Function Analysis that included all clinical variables and controls/hypertensives as the dependent variable. Discriminant Function Analysis is useful in deciding which set of variables is best in discriminating between groups of subjects and thus suitable for our purpose in isolating those clinical variables that most strongly predicted membership in our groups.

The obtained results revealed that Delta values where the most strongly associated with the clinical state of the subjects (Canonical R: 0.82870; $Chi^2(56) = 67.373$ $p = 0.14224$). This was followed by Alpha2 (Canonical R: 0.78902; $Chi^2(48) = 64.833$ $p = 0.05315$), Gamma (Canonical R: 0.75445; $Chi^2(48) = 53.749$; $p = 0.26380$), Alpha1 (Canonical R: 0.64904; $Chi^2(32) = 32.951$ $p = 0.42043$), and Beta1 (Canonical R: 0.60100; $Chi^2(16) = 22.403$; $p = 0.13073$).

The relevant correlation matrices showing the electrodes involved with correlations higher than 0.3 as derived by the Canonical Analyses are given in Table 9 and in Figures 8, 9, 10, and 11.

5. Discussion

The study explored putative relationships between arterial blood pressure variables (24 hr ABPM) and electrophysiological responsiveness (EEG activity) elicited by exposure to sympathoexcitatory stress/pain induced by the CPT in untreated hypertensives and normotensive controls.

Although the two groups differed significantly in all arterial blood pressure variables, a Discriminant Function Analysis revealed that the most robust group differentiators were four: Maximum Diastolic Blood Pressure of the day (Max DBP day), Minimum Heart Rate of the day (Min HR day), Mean Blood Pressure 24 hours (Mean MBP 24), and Minimum Diastolic Blood Pressure of the day (Min DBP day).

An initial series of ANOVA analyses determined significant group differences in CPT-induced EEG oscillations, which were then covaried with the four most robust cardiovascular differentiators by means of Canonical Analyses. This revealed positive correlations between cardiovascular

TABLE 6

	N	Pretest		Stress unit		Tolerance		Posttest		Interaction
		Mean	SD	Mean	SD	Mean	SD	Mean	SD	
Alpha2 AF3										
Controls	18	38.56	3.93	36.71	4.14	38.82	4.07	38.58	3.70	$F_3 = 8.95, p = 0.000$
Hypertensives	22	38.88	5.52	40.04	4.15	39.22	5.66	39.15	4.55	
Alpha2 F3										
Controls	18	37.13	3.59	35.76	3.48	37.28	3.39	37.20	3.17	$F_3 = 7.39, p = 0.006$
Hypertensives	22	38.11	4.44	38.72	4.23	38.51	4.22	38.57	3.93	
Alpha2 AF4										
Controls	18	38.23	4.16	36.69	3.73	38.52	4.43	38.28	4.77	$F_3 = 6.00, p = 0.001$
Hypertensives	22	40.01	5.69	40.73	4.58	40.43	5.20	39.97	4.79	

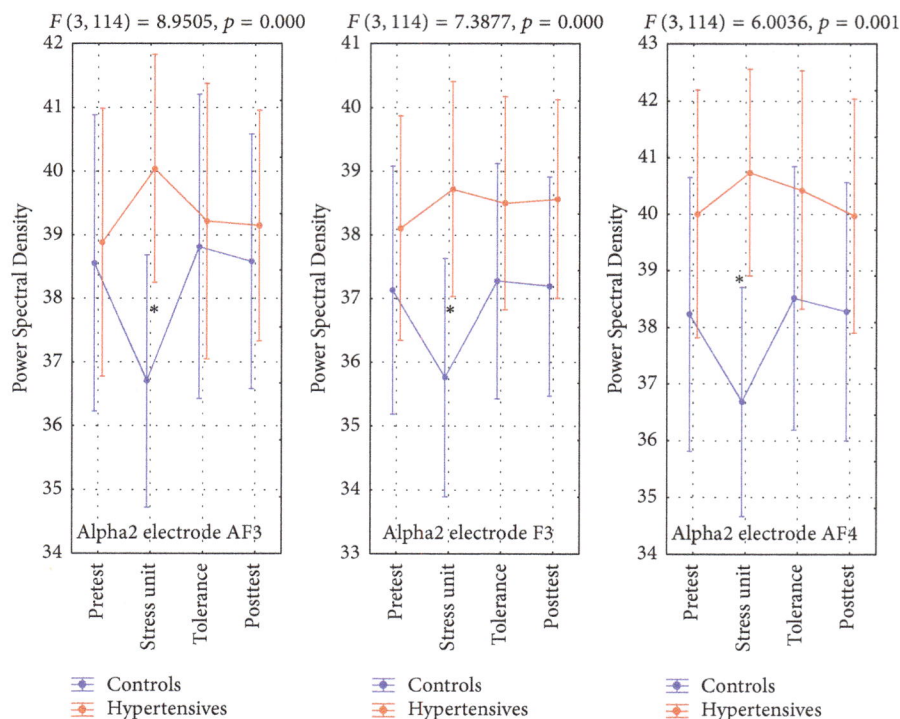

FIGURE 4: Alpha2 brain activity (A2BA). ∗ refers to statistically significant differences.

variables and Delta oscillations (1–4 Hz) during the tolerance phase; in high-alpha oscillations (10–12 Hz) during the stress unit and posttest phase; and in low-alpha oscillations (8–10 Hz) during all four CPT phases.

In contrast, negative correlations were noted between cardiovascular variables and Beta2 oscillations (16.5–20 Hz) during the posttest phase and Gamma oscillations (28.5–45 Hz) during all four CPT phases.

These associations were localised at several sites across the cerebral hemispheres, predominantly in the right one, and in left frontal lobe.

On the behavioural level, pain tolerance measured in terms of self-determined exposure to the CPT ice bath beyond the obligatory 1 min stress unit phase revealed a tendency towards greater tolerance in hypertensives, although this did not reach statistical significance ($p = 0.059$).

This is in line with previous findings indicating hypoalgesia in hypertensives. Hypertension-associated hypoalgesia has important clinical implications, the first of which relates to the phenomenon of silent myocardial ischemia and infarcts which are significantly more common in hypertensives than in normotensives [7, 25].

Given the multiplicity of electrophysiological observations based on the initial ANOVAs analyses, for the purposes of this discussion we have focused on the instances where the Canonical Correlation Analysis revealed strong relationships between the cardiovascular and electrophysiological group differentiators of the study.

5.1. Delta Brain Activity (1–4 Hz). The correlations identified between cardiovascular group differentiators and Delta brain activity (DBA) appear compatible with previous human and

TABLE 7

	N	Pretest		Stress unit		Tolerance		Posttest		Interaction
		Mean	SD	Mean	SD	Mean	SD	Mean	SD	
Beta2 T8										
Controls	18	36.26	4.70	36.12	4.77	36.60	5.10	36.88	5.36	$F_3 = 2.84, p = 0.041$
Hypertensives	22	35.72	6.56	36.06	6.47	36.00	6.75	35.55	6.22	

TABLE 8

	N	Pretest		Stress unit		Tolerance		Posttest		Interaction
		Mean	SD	Mean	SD	Mean	SD	Mean	SD	
Gamma AF3										
Controls	18	33.39	2.41	33.24	2.40	33.58	2.239	33.49	3.20	$F_3 = 3.54, p = 0.017$
Hypertensives	22	31.90	4.19	33.13	3.92	33.37	3.943	32.25	3.46	
Gamma T8										
Controls	18	33.70	3.44	33.49	4.24	31.73	4.16	33.69	4.96	$F_3 = 12.41, p = 0.000$
Hypertensives	22	32.46	4.90	32.83	5.24	34.70	3.44	31.77	4.89	
Gamma FC6										
Controls	18	32.81	3.32	32.85	3.83	34.24	2.02	33.28	4.21	$F_3 = 4.14, p = 0.008$
Hypertensives	22	31.57	3.74	32.10	4.40	31.47	3.90	30.97	3.44	

animal studies suggesting that increased cerebral activity in the spectrum of DBA is associated with increased arterial pressure, probably mediated through suppressed baroreflex control of heart rate [26, 27]. DBA enhancement during perceptual tasks has been associated with functional cortical "deafferentation," that is, inhibition of sensory bottom-up interferences with internal concentration. It has been proposed that this is a sign of neuronal rearrangement phenomena in the acute and chronic phases of recovery [28]. The sustained increase in DBA activity noted in our hypertensive group is compatible with previous findings suggesting "super efforts" in untreated essential hypertension, possibly due to hypoactivation of the reinforcement system combined with compromised functioning of the brain serotonin system [29, 30].

DBA correlations were noted in the left frontal and the right occipital areas. This is consistent with evidence that DBA is involved in cortical communication over long distances [31]. Yener and colleagues [32] suggested that there were two different networks activated in DBA in response to different stimulus modalities, according to the stimulation characteristics and sensory or cognitive demands.

5.2. Alpha Brain Activity, High (10–12 Hz: A2BA) and Low (8–10 Hz: A1BA).

Our findings revealed positive correlations between cardiovascular variables and high (10–12 Hz) alpha oscillations during the CPT stress unit and posttest phases and in low (8–10 Hz) alpha oscillations during the 4 CPT phases overall. The high-alpha subband (A2BA) is considered an index of task-specific sensorimotor activity regulation [33], mainly related to attentional processes [34]: optimal task performance requires inhibition of task-irrelevant areas, which is reflected as high-alpha oscillatory activity facilitating better resource allocation to task-relevant areas [35, 36]. The lower the amplitude of alpha oscillations the better the information transfer through sensorimotor thalamocortical

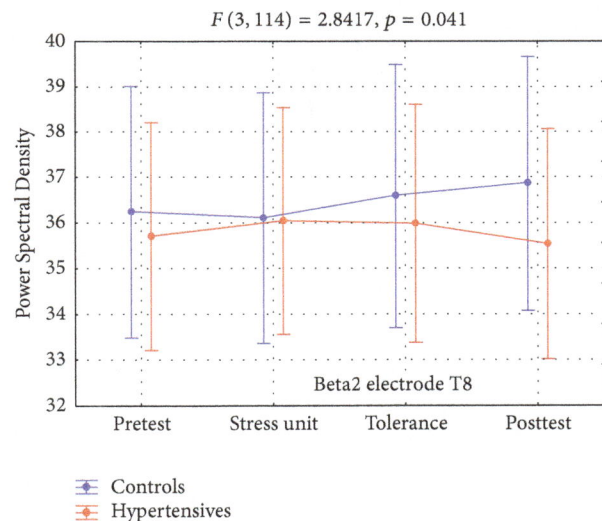

$F(3, 114) = 2.8417, p = 0.041$

FIGURE 5: Beta2 brain activity (B2BA).

and corticocortical pathways [37]. The CPT is a commonly used method for eliciting primarily sympathetic activation during periods of stress. Hence our finding regarding high-alpha power may underline the positive link between stress and a top-down inhibitory mechanism which, in our study, appears deficient in hypertensives. In line with this view there are findings of increased heart rate and blood pressure in high hostile individuals when exposed to stressful conditions such as the CPT [38].

The low-alpha subband (A1BA) is considered an index of general tonic alertness [33]. The different response of our two groups to pain-related processing may reflect changes of cortical excitability related to the special alerting function of preceding pain [38].

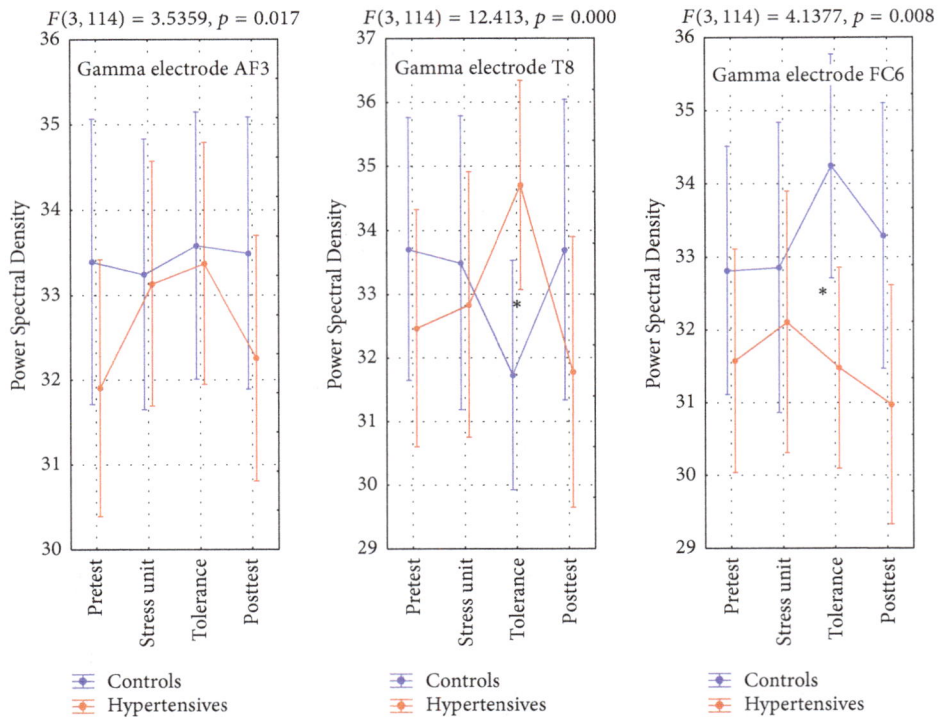

FIGURE 6: Gamma brain activity (GBA). ∗ refers to statistically significant differences.

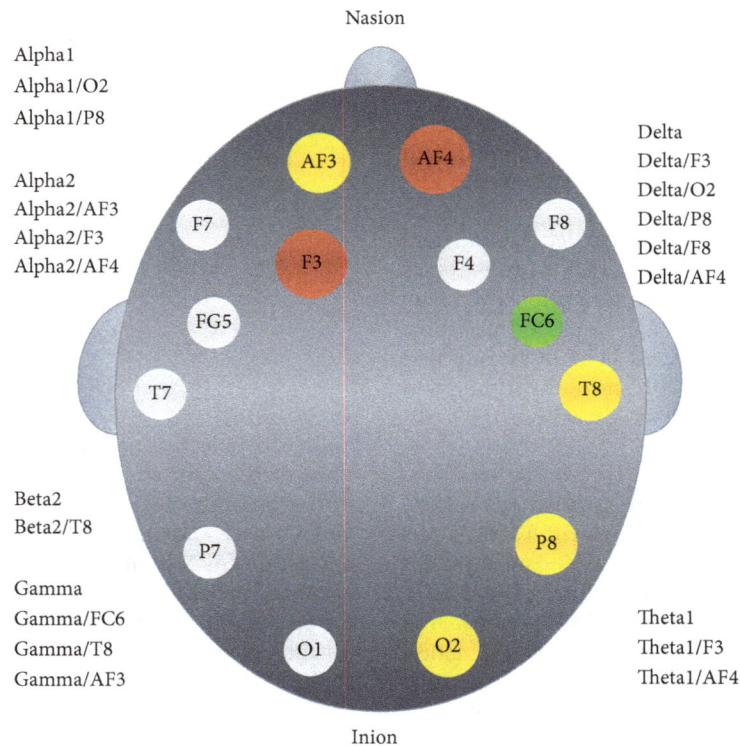

FIGURE 7: EEG oscillations based on the EMOTIV Epoc EEG apparatus; coloured sites indicate significant group differences.

TABLE 9

Correlations left set with right set	Mean MBP24[1]	Max DBP day[2]	Min HR day[3]	Min MBP day[4]
Delta tolerance F3	*0.32*	0.27	−0.11	0.26
Delta tolerance O2	*0.37*	0.15	0.26	*0.40*
Alpha1 pretest resting O2	0.22	0.07	*0.33*	0.35
Alpha1 stress unit O2	0.25	0.12	0.27	*0.38*
Alpha1 tolerance O2	0.24	0.09	0.27	*0.34*
Alpha1 posttest resting O2	*0.30*	0.17	*0.37*	0.39
Alpha2 stress unit AF3	0.24	0.11	0.11	*0.32*
Alpha2 stress unit F3	*0.34*	0.22	0.23	*0.39*
Alpha2 posttest resting F3	0.26	0.17	0.12	*0.34*
Beta2 posttest resting T8	*−0.32*	*−0.31*	−0.02	−0.15
Gamma pretest resting FC6	−0.27	*−0.33*	−0.18	−0.12
Gamma stress unit T8	−0.24	*−0.32*	−0.12	−0.09
Gamma tolerance FC6	*−0.38*	*−0.37*	−0.27	−0.23
Gamma posttest resting AF3	−0.24	*−0.34*	−0.14	*−0.31*
Gamma posttest resting T8	*−0.41*	*−0.41*	−0.17	−0.27
Gamma posttest resting FC6	*−0.39*	*−0.38*	−0.21	−0.27

[1] Figure 8, [2] Figure 9, [3] Figure 10, and [4] Figure 11.

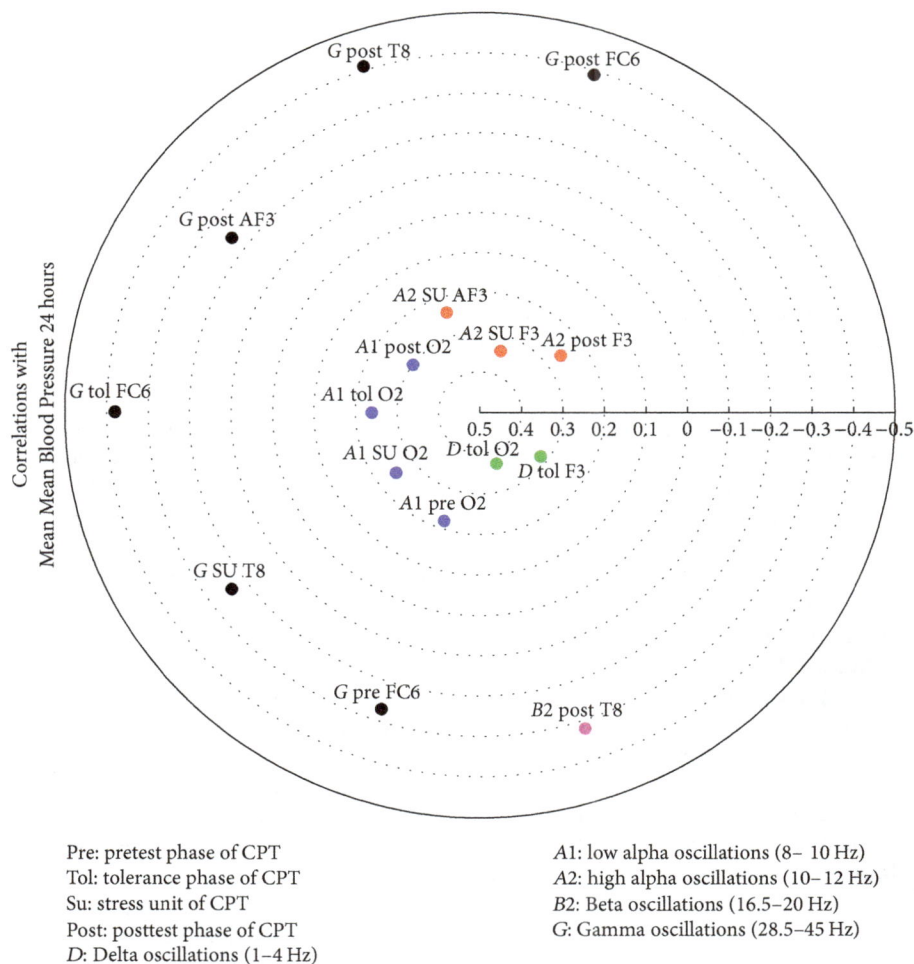

Pre: pretest phase of CPT
Tol: tolerance phase of CPT
Su: stress unit of CPT
Post: posttest phase of CPT
D: Delta oscillations (1–4 Hz)

A1: low alpha oscillations (8– 10 Hz)
A2: high alpha oscillations (10– 12 Hz)
B2: Beta oscillations (16.5–20 Hz)
G: Gamma oscillations (28.5–45 Hz)

FIGURE 8: Heliograph of the correlations between Mean Mean Blood Pressure 24 hours and the statistically significant different CPT-induced EEG oscillations depicted by concentric circles in the (−1)-(0)-(+1) continuum.

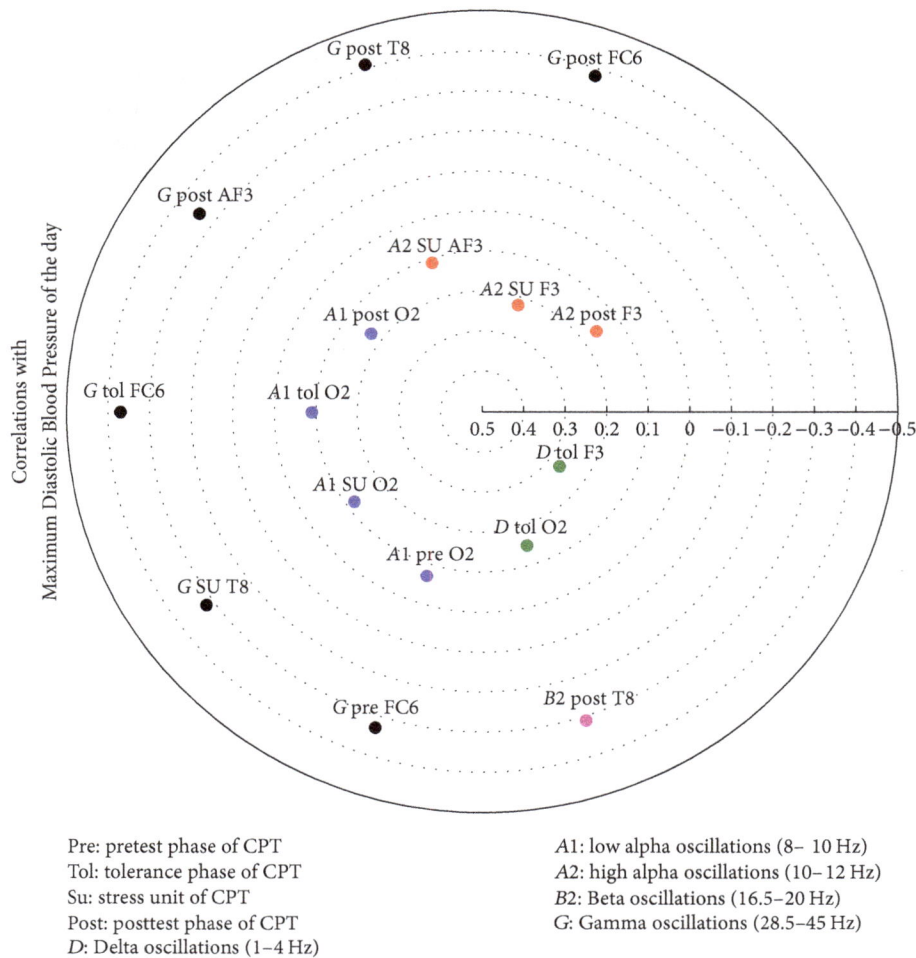

FIGURE 9: Heliograph of the correlations between Maximum Diastolic Blood Pressure of the day and the statistically significant different CPT-induced EEG oscillations depicted by concentric circles in the (−1)-(0)-(+1) continuum.

It is a reasonable assumption that the pretest brain oscillations noted in our study may be explained in terms of anticipation of pain. Such anticipation can cause mood changes and behavioural adaptations which may influence subsequent pain perception [39, 40]. It has been shown [34] that the magnitude of a nociceptively induced alpha oscillation related desynchronization (a-ERD) was significantly more dependent on prestimulus than on poststimulus alpha power. A more recent study [41] showed that prestimulus EEG oscillations in the alpha frequency band modulated the subjective perception of painful stimuli: prestimulus alpha oscillatory activities in fact assisted in predicting subjective pain perception. This notion is in line with reports indicating that decreased low-alpha brain oscillations are correlated with higher numerical pain scores collected during both resting-state and noxious conditions by the application of tonic noxious stimuli [42].

5.3. Beta2 Brain Activity (16.5–20 Hz, B2BA). A negative correlation was noted between cardiovascular variables and B2BA during the posttest phase. Given that Beta brain activity plays a role in motor processing, a possible interpretation

of this correlation is that pain-related B2BA modulations reflect the preparation and execution of a defensive response [43]. This view is consistent with recent reports showing negative correlations between Beta oscillations and sympathetic activity subserving the interaction between brain neural populations involved in somatomotor control and brain neural populations regulating ANS signals to heart [44].

5.4. Gamma Brain Activity (GBA). A negative correlation between GBA and cardiovascular group differentiators emerged from our study. GBA is considered to play a crucial role in cortical integration and perception [45]. Brief painful stimuli induce GBA in somatosensory cortices [10, 46], probably reflecting local sensory processing in the somatosensory cortex [47].

In contrast, longer-lasting painful stimulation (perception of tonic pain) does not appear to be encoded by GBA in the somatosensory cortex, but rather in the medial prefrontal cortex, close to premotor and cingulate cortices [48]. This GBA encoding of tonic pain might indicate that the subjective perception of longer-lasting pain is more dependent on

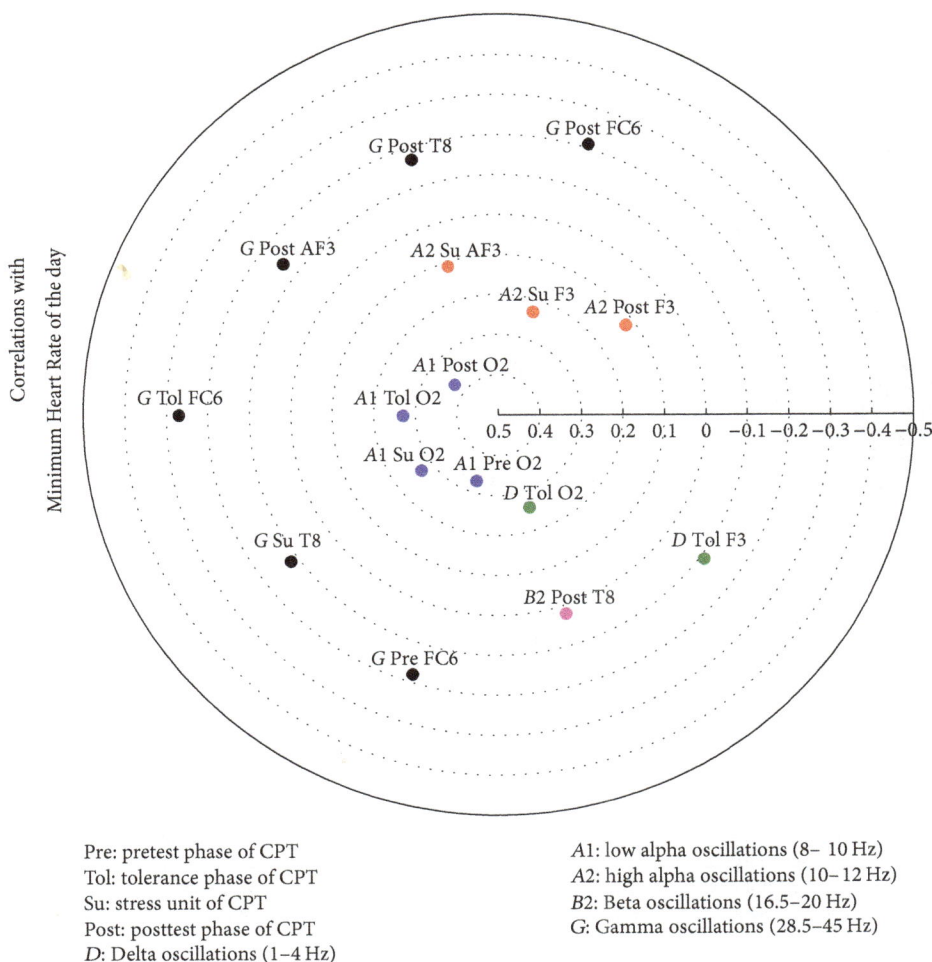

Pre: pretest phase of CPT
Tol: tolerance phase of CPT
Su: stress unit of CPT
Post: posttest phase of CPT
D: Delta oscillations (1–4 Hz)

A1: low alpha oscillations (8–10 Hz)
A2: high alpha oscillations (10–12 Hz)
B2: Beta oscillations (16.5–20 Hz)
G: Gamma oscillations (28.5–45 Hz)

FIGURE 10: Heliograph of the correlations between Minimum Heart Rate of the day and the statistically significant different CPT-induced EEG oscillations depicted by concentric circles in the (−1)-(0)-(+1) continuum.

contextual/emotional processes than on the sensory ones which determine perception of brief painful stimuli. The GBA modulation in our study may be considered in this light.

Previous studies have shown that GBA is enhanced during attentional selection of sensory information [49]. Additionally GBA modulations over the somatosensory cortex are enhanced by attention and vary with pain processing [10, 38, 49]. Thus the enhancement of GBA in our hypertensive group, over the contralateral somatosensory cortex may be related to subjective pain intensity and reflect the internal representations of behaviourally relevant stimuli that should receive enhanced/preferred processing [10, 38]. GBA observed in the pretest (anticipatory) phase of our procedure may be explained in terms of anticipation of pain, causing mood changes and behavioural adaptations which may then influence perception of subsequent pain [50].

In the service of adaptive environmental engagement low coping capacity has been associated with a more pronounced decrease in GBA [51]. Hence the negative correlations obtained between GBA and cardiovascular variables across CPT phases would seem to confirm this perspective.

It is compatible with converging evidence which consistently indicates significant involvement of GBA in hemodynamic fluctuations being mediated by the bidirectional connections between neuronal substrates underlying GBA and autonomic responses [52, 53].

As a whole, the correlations we noted between brain oscillations and cardiovascular parameters may be better understood in the light of reports suggesting that cognitive alterations depend upon the degree of hypertension. It is established that the systolic and diastolic blood pressures have effects on distinct cognitive domains [54, 55]. Anson and Paran [56] and Gupta et al. [57] endorsed the view that systolic and diastolic hypertension may also affect cognitive measures in a different way.

Furthermore, the relative scalp locations of differences in magnitude of cerebral activation between the two hemispheres could determine the overall changes in blood pressure and heart rate. This idea is supportive to the view, which states that the two cerebral hemispheres act in concert to promote changes in cardiovascular functioning; however, the right hemisphere predominantly modulates sympathetic efferents, while the left hemisphere predominantly modulates

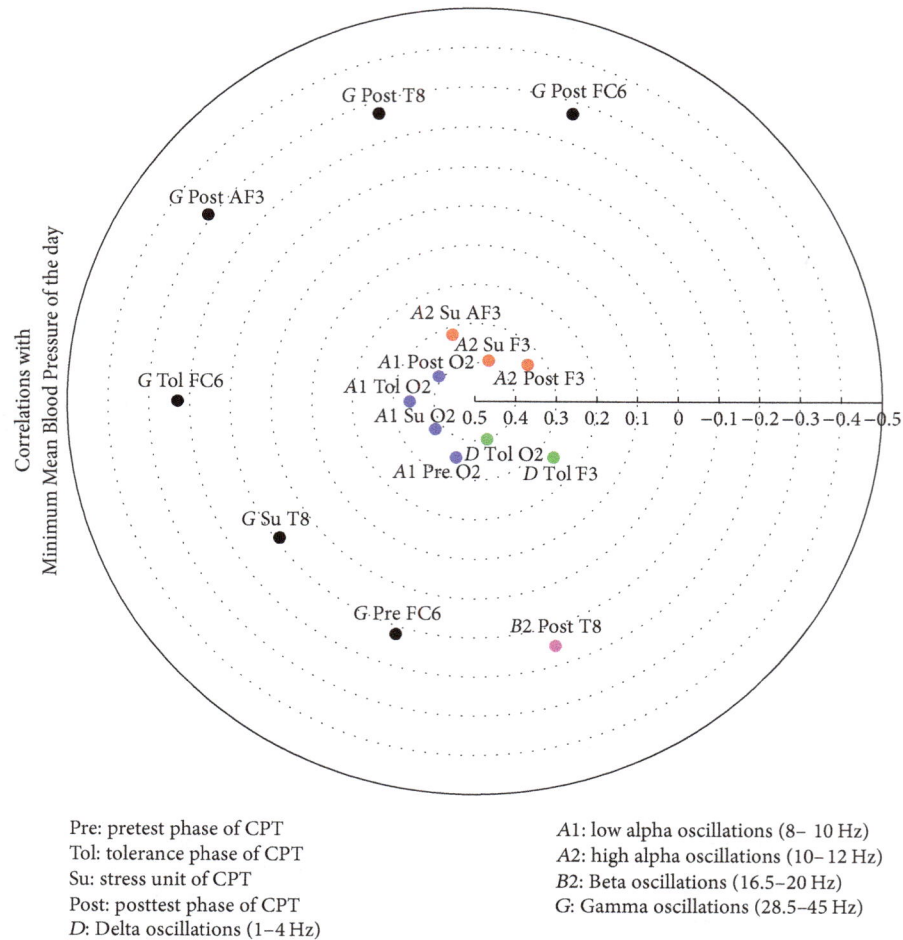

Pre: pretest phase of CPT
Tol: tolerance phase of CPT
Su: stress unit of CPT
Post: posttest phase of CPT
D: Delta oscillations (1–4 Hz)

A1: low alpha oscillations (8– 10 Hz)
A2: high alpha oscillations (10–12 Hz)
B2: Beta oscillations (16.5–20 Hz)
G: Gamma oscillations (28.5–45 Hz)

FIGURE 11: Heliograph of the correlations between Minimum Mean Blood Pressure of the day and the statistically significant different CPT-induced EEG oscillations depicted by concentric circles in the (−1)-(0)-(+1) continuum.

parasympathetic efferents, of the autonomic nervous system [58].

In conclusion, our results add to a growing body of evidence that the brain is implicated in the initiation of high blood pressure while it is itself altered by early disease processes. Thus the brain and vasculature may be independently and concurrently targeted by the factors inducing essential hypertension [59].

Previous studies have thoroughly evaluated the impact of TR of BP variation on target organ damage. A cross-sectional study in 514 normotensive and uncomplicated hypertensive patients demonstrated that the 24-hour rate of systolic BP variation was greater in hypertensive than in normotensive subjects and was the only office or ambulatory BP monitoring parameter that was linearly and independently associated with carotid intima-media thickening [14]. Moreover, another study of our group illustrated that the TR of BP variation, derived from computerized analysis of ambulatory BP monitoring data, is superior to central hemodynamics as an associate of carotid intima-media thickness in hypertensive and normotensive individuals [60]. Additionally, a marker of increased cardiovascular risk, left ventricular mass was

linearly and independently related to the daytime rate of SBP variation in hypertensive patients [61]. The former correlation persisted after adjustment for vascular risk factors, body habitus, BP and HR levels, BPV, and nocturnal BP dipping. Furthermore, Manios et al. demonstrated that increased TR of BP variation was independently associated with impaired renal function and coronary atherosclerosis in hypertensive and normotensive subjects, respectively [62, 63]. Moreover, recent studies in acute stroke patients showed that higher TR of BP variation values were associated with brain edema formation and poor outcome [64, 65]. These findings indicate that steeper BP variations may produce a greater stress on the arterial wall and may have an additive role to vascular risk factors and BP parameters in the detection of target organ damage development.

Our results also demonstrate the advantage of simultaneous EEG recording under well-defined pain inducing conditions. Our approach of factoring contributions from multiple, interconnected brain processes is relevant to all studies which attempt to link evoked brain responses with behaviour and demonstrates that exploiting these interactions leads to a more complete understanding of brain response to stimulation and the psychophysiological emergence of the experience of pain.

5.5. Limitations. A number of limitations must be considered when interpreting the findings of the current study. First, the study relied on a relatively small sample. Second, we employed CPT as a measure of pain. Although this approach is consistent with the literature, we cannot necessarily generalize the current results to other types of painful stimuli, such as thermal stimuli. Third, an additional limitation relates to the fact that EEG and cardiovascular measurements were noncontemporaneous. This potentially limits the findings in that the two measures were not precisely coupled. Fourth, data were collected in a single testing session. Therefore, we cannot comment on the stability of the relation between hypertension and EEG activity over time.

Nevertheless, the study adds to the understanding of the role of brain oscillations evoked by stress and/or pain stimulation in the underlying mechanisms of hypertension. Our data suggest that brain oscillations in response to stress and/or pain challenge may give greater insight into underlying systems and the mechanisms of hypertension.

6. Conclusions

EEG recorded in the course of the CPT provides a measure of cortical activity, on the basis of which untreated hypertensives may be differentiated from healthy controls. Furthermore, the method utilized in this study helps isolate pain-related features in the EEG during CPT in association with cardiovascular variables. This lends credibility to the hypothesis that top-down and bottom-up control mechanisms are implicated in the development of hypertension. Future applications of the methodology may help identify specific EEG features related to the neuronal processing of pain perception in hypertension.

Acknowledgments

The authors gratefully appreciate Professor Antonio T. Alexandridis and Ph.D. student Panos Papageorgiou of the Department of Electrical and Computer Engineering, University of Patras, Greece, for their valuable contribution of biosignal processing and analyzing. The authors would also like to thank Emmanouil A. Kitsonas, Electrical Engineer, Ph.D. Technical Director, Eugenides Foundation Member TCG, IEEE, IPS Council, for his technical support in the experimental procedure.

References

[1] G. Mancia, R. Fagard, K. Narkiewicz et al., "2013 ESH/ESC Guidelines for the management of arterial hypertension: the Task Force for the management of arterial hypertension of the European Society of Hypertension (ESH) and of the European Society of Cardiology (ESC)," *Journal of Hypertension*, vol. 31, no. 7, pp. 1281–1357, 2013.

[2] H. D. Critchley and S. N. Garfinkel, "Interactions between visceral afferent signaling and stimulus processing," *Frontiers in Neuroscience*, vol. 9, article 286, 2015.

[3] M. P. Schlaich, E. Lambert, D. M. Kaye et al., "Sympathetic augmentation in hypertension: role of nerve firing, norepinephrine reuptake, and angiotensin neuromodulation," *Hypertension*, vol. 43, no. 2 I, pp. 169–175, 2004.

[4] H. D. Critchley, "Neural mechanisms of autonomic, affective, and cognitive integration," *Journal of Comparative Neurology*, vol. 493, no. 1, pp. 154–166, 2005.

[5] K. Heusser, J. Tank, S. Engeli et al., "Carotid baroreceptor stimulation, sympathetic activity, baroreflex function, and blood pressure in hypertensive patients," *Hypertension*, vol. 55, no. 3, pp. 619–626, 2010.

[6] S. Duschek, I. Mück, and G. A. Reyes del Paso, "Relationship between baroreceptor cardiac reflex sensitivity and pain experience in normotensive individuals," *International Journal of Psychophysiology*, vol. 65, no. 3, pp. 193–200, 2007.

[7] M. Saccò, M. Meschi, G. Regolisti et al., "The relationship between blood pressure and pain," *Journal of Clinical Hypertension*, vol. 15, no. 8, pp. 600–605, 2013.

[8] A. Tsutsumi, "Prevention and management of work-related cardiovascular disorders," *International Journal of Occupational Medicine and Environmental Health*, vol. 28, no. 1, pp. 4–7, 2015.

[9] J. Gross, A. Schnitzler, L. Timmermann, and M. Ploner, "Gamma oscillations in human primary somatosensory cortex reflect pain perception," *PLoS Biology*, vol. 5, no. 5, pp. 1168–1173, 2007.

[10] Z. G. Zhang, L. Hu, Y. S. Hung, A. Mouraux, and G. D. Iannetti, "Gamma-band oscillations in the primary somatosensory cortex-A direct and obligatory correlate of subjective pain intensity," *Journal of Neuroscience*, vol. 32, no. 22, pp. 7429–7438, 2012.

[11] R. Dowman, D. Rissacher, and S. Schuckers, "EEG indices of tonic pain-related activity in the somatosensory cortices," *Clinical Neurophysiology*, vol. 119, no. 5, pp. 1201–1212, 2008.

[12] M. Gram, C. Graversen, S. S. Olesen, and A. M. Drewes, "Dynamic spectral indices of the electroencephalogram provide new insights into tonic pain," *Clinical Neurophysiology*, vol. 126, no. 4, pp. 763–771, 2015.

[13] N. A. Zakopoulos, G. Tsivgoulis, G. Barlas et al., "Impact of the time rate of blood pressure variation on left ventricular mass," *Journal of Hypertension*, vol. 24, no. 10, pp. 2071–2077, 2006.

[14] N. A. Zakopoulos, G. Tsivgoulis, G. Barlas et al., "Time rate of blood pressure variation is associated with increased common carotid artery intima-media thickness," *Hypertension*, vol. 45, no. 4, pp. 505–512, 2005.

[15] L. Mourot, M. Bouhaddi, and J. Regnard, "Effects of the cold pressor test on cardiac autonomic control in normal subjects," *Physiological Research*, vol. 58, pp. 83–91, 2009.

[16] L. Wang, L. Hou, H. Li et al., "Genetic variants in the renin-angiotensin system and blood pressure reactions to the cold pressor test," *Journal of Hypertension*, vol. 28, no. 12, pp. 2422–2428, 2010.

[17] S. Debener, F. Minow, R. Emkes, K. Gandras, and M. de Vos, "How about taking a low-cost, small, and wireless EEG for a walk?" *Psychophysiology*, vol. 49, no. 11, pp. 1617–1621, 2012.

[18] A. Rodríguez, B. Rey, and M. Alcañiz, "Validation of a low-cost EEG device for mood induction studies , Stud Health Technol Inform," *Stud Health Technol Inform*, vol. 191, pp. 43–47, 2013.

[19] P. de Lissa, S. Sörensen, N. Badcock, J. Thie, and G. McArthur, "Measuring the face-sensitive N170 with a gaming EEG system: a validation study," *Journal of Neuroscience Methods*, vol. 253, pp. 47–54, 2015.

[20] R. Ramirez, M. Palencia-Lefler, S. Giraldo, and Z. Vamvakousis, "Musical neurofeedback for treating depression in elderly people," *Frontiers in Neuroscience*, vol. 9, article 354, 2015.

[21] A. Delorme and S. Makeig, "EEGLAB: an open source toolbox for analysis of single-trial EEG dynamics including independent component analysis," *Journal of Neuroscience Methods*, vol. 134, no. 1, pp. 9–21, 2004.

[22] V. J. Samar, A. Bopardikar, R. Rao, and K. Swartz, "Wavelet analysis of neuroelectric waveforms," *Brain and Language*, vol. 66, pp. 7–60, 1999.

[23] R. Princy, P. Thamarai, and B. Karthik, "Denoising EEG signal using wavelet transform," *International Journal of Advanced Research in Computer Engineering & Technology*, p. 3, 2015.

[24] E. S. Dos Santos Pinheiro, F. C. De Queirós, P. Montoya et al., "Electroencephalographic patterns in chronic pain: A systematic review of the literature," *PLoS ONE*, vol. 11, no. 2, Article ID e0149085, 2016.

[25] W. B. Kannel, A. L. Dannenberg, and R. D. Abbott, "Unrecognized myocardial infarction and hypertension: The Framingham Study," *American Heart Journal*, vol. 109, no. 3, pp. 581–585, 1985.

[26] S. Masuki and H. Nose, "Increased cerebral activity suppresses baroreflex control of heart rate in freely moving mice," *Journal of Physiology*, vol. 587, no. 23, pp. 5783–5794, 2009.

[27] L.-M. Liou, D. Ruge, M.-C. Kuo et al., "Functional connectivity between parietal cortex and the cardiac autonomic system in uremics," *Kaohsiung Journal of Medical Sciences*, vol. 30, no. 3, pp. 125–132, 2014.

[28] V. Di Lazzaro, P. Profice, F. Pilato et al., "Motor cortex plasticity predicts recovery in acute stroke," *Cerebral Cortex*, vol. 20, no. 7, pp. 1523–1528, 2010.

[29] L. I. Aftanas, I. V. Brak, O. M. Gilinskaya, V. V. Korenek, S. V. Pavlov, and N. V. Reva, "Hypoactivation of reward motivational system in patients with newly diagnosed hypertension grade I-II," *Bulletin of Experimental Biology and Medicine*, vol. 157, no. 4, pp. 430–435, 2014.

[30] G. G. Knyazev, "EEG delta oscillations as a correlate of basic homeostatic and motivational processes," *Neuroscience and Biobehavioral Reviews*, vol. 36, no. 1, pp. 677–695, 2012.

[31] A. Bruns and R. Eckhorn, "Task-related coupling from high-to low-frequency signals among visual cortical areas in human subdural recordings," *International Journal of Psychophysiology*, vol. 51, no. 2, pp. 96–116, 2004.

[32] G. G. Yener, B. Güntekin, D. N. Örken, E. Tülay, H. Forta, and E. Başar, "Auditory delta event-related oscillatory responses are decreased in Alzheimer's disease," *Behavioural Neurology*, vol. 25, no. 1, pp. 3–11, 2012.

[33] C. Babiloni, C. Del Percio, L. Arendt-Nielsen et al., "Cortical EEG alpha rhythms reflect task-specific somatosensory and motor interactions in humans," *Clinical Neurophysiology*, vol. 125, no. 10, pp. 1936–1945, 2014.

[34] W. Klimesch, P. Sauseng, and S. Hanslmayr, "EEG alpha oscillations: the inhibition-timing hypothesis," *Brain Research Reviews*, vol. 53, pp. 63–88, 2007.

[35] J. J. Foxe and A. C. Snyder, "The role of alpha-band brain oscillations as a sensory suppression mechanism during selective attention, front psychol," *Front Psychol*, vol. 2, p. 154, 2011.

[36] O. Jensen and A. Mazaheri, "Shaping functional architecture by oscillatory alpha activity: gating by inhibition," *Frontiers in Human Neuroscience*, vol. 4 article 186, 2010.

[37] H. A. Demaree and D. W. Harrison, "A neuropsychological model relating self-awareness to hostility," *Neuropsychology Review*, vol. 7, no. 4, pp. 171–185, 1997.

[38] L. Hu, P. Xiao, Z. G. Zhang, A. Mouraux, and G. D. Iannetti, "Single-trial time-frequency analysis of electrocortical signals: Baseline correction and beyond," *NeuroImage*, vol. 84, pp. 876–887, 2014.

[39] C. F. Beckmann, M. DeLuca, J. T. Devlin, and S. M. Smith, "Investigations into resting-state connectivity using independent component analysis," *Philosophical Transactions of the Royal Society of London B: Biological Sciences*, vol. 360, pp. 1001–1013, 2005.

[40] J. S. Damoiseaux, S. A. R. B. Rombouts, F. Barkhof et al., "Consistent resting-state networks across healthy subjects," *Proceedings of the National Academy of Sciences of the United States of America*, vol. 103, no. 37, pp. 13848–13853, 2006.

[41] Y. Tu, Z. Zhang, A. Tan et al., "Alpha and gamma oscillation amplitudes synergistically predict the perception of forthcoming nociceptive stimuli," *Human Brain Mapping*, vol. 37, no. 2, pp. 501–514, 2016.

[42] R.-R. Nir, A. Sinai, R. Moont, E. Harari, and D. Yarnitsky, "Tonic pain and continuous EEG: prediction of subjective pain perception by alpha-1 power during stimulation and at rest," *Clinical Neurophysiology*, vol. 123, pp. 605–612, 2012.

[43] D. Senkowski, M. Höfle, and A. K. Engel, "Crossmodal shaping of pain: a multisensory approach to nociception," *Trends in Cognitive Sciences*, vol. 18, no. 6, pp. 319–327, 2014.

[44] Triggiani A. I., Valenzano A., Del Percio C. et al., "Resting state rolandic mu rhythms are related to activity of sympathetic component of autonomic nervous system in healthy humans," *International Journal of Psychophysiology*, vol. 103, pp. 79–87, 2016.

[45] P. Fries, "Neuronal gamma-band synchronization as a fundamental process in cortical computation," *Annual Review of Neuroscience*, vol. 32, pp. 209–224, 2009.

[46] H. E. Rossiter, S. F. Worthen, C. Witton, S. D. Hall, and P. L. Furlong, "Gamma oscillatory amplitude encodes stimulus intensity in primary somatosensory cortex," *Frontiers in Human Neuroscience*, 2013.

[47] T. H. Donner and M. Siegel, "A framework for local cortical oscillation patterns," *Trends in Cognitive Sciences*, vol. 15, no. 5, pp. 191–199, 2011.

[48] E. Schulz, E. S. May, M. Postorino et al., "Prefrontal gamma oscillations encode tonic pain in humans," *Cerebral Cortex*, vol. 25, no. 11, pp. 4407–4414, 2015.

[49] E. Schulz, L. Tiemann, V. Witkovsky, P. Schmidt, and M. Ploner, "Gamma oscillations are involved in the sensorimotor transformation of pain," *Journal of Neurophysiology*, vol. 108, no. 4, pp. 1025–1031, 2012.

[50] L. Tiemann, E. Schulz, J. Gross, and M. Ploner, "Gamma oscillations as a neuronal correlate of the attentional effects of pain," *Pain*, vol. 150, no. 2, pp. 302–308, 2010.

[51] R. Luijcks, C. J. Vossen, H. J. Hermens, J. Van Os, and R. Lousberg, "The influence of perceived stress on cortical reactivity: a proof-of-principle study," *PLoS ONE*, vol. 10, no. 6, Article ID e0129220, 2015.

[52] J. B. M. Goense and N. K. Logothetis, "Neurophysiology of the BOLD fMRI signal in awake monkeys," *Current Biology*, vol. 18, no. 9, pp. 631–640, 2008.

[53] J. J. Riera and A. Sumiyoshi, "Brain oscillations: ideal scenery to understand the neurovascular coupling," *Current Opinion in Neurology*, vol. 23, no. 4, pp. 374–381, 2010.

[54] D. Knopman, L. L. Boland, T. Mosley et al., "Cardiovascular risk factors and cognitive decline in middle-aged adults," *Neurology*, vol. 56, no. 1, pp. 42–48, 2001.

[55] M. C. Morris, P. A. Scherr, and L. E. Hebert, "Association between blood pressure and cognitive function in a biracial community population of older persons," *Neuroepidemiology*, vol. 21, pp. 123–130, 2002.

[56] O. Anson and E. Paran, "Hypertension and cognitive functioning among the elderly: an overview," *American Journal of Therapeutics*, vol. 12, pp. 359–365, 2005.

[57] R. Gupta, R. Solanki, and V. Pathak, "Blood pressure is associated with cognitive impairment in young hypertensives," *World Journal of Biological Psychiatry*, vol. 9, pp. 43–50, 2008.

[58] J. J. Mcginley and B. H. Friedman, "Autonomic responses to lateralized cold pressor and facial cooling tasks," *Psychophysiology*, vol. 52, no. 3, pp. 416–424, 2015.

[59] J. R. Jennings and Y. Zanstra, "Is the brain the essential in hypertension?" *NeuroImage*, vol. 47, no. 3, pp. 914–921, 2009.

[60] K. S. Stamatelopoulos, E. Manios, G. Barlas et al., "Time rate of blood pressure variation is superior to central hemodynamics as an associate of carotid intima-media thickness," *Journal of Hypertension*, vol. 28, no. 1, pp. 51–58, 2010.

[61] N. A. Zakopoulos, G. Tsivgoulis, G. Barlas et al., "Impact of the time rate of blood pressure variation on left ventricular mass," *Journal of Hypertension*, vol. 24, no. 10, pp. 2071–2077, 2006.

[62] E. Manios, G. Tsagalis, G. Tsivgoulis et al., "Time rate of blood pressure variation is associated with impaired renal function in hypertensive patients," *Journal of Hypertension*, vol. 27, no. 11, pp. 2244–2248, 2009.

[63] E. Manios, K. Stamatelopoulos, G. Tsivgoulis et al., "Time rate of blood pressure variation: a new factor associated with coronary atherosclerosis," *Journal of Hypertension*, vol. 29, no. 6, pp. 1109–1114, 2011.

[64] S. J. Skalidi, E. D. Manios, K. S. Stamatelopoulos et al., "Brain edema formation is associated with the time rate of blood pressure variation in acute stroke patients," *Blood Pressure Monitoring*, vol. 18, no. 4, pp. 203–207, 2013.

[65] P. Zis, K. Vemmos, K. Spengos et al., "Ambulatory blood pressure monitoring in acute stroke: pathophysiology of the time rate of blood pressure variation and association with the 1-year outcome," *Blood Pressure Monitoring*, vol. 18, no. 2, pp. 94–100, 2013.

20

Predictors of Hypertension in a Population of Undergraduate Students in Sierra Leone

Aiah Lebbie,[1] Richard Wadsworth,[1] Janette Saidu,[2] and Camilla Bangura[1]

[1]Department of Biological Sciences, Njala University, PMB, Freetown, Sierra Leone
[2]Institute of Food Technology, Nutrition & Consumer Studies, Njala University, PMB, Freetown, Sierra Leone

Correspondence should be addressed to Aiah Lebbie; aiahlebbie@gmail.com

Academic Editor: Tomohiro Katsuya

We report on the first survey of hypertension in undergraduates in Sierra Leone. Levels of hypertension (12%) and obesity (4%) appear low compared to the general population but given the rapid increase of both and the expectation that many graduates will enter the formal employment sector and a sedentary lifestyle, there is still cause for concern. We measured their BMI (body mass index) and used a questionnaire to investigate demographic and lifestyle choices. In agreement with most authorities, we found that BMI and age were statistically significant predictors of systolic and diastolic blood pressure but that the explanatory power was low ($r = 0.21$ to 0.27). Men may be more sensitive than women to an increase in BMI on blood pressure ($p < 0.1$). We failed to find statistically significant relationships with ethnicity, religion, stress, course of study, levels of physical activity, diet, smoking, or consumption of caffeine and alcohol. Family history of hypertension, consumption of red palm oil, and self-diagnosed attacks of typhoid fever were close to conventional levels of significance ($p < 0.1$). We intend to use this as a baseline for longitudinal studies to assess risks and suggest appropriate public health action.

1. Introduction

Most investigations into public health in Sierra Leone have concentrated on "exciting" diseases, such as Ebola virus disease (EVD), and on acute problems associated with perinatal and maternal mortality; these continue to receive national and international attention. Research into noncommunicable chronic health problems such as hypertension and obesity has been limited, and we have found only four papers in the PubMed database [1–4]; in addition there is the WHO [5] country profile. From these papers, the rate of adult hypertension is somewhere from a low of 15% [2] to over 44% [4] with the WHO [5], settling on a prevalence of adult (over 25 years) hypertension of 36.7% and 36.0%, for men and women, respectively. This is higher than the nearby country of Ghana (28.3% and 32.8% for urban and rural populations) [6, 7] or the year 2000 survey of Sub-Saharan Africa (SSA) (28.3% and 26.9% for men and women) [8], but lower than rates in rural southeast Nigeria (50.2% and 44.8% for men and women) [9]. Recent levels in Nigeria are much higher than ten years previously [10, 11] when levels of only 10% and 11.2%

were recorded. Comparison of rates is hampered by different methodologies and selection biases. Where the sample size is large and methodology is consistent, others have shown that rates of hypertension can increase rapidly, for example, in China from 18% in 2002 to 33.6% in 2010 [12].

Of the four papers on blood pressure (BP) in Sierra Leone, recorded in PubMed, two of the papers [1, 2] utilize data collected during the civil war and may reflect a population under a variety of severe psychological and physiological stresses and one paper [3] relates to patients attending a medical clinic. Lisk and others [2] found a significant relation with age and gender but not rural or urban location. Other researchers [1, 3] only found age to be significant, and data collected on demographic, dietary, and social factors, including smoking and consumption of alcohol, salt, palm oil, and kola nuts were not statistically significant predictors [2]. In a cross-sectional study conducted in the Gambia and Sierra Leone, over 40% prevalence rates of hypertension were recorded in both male and female patients [4].

West Africa is noted as a location where many people have high blood pressure; anecdotally hypertension is a major cause of early death, especially among men, but few autopsies are performed and national statistics are of variable quality. In Sierra Leone, no studies have examined the prevalence of and associated risks of hypertension among young university students, despite the evidence that hypertension is a risk for undergraduates in other countries in the region [13]. Given the asymptomatic nature of hypertension, there is a need to determine populations that would be most vulnerable and to identify appropriate risk factors to provide the needed public health support. One of the problems with studying hypertension is the large number of factors that can influence blood pressure. With this in mind, we measured and interviewed 345 undergraduates on the main campus of Njala University to try and determine what physical and environmental features best predicted systolic blood pressure (BP-S) and diastolic blood pressure (BP-D) and whether there are public health implications or recommendations that needed to be made.

2. Materials and Methods

2.1. Study Site and Approach. The study was conducted on the main campus of Njala University, located in a rural setting in the Moyamba District of Southern Sierra Leone, and attracts students from across the country primarily interested in pursuing university degrees in agriculture, science, and technology. Data collection began in March and ended in May 2016 and was intended to establish a baseline data for a long-term longitudinal study with the students.

2.2. Blood Pressure and Anthropometric Measurements. Blood pressure and anthropometric measurements were done with the assistance of one trained nurse and 3 student volunteers. Measurements for blood pressure, height, and weight, as well as circumferences for arm, chest/bust, hip, and waist, were made. A digital sphygmomanometer (OMROM Blood Pressure Monitor, Model: BP765) with two different cuff sizes was used to record the conventional blood pressure (systolic and diastolic) from the distal part of the left arm of the students after resting for at least 10 minutes in a resting position [14]. The average of two BP measurements of between 5 and 6 minutes' interval was taken and recorded. This equipment consistently gave the same readings when used on different sets of people on different occasions before we commenced actual BP recording of the students. Participants' weights were measured on a manual scale to one decimal figure in kilograms, and they were encouraged to put on light clothing and put aside phones and step out of their shoes before the measurement was done. A marked "height wall" was used to measure the heights in the nearest centimetre, while a nonelastic tape measured the circumferences of the arm, chest/bust, waist, and hip.

2.3. Questionnaire and Sociodemographic Characteristics. A questionnaire divided into four sections covering basic sociodemographic information, food recall data, personal and family health, and physical exercise and lifestyle was given to each study participant to fill out. Upon completion of the questionnaire, each participant was given the equivalent amount of $1 (Le 5,000) to buy telephone credit to call the PI should they have any questions or desire to opt out of the study.

2.4. Data Analyses and Statistical Approach. Data from the questionnaires was recorded onto an Excel spreadsheet primarily as a mixture of ordinal and categorical data (e.g., gender, preferred type of alcohol) with some continuous variables (e.g., frequency of playing sports) categorised into a limited number of choices (e.g., "every day," "3-4 times per week," "once a week," "occasionally," etc.). Anthropometric measurements (e.g., body mass index (BMI)) are treated as continuous variables.

The simplest relevant statistical approach was adopted for each analysis. Statistical significance was mainly tested using ANOVA (analysis of variance) and linear regression with some use of mixed models (e.g., using BMI, age, and gender to predict BP). Quantile and median regression gave similar results to linear regression using maximum likelihood and are not therefore reported. Sample size (and degrees of freedom) varies slightly with the different variables being analysed as not all respondents answered all questions in a usable manner.

2.5. Ethical Approval Process. In February 2016, ethical approval to conduct the study was sought and obtained from the Njala University Institutional Review Board. We first publicized the study on the Njala campus, and students were encouraged to participate in a campus-wide briefing on the study objectives and data collection process in the university auditorium. A question and answer session was followed by information sharing on ethical approval and consent process before data collection commenced. Interested students were given a prepared consent form to take home and read; 345 (82.7%) completed forms were returned (after collecting and cleaning the data, 332 usable responses were obtained). The consent forms were countersigned and witnessed by the first and third authors. Students who agreed to participate had their BP measured and then had their anthropometric measurements recorded and completed a "lifestyle" and sociodemographic questionnaire.

3. Results

3.1. General Characteristics of the Population. The general characteristics of the sample are shown in Table 1 for selected demographic and biological attributes. More male students participated in the study than female students, with the median age of males being 25 years (quartile 22–27) and that of the female students being 23 years (quartile 21–25). Male students were generally taller than female students, and median BMI for male students was 2.1 kg/m^2 less than that of female students (Table 1). The percentage of obesity was higher among female students than male students, with the number of siblings higher for male than female students. Religious beliefs and practices were more engendered, with female students likely to be Christian than Muslim. Most of the students were single, with slightly more married female than male students.

TABLE 1: Selected characteristics of the student population on Njala campus.

Characteristic	Male Median or percentage	Quartiles	Female Median or percentage	Quartiles
Number of respondents	252		80	
Age (years)	25	22 : 27	23	21 : 25
Height (cm)	172	167 : 176	161	155 : 165
Weight (kg)	62.5	58 : 69	61.0	53.0 : 70.3
BMI (kg/m^2)	21.3	20.0 : 23.3	23.4	21.1 : 26.7
Obese (BMI > 30)	2.0%		4.0%	
Number of siblings	4	3 : 6	3	2 : 4
Christian	49.4%		62.5%	
Muslim	50.6%		37.5%	
Married	6.4%		7.5%	

BMI: body mass index.

3.2. Risk Factors and Blood Pressure. Factors that were significantly predictors of either BP-S or BP-D and factors that are close to conventional levels of statistical significance ($p < 0.1$) are shown in Table 2. Factors that were not significant are listed briefly in Table 3.

3.2.1. Body Morphology. We measured the weight, height, waist, and hip circumferences of each respondent. Median BMI is 21.7 (interquartile range 20.1 to 23.8). The majority (251, 76%) were in the "normal" range (BMI of 18.5 to 25), 18 were "underweight" and 46 "overweight", 14 were "obese," and only one individual was categorised as "extremely obese" (with a BMI greater than 40). Women were on average 2.1 BMI units larger than the men (median values 23.4 versus 21.3) and this was statistically significant (one-way ANOVA, $p < 0.001$, $F = 26.0$, $df = 328$).

BMI is a significant predictor of BP-S and BP-D but the relationships for BP-S ((1) and (3)) are different for men and women, with an increase in BMI having a greater effect on BP-S for men than for women (see Figure 1); the relationship for BP-D ((2) and (4)) is virtually the same for both genders (Figure 2). Unfortunately, while being statistically significant, linear regression has only a weak explanatory capability with adjusted r^2 values of less than 10%.

Men:

$$BP\text{-}S = 91.7 + 1.38 * BMI$$
$$\left(\text{adjusted } r^2 = 0.072, \ F = 20.4, \ df = 251, \ p < 0.001\right) \quad (1)$$

$$BP\text{-}D = 61.5 + 0.60 * BMI$$
$$\left(\text{adjusted } r^2 = 0.023, \ F = 7.11, \ df = 251, \ p < 0.01\right). \quad (2)$$

Women:

$$BP\text{-}S = 95.5 + 0.73 * BMI$$
$$\left(\text{adjusted } r^2 = 0.044, \ F = 4.56, \ df = 77, \ p < 0.05\right) \quad (3)$$

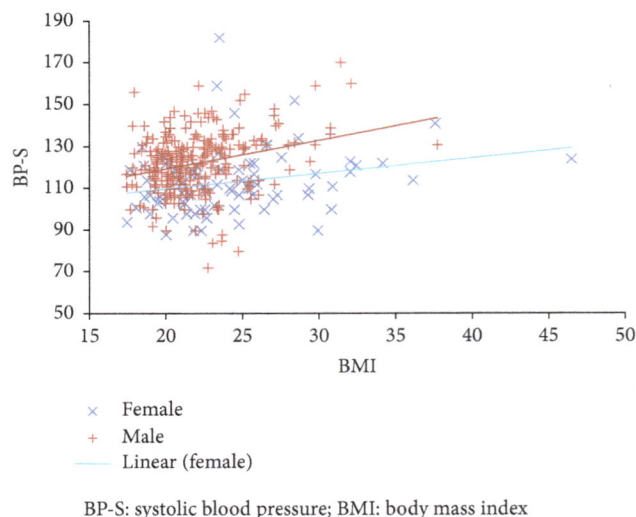

BP-S: systolic blood pressure; BMI: body mass index

FIGURE 1: Systolic blood pressure (BP-S) and BMI for men and women.

$$BP\text{-}D = 61.3 + 0.58 * BMI$$
$$\left(\text{adjusted } r^2 = 0.062, \ F = 6.09, \ df = 77, \ p < 0.05\right). \quad (4)$$

The difference in slope in (1) and (3) is not quite statistically significant ($p = 0.078$, $t = 1.768$, and $df = 341$). The difference between (2) and (4) (for BP-D) is not significant. Adding the variable "age" (of student) into the equations does not improve either the statistical significance or explanatory power of the equations for BP-S, but it does slightly in a combined equation for BP-D for men and women (5).

Men and women:

$$BP\text{-}D = 56.5 + 0.434 * BMI + 0.344 * Age$$
$$\left(\text{adjusted } r^2 = 0.062, \ F = 11.9, \ p < 0.001, \ df = 329\right). \quad (5)$$

3.2.2. Food Intake Recall. One feature of West African cuisine is a heavy reliance on red palm oil, and this is considered

Table 2: Potential risk factors for the student population on Njala campus (probabilities from single factor ANOVA or linear regression).

Attribute	Number	Median BP-S (interquartile)	Significance	Median BP-D (interquartile)	Significance
Sociodemographic					
Sex					
Male	250	122 (112 : 131)	$p < 0.001$	75 (67 : 82)	NS
Female	80	112 (103 : 121)		76 (68 : 82)	
Age range					
Age < 25 years	171	118 (108 : 130)	$p = 0.026$	72 (65 : 80)	$p < 0.001$
Age ≥ 25 years	159	121 (111 : 130)		77 (70 : 83)	
Biological variables					
BMI					
Obese (I & II)	15	123 (118 : 137)	Regression	84 (74 : 91)	$p = 0.017$
Overweight	46	124 (111 : 132)	$p = 0.003$	77 (70 : 84)	
Normal	251	119 (109 : 128)		73 (67 : 81)	
Marital status					
Married	22	124 (115 : 130)	NS	77 (72 : 87)	NS
Single	305	120 (109 : 129)		74 (67 : 82)	($p = 0.093$)
Health behaviour					
Alcoholic intake					
Drink alcohol	109	120 (111 : 129)	NS	72 (66 : 80)	NS
No alcohol	238	119 (109 : 130)		76 (68 : 82)	($p = 0.089$)
Palm oil intake					
Palm oil > 4 d/w	158	123 (110 : 131)	Regression	75 (67 : 83)	NS
Palm oil 3-4 d/w	153	118 (110 : 128)	$p = 0.073$	73 (67 : 81)	
Palm oil 1-2 d/w	33	115 (108 : 128)		76 (67 : 82)	
Palm oil, never	3	123 (122 : 129)		87 (83 : 87)	
Vegetable intake					
Fresh tomato	83	120 (111 : 130)	NS	79 (69 : 84)	$p = 0.034$
No fresh tomato	263	119 (109 : 129)		73 (67 : 81)	
Self-reported					
Typhoid					
Typhoid recently	38	112 (102 : 122)	$p = 0.020$	69 (65 : 78)	$p = 0.011$
No typhoid	308	120 (110 : 130)		76 (68 : 82)	
Self-reported					
Malaria					
Malaria recently	147	118 (109 : 129)	NS	73 (66 : 81)	NS
No malaria	199	120 (110 : 130)		76 (68 : 83)	($p = 0.097$)

BP-S: systolic blood pressure; BP-D: diastolic blood pressure; NS: not significant; d/w = days per week.

one of the least healthy vegetable oils but is consumed by most of our respondents on a daily or weekly basis (Table 2). Frequency of consumption of palm oil was not significant at a conventional level of 0.05 but was positively related to increased BP-S ($p = 0.068$). We could not measure actual consumption, only approximate frequency ("every day," "3 to 4 times per week," "once per week," "occasionally," and "never"). Consumption of other vegetable oils (used for frying foods) does not appear related to BP (or BMI). Sierra Leone produces many types of leafy green vegetables and we enquired as to peoples favourite foods, taboo foods, allergies, and consumption of vegetables (which was generally interpreted by our respondents as being "western" foods such as lettuce, carrots, and cabbage and relatively few classed okra, garden eggs, or any of the "leafy green vegetables"

as vegetables). By far the favourite meal of our sample is cassava leaf sauce (62%, 215) (although 22 people reported being allergic to some forms of cassava). There was no statistically significant relationship between favourite foods, taboo foods, allergies, and consumption of vegetables and BP, although consumption of tomatoes was significant ($p = 0.034$) (Table 2).

3.2.3. Lifestyle and General Health. At Njala, only 17 respondents (5%) admitted smoking and this is much lower than the 43% (male) and 11% (female) levels given by the WHO [15] for Sierra Leone adults. Contrary to expectation, there was no statistical difference in BP. Alcohol consumption seems relatively low by European standards and those that consumed alcohol had a slightly lower BP-D than

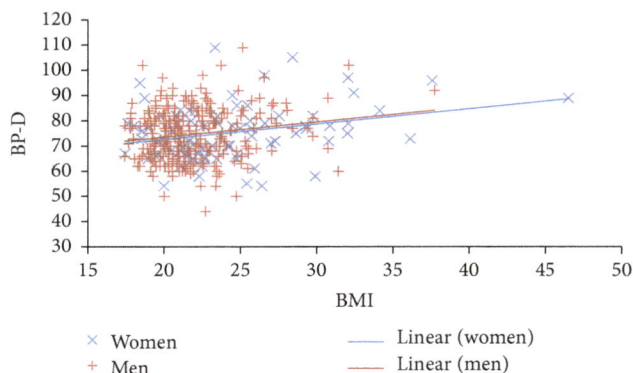

Figure 2: Diastolic blood pressure (BP-D) and BMI for men and women.

nonconsumers but this was not significant at conventional levels.

Most undergraduates consider themselves to be healthy (303 consider they are "very" or "moderately" heathy); however, many (42%) have been affected by malaria since coming to Njala campus. Reported attacks of malaria had no effect on BP-S; however, those reporting an attack of typhoid (often as "typhoid-malaria") had lower median BP-S (117 versus 126) but this is not quite significant at the 0.05 level ($p = 0.08$, one-way ANOVA, $F = 3.04$, and $df = 332$), and reports of other illnesses had no statistical significance. Family health in terms of parents and grandparents diagnosed with diabetes, heart attacks, and obesity had no statistical effect on BP with the exception of a recent death from "high blood pressure." Married respondents had slightly higher BP-D than singles but this was not quite significant at conventional levels ($p = 0.093$).

3.3. Factors with No Significant Relation to Blood Pressure. Table 3 lists those factors that were tested and where the "p" values were always greater than 0.1. We performed one-way ANOVA on many sociodemographic and lifestyle attributes to determine their possible impact on blood pressure including the following:

  (i) place of origin (northern, southern, or eastern province and western area) in Sierra Lone,

  (ii) ethnicity (tribe) of father and mother separately, and for a subset where the tribe of both parents was the same,

  (iii) number of siblings and birth order,

  (iv) religion (males split almost equally between Islam and Christianity (125 : 119); women were more likely to be Christian (50–30); only three "preferred not to answer").

There were no statistically significant relationships with place of origin or ethnicity with BP. We had hypothesised that ethnicity (as a surrogate for genetics) and place of birth (as a surrogate for environment, e.g., coastal versus inland)

might be factors affecting either early diet (e.g., relative availability of fish on the coast or meat in the interior) or levels of activity (e.g., plains versus mountains) and hence BP.

We asked about the spacing of siblings (number of years between them and siblings) but the quality of responses prevented detailed analysis. Large family size and a short period between siblings (less than 18 months) are known to have an adverse effect on some aspects of health and mortality, but we found no statistically significant effect on blood pressure (possibly because less healthy siblings are less likely to do well enough in school to get to university?).

Periodic fasting, a feature for observant Muslims might affect metabolism, but we found no effect on mean BP. An F-test showed significantly more variance in the Christian population than in the Muslim population for both men and women (women $F = 2.45$, $p < 0.01$, $df = 49, 29$; men $F = 2.04$, $p < 0.001$, $df = 121, 125$); we are uncertain why this might be the case.

In our sample, less than one-third of undergraduates (31.4%) reported drinking alcohol, and for the purpose of analysis alcohol was grouped into "beers and wine," "spirits," and "palm wine" and consumption as "every day," "3 to 4 times per week," and so forth. Consumption of stimulants was categorised into "energy drinks," "coffee, kola nuts, and coca cola," and noncaffeinated "soft drinks" (mostly locally produced ginger beer and synthetic apple juice). Consumption of energy drinks was very widespread (83% of male and 70% of female students). There was no significant relationship (one-way ANOVA) with alcohol or caffeine (BP for men was higher for those that took energy drinks, but lower for women; neither relationship was close to significance with $p > 0.1$).

Levels of physical activity were assessed through frequency of participating in organised sports (football and volley ball). Male students at Njala reported much more sporting activity than female students and had lower BMI on average than nonsports players, but this was not sufficient to result in a significantly lower BP.

Anecdotally some university courses are harder than others, and we hypothesised that there would be a change in the levels of stress as the undergraduates passed through the four years of the degree course or whether certain schools (e.g., agriculture, education, technology, and environmental sciences) were inherently more stressful than others. One-way ANOVA revealed no significant differences between the seven schools represented by the male respondents and the four schools represented by the female students.

Students reported a wide range of stresses relating to student life, such as poor accommodation (excessive noise, limited water supply), exams and essays, money, and relationships. These stresses on their own and in aggregate did not statistically affect BP. One symptom of stress can be problems sleeping, and a large proportion (151, 44%) reported only sleeping 5 hours per night (and just 6% reported sleeping 8 hours per night). Lack of sleep was not a predictor of BP. Ulcers can also be related to stress and 30 (8.6%) reported they had ulcers (although whether this has been formally diagnosed is unknown). Ulcers might lead to a reduction

TABLE 3: Risk Factors with no conventionally statistically significant relations to blood pressure in our sample.

Factor	Categories
Religion	Christian, Muslim, "prefer not to say"
Marital status	Married, single
Place of birth	Northern, southern, eastern province, western area
Place of birth	14 districts
Ethnicity of mother, father	Fula, Koranko, Limba, Mandingo, Mende, Susu, Temne, others
Number of siblings	Only child, 1, 2, 3, 4, 5, 6, 7, 8, 9, more than 9
Birth order	1 (first) through 9 (ninth)
Years to nearest sibling	Insufficient quality data for analysis
School of study	Agriculture, education, environment, health, natural resources, physics/technology, social sciences
Year of study	1st, 2nd, 3rd, or 4th
Physical activity	Play sports (football, volleyball, running), do not play sports
Watch TV	More than 4 days/week, 3-4 days/week, 1-2 days/week, occasionally
Smoker	Yes, no
Drink alcohol	Yes (spirits, wine, beer, palm wine), no
High caffeine intake	Yes (energy drinks, caffeinated drinks, cola nuts), no
Favourite food	Cassava leaf, other leafy green vegetables, beans, "soup," other
Food allergies and taboos	Cassava, pumpkin, lizard, pig, other
Fresh fruit consumption	More than 4 days/week, 3-4 days/week, 1-2 days/week, occasionally
Green vegetables	More than 4 days/week, 3-4 days/week, 1-2 days/week, occasionally
Number of meals per day	1, 2, or 3
Go to bed hungry	Sometimes, never
Go to bed bloated	Sometimes, never
General health	Very good, moderate, ok, poor
Malaria recently (3 months)	Yes, no
Stressed	Yes (money, relationships, exams, accommodation, water supply, noise), no
Number of hours of sleep	4, 5, 6, 7, or 8
Family deaths (last 2 years)	None, heart failure, high blood pressure, diabetes, other

in consumption of oil and chili pepper, but this was not detectable in our data.

4. Discussion

Values of BMI (body mass index) in the student population are broadly consistent with estimates for adults made by the WHO between 1980 and 2009, which shows a monotonic increase from 21.4 to 24.1 for women (median 23.4 in our sample) and from 21.4 to 22.7 for men [5] (median 21.3 in our sample). The WHO data does not indicate any interruption of the increase in BMI during the Sierra Leone civil war, but a slight increase in slope after the end of the war in 2001. The BMI of male students was remarkably consistent by year of study. For the women (a smaller sample) there was a significant difference between years, due to a high average value for first-year students (who constituted 56% of the female sample).

In our study population, BMI was a significant predictor of both diastolic and systolic blood pressure, though the increase in BMI had a greater effect on systolic pressure for men than women, and when age was included together with BMI for a combined male and female diastolic pressure, the difference was statistically significant. Body mass index is reported to be positively and independently associated with morbidity and mortality from hypertension, cardiovascular disease, type II diabetes mellitus, and other chronic diseases [16]. In Caucasian populations, a strong association has been depicted between BMI and mortality [17], and positive relationship between BMI and BP has also been reported among African and Asian populations [18–21]. In West Africa, a meta-analysis conducted on 55 articles from 5 countries includes obesity, age, and gender as significant predictors [22] and is similar to studies of adults in Sierra Leone [2, 3]. Significant relationships have also been reported between age and BMI among adolescents in northeast Nigeria [23, 24], in which BMI was found to be a significant factor in predicting hypertension in rural Nigeria. In a small sample (60 students) of obese Nigerian students, Ibhazehiebo and others [25] found a strong, significant correlation ($r = 0.60$) between BMI and blood pressure. Others have also observed statistically significant relationship between BMI and blood pressure in undergraduates in three Nigerian universities [26, 27].

In Europe, the waist-to-hip ratio is sometimes used as an alternative to the BMI to assess risk. Within our dataset, the waist-to-hip ratio was not significantly correlated with BP, possibly due to different patterns of where fat accumulates. The waist-to-height ratio was statistically significant but resulted in regression equations with a lower r^2 than BMI; however, it requires one less piece of equipment to measure it (hip-to-height ratio was not significant). Studies done on populations in Haiti and Benin found the waist-to-height ratio to be a significant predictor of cardiovascular risk [28]; unfortunately, they did not report if this was as effective a predictor as BMI.

Although high blood pressure is common in SSA, a study from Brazil [29] supports a view that it is socioeconomic factors (such as low levels of education and income) and not genetic composition (African, European, or Native American) that are the important predictors. No significant difference between adults in Sierra Leone and the Gambia was found [4], and a meta-analysis also failed to find a consistent relationship with ethnicity [22].

Diet is often considered as a predictor of health; however, comparisons of BP for a small sample of vegetarians (who were all Seventh Day Adventists) with nonvegetarians in Nigeria found no difference [30]. There are very few vegetarians in Sierra Leone; however, consumption of meat is low and the majority of animal protein is provided in the form of marine fish. As Njala University has demonstration units for pigs, chickens, goats, and cattle, meat consumption might be above the national average among the university students. In rural Nigeria [24], a liking for fried chicken was found to be a significant risk factor for high blood pressure among females. In school children in the Democratic Republic of Congo boys with chronic malnutrition had significant higher blood pressure levels, but only low socioeconomic status was identified as a significant risk factor of arterial hypertension [31]. In our study group, the frequency of consumption of palm oil was high and, while being not significant, was positively related to increased systolic blood pressure ($p = 0.068$).

The nicotine in tobacco is capable of increasing blood pressure in otherwise healthy individuals [32], and studies of smoking among West African students reported that smoking is low in a sample of 1,800 Nigerian students, as only 5.7% smoked (7.7% in males and 2.0% in females), and unfortunately, few of them (32%) believed they were incurring any health risk and hence were willing to consider giving up [33]. At Njala University, approximately 5% of the students admitted smoking, a much lower frequency than the 43% (male) and 11% (female) levels given by the WHO [15] for adults in Sierra Leone, but differences in BP are not statistically significant. In a small sample of undergraduate students at Benin University in Nigeria, blood pressure measurements results were similar to studies of Black Americans [34], despite the observation that levels of smoking and alcohol intake among the Nigerian students were lower. While alcohol consumption has been found to be significantly related to higher blood pressure [22], no significant relationship was found in our study population,

although men who drank energy drinks had a higher BP than women.

Male students showed more involvement in physical activities such as sports than their female colleagues. Watching of movies (mostly "Nigerian Soap Opera") was more common among the female students who also showed less preference for sports that were physically challenging. Studies done in South Africa found that male South African students were more physically active than the females but had poorer eating habits [35]. They, however, worry that hypertension is becoming an increasing problem and health problems were starting earlier than expected.

Our study population reported a wide range of stressful experiences, including money, exams and essays, noise, health of family members and themselves, water supply, and relationships. By far, stress related to lack of money is more prevalent among male and female students, given that most of them have to finance their own education, feeding, transportation for getting around the campus, and paying for educational materials and medical treatment when they are sick. While we could not find any significant relationship between any of the observed stress categories and blood pressure, others [36] observed a statistically significant relationship between blood pressure and women with premenstrual syndrome. A recent study has also observed that emotional stress is often ignored as a cause of high blood pressure in SSA [37]. In a behavioural study of under- and postgraduates in 208 Lagos students (equally split male : female, mean age 20.2), Agbu [38] found that the female students were more motivated and felt under greater pressure to get things done and find a job.

5. Conclusions

The standard of living in Sub-Sahara Africa (SSA) is on the rise, and families are taking on lifestyles of the developed world with attendant health implications, including weight gain/obesity and hypertension, arising from a higher calorie intake coupled with less physical activity [39, 40]. The magnitude of these changes in most countries across the region is not clear as there are thoughts to be high levels of underdiagnoses and reporting. Odili and others [41] using the "International Database on Home Blood Pressure in Relation to Cardiovascular Outcome" (IDHOCO) consider that hypertension is both underdiagnosed and a major cause of death in SSA. The extent of "masked" hypertension in SSA is described as being "alarming" [42] and a "silent killer" [13].

Levels of hypertension are high in the Sierra Leone adult population and appear to have increased over the last few decades; but the student population at Njala is currently quite healthy with 12% having either high BP-S or BP-D and only 7 (2.1%) having both high BP-S and BP-D. Levels of obesity are low (4%) but likely to increase as they age and with the expectation that they will enter the formal employment sector and a sedentary lifestyle.

Like most other studies, we found a statistically significant correlation between BMI and BP. Work done in South Africa suggests that the critical "cut-off" points for BMI in relation to public health advice on the risks of high blood pressure should be considerably lower than those currently used [43]. Gender and BMI are significant predictors of BP-S. For the combined BP-D equation age is also a significant predictor, but we noted that the age range of our sample is small (interquartile range 22 to 27 years). There is some indication that men are more sensitive to increases in BMI than women (but the difference in slopes of the linear regression equations is not significant at conventional levels, $p = 0.08$).

Consumption of palm oil (increase BP) and recent attacks of "typhoid" fever (decrease BP) are close to conventional levels of statistical significance ($p < 0.1$). Red palm oil is known to be less healthy than some other vegetable oils. In laboratory experiments involving rats, repeatedly heated palm oil was reported to have caused elevation in BP [44]. We have not been able to trace any existing literature on typhoid fever that ties in any relationship with BP, and the self-reported "typhoid fever" by students did not accompany any proof that they had typhoid fever or "malaria fever" (as people in Sierra Leone generally use both terms synonymously until proven otherwise). However, we can only speculate that malaria fever which affects normal blood cell counts might impact on BP. In fact, it has been shown that there is a decrease in blood pressure with malaria attacks [45].

We are tempted to speculate that fasting among the Muslim students might reset their metabolic rates over that of the Christian students, hence the variance in BP. Restrictions on caloric intake have been shown to have favourable outcome for blood pressure and other health outcomes [46]. We were unable to ask about strict adherence to religious tenets to ascertain whether reported religious affiliations of the students actually translated into practices that might influence metabolic rates and hence health-related outcomes. This issue will be included in our long-term studies with the students and develop hypotheses for testing it.

Levels of alcohol consumption and smoking (if honestly reported) are low with less than one-third drinking and just 5% smoking, neither is a statistically significant predictor of BP in our sample. Physical activity slightly reduces BMI but does not significantly improve BP. Students report many sources of stress but these do not significantly increase BP. We did not identify ethnicity, religion, place of birth, or a family history of ill-health as significant predictors of BP.

The Njala campus is a relatively calm and peaceful rural environment; the University has some departments located in the cities of Bo and Freetown, and we would like to conduct a similar survey to see whether the urban environment has a measurable effect on BP. Our sample generally comes from better off sections of society; it would be interesting to conduct similar surveys in more typical communities. We expect many of our undergraduates to enter the formal economy and probably adopt a more sedentary existence thereby increasing their risk factors; whether they can be influenced now before they start to spread out is something we must address.

As the levels of smoking at 5% are much lower than the national statistics (40% for men), it would be interesting to follow this up and see whether students have been influenced by public health messages. This is especially important as relying on conventional medical treatment for chronic conditions like hypertension once someone is affected is unlikely to be effective; in Ghana 93% of patients did not take their prescribed medication, most (96%) stating that the medicines were unaffordable [47].

Abbreviations

BP: Blood pressure
BP-S: Systolic blood pressure
BP-D: Diastolic blood pressure
BMI: Body mass index
D/W: Days per week
EVD: Ebola virus disease
HF: High fever
HBP: High blood pressure
LGV: Leaf green vegetables
NS: Not significant
PI: Principal investigator
SSA: Sub-Sahara Africa.

Acknowledgments

The authors wish to thank all the students who willingly volunteered to participate in the study. They also extend their appreciation to the following students for helping out with the data collection: Emmauel Saidu, Augustus Osborne, Joseph Bangura, Richard Suluku, and Josephine Lansana.

References

[1] D. E. Williams and D. R. Lisk, "A High Prevalence of Hypertension in Rural Sierra Leone," *West African Journal of Medicine*, vol. 7, no. 2, pp. 85–90, 1998.

[2] D. R. Lisk, D. E. Williams, and J. Slattery, "Blood Pressure and Hypertension in Rural and Urban Sierra Leoneans," *Ethnicity & Disease*, vol. 9, no. 2, pp. 254–263, 1999.

[3] K. A. Meehan, A. J. Bankoski, E. Tejan et al., "Hypertension in Bo, Sierra Leone," *Ethnicity and Disease*, vol. 21, no. 2, pp. 237–242, 2011.

[4] M. Awad, A. Ruzza, J. Mirocha et al., "Prevalence of Hypertension in The Gambia And Sierra Leone, Western Africa: A Cross-Sectional Study," *Cardiovascular Journal of Africa*, vol. 25, no. 6, pp. 269–278, 2014.

[5] WHO, *World Health Organisation – Non-communicable Diseases (NCD) Country Profiles*, 2014.

[6] A. G. Amoah, "Hypertension in Ghana: A Cross-Sectional Community Prevalence Study in Greater Accra," *Ethnicity & Disease*, vol. 13, no. 3, pp. 310–315, 2003.

[7] B. A. Burket, "Blood Pressure Survey in Two Communities in The Volta Region, Ghana, West Africa," *Ethnicity and Disease*, vol. 16, pp. 292–294, 2006.

[8] P. M. Kearney, M. Whelton, K. Reynolds, P. Muntner, P. K. Whelton, and J. He, "Global Burden of Hypertension: Analysis of Worldwide Data," *The Lancet*, vol. 365, no. 9455, pp. 217–223, 2005.

[9] B. J. C. Onwubere, E. C. Ejim, C. I. Okafor et al., "Pattern of Blood Pressure Indices among the Residents of a Rural Community in South East Nigeria," *International Journal of Hypertension*, vol. 2011, Article ID 621074, 6 pages, 2011.

[10] O. O. Akinkugbe, "Current Epidemiology of Hypertension in Nigeria," *Archives of Ibadan Medicine*, vol. 1, pp. 3–7, 2001.

[11] A. F. B. Mabadeje, "WHO-ISH Guidelines for The Management of Hypertension: Implementation in Africa—The Nigerian Experience," *Clinical and Experimental Hypertension*, vol. 21, no. 5-6, pp. 671–681, 1999.

[12] J. He, "Hypertension in China," *Journal of Hypertension*, vol. 34, no. 1, pp. 29–31, 2016.

[13] M. M. M. Moussa, R. I. El-mowafy, and H. H. El-Ezaby, "Prevalence of Hypertension and Associated Risk Factors among University Students: Comparative Study," *Journal of Nursing Education and Practice*, vol. 6, no. 5, pp. 19–27, 2016.

[14] L. S. Acree, J. Longfors, A. S. Fjeldstad et al., "Physical Activity Is Related to Quality of Life in Older Adults," *Health and Quality of Life Outcomes*, vol. 4, no. 37, 2006.

[15] WHO, "Non-Communicable Disease," 2016, http://www.aho.afro.who.int/profiles_information/images/1/19/Sierra_Leone-Statistical_Factsheet.pdf.

[16] F. X. Pi-Sunyer, "Medical Hazards of Obesity," *Annual International Medicine*, vol. 119, no. 7, pp. 655–660, 1993.

[17] J. Stevens, J. Cai, E. R. Pamuk, D. F. Williamson, M. J. Thun, and J. L. Wood, "The Effect of Age on The Association between Body-Mass Index and Mortality," *The New England Journal of Medicine*, vol. 338, no. 1, pp. 1–7, 1998.

[18] K. Tandon, *Obesity, Its Distribution Pattern and Health Implications among Khatri Population [Ph.D. thesis]*, Department of Anthropology, University of Delhi, Delhi, India, 2006.

[19] S. S. Kapoor, "Blood pressure, waist to hip ratio and body mass index among affluent Punjabi girls of Delhi," *Acta Medica Auxologica*, vol. 32, no. 3, pp. 153–157, 2000.

[20] N. K. Mungreiphy, S. Kapoor, and R. Sinha, "Association between BMI, blood pressure, and age: study among Tangkhul Naga tribal males of northeast India," *Journal of Anthropology*, vol. 2011, Article ID 748147, 6 pages, 2011.

[21] F. Kidy, D. Rutebarika, S. A. Lule et al., "Blood pressure in primary school children in Uganda: a cross-sectional survey," *BMC Public Health*, vol. 14, no. 1223, 2014.

[22] W. K. Bosu, "Determinants of mean blood pressure and hypertension among workers in west africa," *International Journal of Hypertension*, vol. 2016, Article ID 3192149, 19 pages, 2016.

[23] A. Y. Oyeyemi, M. A. Usman, A. L. Oyeyemi, and O. A. Jaiyeola, "Casual blood pressure of adolescents attending public secondary schools in Maiduguri, Nigeria," *Clinical Hypertension*, vol. 21, no. 16, 2015.

[24] N. A. Odunaiya, Q. A. Louw, and K. A. Grimmer, "Are lifestyle cardiovascular disease risk factors associated with prehypertension in 15–18 years rural Nigerian youth? A cross sectional study," *BMC Cardiovascular Disorders*, vol. 15, no. 144, 2015.

[25] K. Ibhazehiebo, U. I. Dimkpa, and V. I. Iyawe, "Hypertension, and blood pressure response to graded exercise in young obese and non-athletic Nigerian university students," *Nigerian Journal of Physiological Sciences*, vol. 22, no. 1-2, pp. 37–42, 2007.

[26] D. C. Nwachukwu, U. I. Nwagha, E. N. Obikili et al., "Assessment of body mass index and blood pressure among university students in, Enugu, South East, Nigeria," *Nigerian Journal of Medicine*, vol. 19, no. 2, pp. 148–152, 2010.

[27] M. U. Nwankwo, L. L. Adams-Campbell, F. A. Ukoli, I. N. Olomu, C. O. Ukoli, and E. Ugwu, "Blood pressure in Nigerian college males," *Journal of Human Hypertension*, vol. 4, no. 2, pp. 72-73, 1990.

[28] A. El Mabchour, H. Delisle, C. Vilgrain, P. Larco, R. Sodjinou, and M. Batal, "Specific cut-off points for waist circumference and waist-to-height ratio as predictors of cardiometabolic risk in Black subjects: a cross-sectional study in Benin and Haiti," *Diabetes, Metabolic Syndrome and Obesity: Targets and Therapy*, vol. 8, pp. 513–523, 2015.

[29] M. F. Lima-Costa, J. V. Mambrini, M. L. Leite et al., "Socioeconomic position, but not african genomic ancestry, is associated with blood pressure in the bambui-epigen (Brazil) cohort study of aging," *Hypertension*, vol. 67, no. 2, pp. 349–355, 2016.

[30] A. A. Famodu, O. Osilesi, Y. O. Makinde et al., "The influence of a vegetarian diet on haemostatic risk factors for cardiovascular disease in Africans," *Thrombosis Research*, vol. 95, no. 1, pp. 31–36, 1999.

[31] B. Longo-Mbenza, E. Lukoki Luila, and J. R. M'Buyamba-Kabangu, "Nutritional status, socio-economic status, heart rate, and blood pressure in African school children and adolescents," *International Journal of Cardiology*, vol. 121, no. 2, pp. 171–177, 2007.

[32] C. O. Timothy and R. O. Nneli, "The effects of cigarette smoking on intraocular pressure and arterial blood pressure of normotensive young Nigerian male adults," *Nigerian Journal of Physiological Sciences*, vol. 22, no. 1-2, pp. 33–36, 2007.

[33] A. E. Fawibe and A. O. Shittu, "Prevalence characteristics of cigarette smokers among undergraduates of the University of Ilorin," *Nigerian Journal of Clinical Practice*, vol. 14, no. 2, pp. 201–205, 2011.

[34] L. L. Adams-Campbell, M. U. Nwankwo, J. A. Omene et al., "Assessment of cardiovascular risk factors in Nigerian students," *Arteriosclerosis, Thrombosis, and Vascular Biology*, vol. 8, no. 6, pp. 793–796, 1988.

[35] N. T. A. Rosendaal, M. E. Hendriks, M. D. Verhagen et al., "Costs and cost-effectiveness of hypertension screening and treatment in adults with hypertension in rural nigeria in the context of a health insurance program," *PLoS ONE*, vol. 11, no. 6, Article ID e0157925, 2016.

[36] B. N. Okeahialam, J. T. Obindo, and C. Ogbonna, "Prevalence of premenstrual syndrome and its relationship with blood pressure in young adult females," *African Journal of Medicine and Medical Sciences*, vol. 37, no. 4, pp. 361–367, 2008.

[37] L. Malan and N. T. Malan, "Emotional stress as a risk for hypertension in sub-saharan africans: are we ignoring the odds?" *Advances in Experimental Medicine and Biology*, 2016.

[38] J.-F. Agbu, "Type A behaviour pattern: a new insight to gender challenges in higher education," *Psychology, Health and Medicine*, vol. 15, no. 5, pp. 528–539, 2010.

[39] C. H. Hennekens, "Increasing burden of cardiovascular disease: current knowledge and future directions for research on risk factors," *Circulation*, vol. 97, no. 11, pp. 1095–1102, 1998.

[40] T. J. Aspray, F. Mugusi, S. Rashid et al., "Rural and urban differences in diabetes prevalence in Tanzania: the role of obesity, physical inactivity and urban living," *Transactions of the Royal Society of Tropical Medicine and Hygiene*, vol. 94, no. 6, pp. 637–644, 2000.

[41] A. N. Odili, L. Thijs, A. Hara et al., "Investigators, International Database on Home Blood Pressure in Relation to Cardiovascular Outcome (IDHOCO)," *Hypertension*, vol. 67, no. 6, pp. 1249–1255, 2016.

[42] J. E. Thompson, W. Smith, L. J. Ware et al., "Masked hypertension and its associated cardiovascular risk in young individuals: The African-PREDICT study," *Hypertension Research*, vol. 39, no. 3, pp. 158–165, 2016.

[43] H. S. Kruger, A. E. Schutte, C. M. Walsh, A. Kruger, and K. L. Rennie, "Body mass index cut-points to identify cardio-metabolic risk in black South Africans," *European Journal of Nutrition*, vol. 56, no. 1, pp. 193–202, 2015.

[44] X.-F. Leong, M. N. M. Najib, S. Das, M. R. Mustafa, and K. Jaarin, "Intake of repeatedly heated palm oil causes elevation in blood pressure with impaired vasorelaxation in rats," *The Tohoku Journal of Experimental Medicine*, vol. 219, no. 1, pp. 71–78, 2009.

[45] C. Anigbogu and O. Olubowale, "Effects of malaria on blood pressure, heart rate, electrocardiogram and cardiovascular response to change in posture," *Nigerian Quarterly Journal of Hospital Medicine*, vol. 12, no. 1-4, pp. 17–20, 2002.

[46] J. F. Trepanowski and R. J. Bloomer, "The impact of religious fasting on human health," *Nutrition Journal*, vol. 9, no. 57, 2010.

[47] K. O. Buabeng, "Unaffordable drug prices: the major cause of non-compliance with hypertension medication in Ghana," *Journal of Pharmacy and Pharmaceutical Sciences*, vol. 7, no. 3, pp. 350–352, 2004.

21

Renal Dysfunction among Ghanaians Living with Clinically Diagnosed Hypertension

Sylvester Yao Lokpo ⓘ,[1] James Osei-Yeboah ⓘ,[1] William K. B. A. Owiredu ⓘ,[2,3] Francis Abeku Ussher,[4] Verner Ndudiri Orish,[5] Felix Gadzeto,[6] Paul Ntiamoah,[6] Felix Botchway,[7] Ivan Muanah,[8] and Romeo Asumbasiya Aduko ⓘ[1]

[1]Department of Medical Laboratory Sciences, School of Allied Health Sciences, University of Health and Allied Sciences, Ho, Ghana
[2]Department of Molecular Medicine, School of Medical Sciences, Kwame Nkrumah University of Science and Technology, Kumasi, Ghana
[3]Department of Clinical Biochemistry, Diagnostic Directorate, Komfo Anokye Teaching Hospital, Kumasi, Ghana
[4]Faculty of Health and Allied Sciences, Koforidua Technical University, Koforidua, Eastern Region, Ghana
[5]Department of Microbiology and Immunology, School of Medicine, University of Health and Allied Sciences, Ho, Ghana
[6]Laboratory Department, St. Elizabeth Hospital, Catholic Health Services, Hwidiem, Brong Ahafo Region, Ghana
[7]Department of Chemical Pathology, University of Ghana, Accra, Ghana
[8]St. Elizabeth Hospital, Catholic Health Services, Hwidiem, Brong Ahafo Region, Ghana

Correspondence should be addressed to Sylvester Yao Lokpo; sylvesteryao34@gmail.com

Academic Editor: Tomohiro Katsuya

Background. This study aimed at evaluating the burden of renal dysfunction among people living with hypertension in the Asutifi-South District of the Brong Ahafo Region, who were attending clinic at the St. Elizabeth Hospital in Hwidiem. *Methodology.* A hospital-based, cross-sectional study was conducted among two hundred (200) hypertensive clients aged between 27 and 88 years who reported for clinical management from January to March, 2018. Data on sociodemography, comorbid disease status, antihypertensive medication, and their duration was obtained using a semistructured questionnaire and patient folders. Blood pressure, weight, and creatinine were measured using standard methods. Kidney function was assessed using Cockcroft Gault (CG), Four-Variable Modification of Diet in Renal Disease (4v-MDRD) and the Chronic Kidney Disease-Epidemiology Collaboration (CKD-EPI) equations. The 2012 Kidney Disease Improvement Global Outcome (KDIGO) Criteria were used to categorize renal function among study participants. *Results.* Renal impairment was observed among 25.00%, 9.50%, and 10.50% of study participants using CG, 4v-MDRD, and CKD-EPI equations, respectively. With the exception of CKD-EPI equation, females significantly recorded higher scores compared to their male counterparts (28.95% vs 12.5%, 11.84%, vs 2.08%) using CG and 4v-MDRD, respectively. Participants aged 50 years or more recorded the highest renal impairment. *Conclusion.* Renal dysfunction is common among people living with hypertension in the Asutifi-South District of the Brong Ahafo Region. Femininity, older age, disease comorbidity with diabetes, Thiazide diuretic and AR Blocker usage, and increasing duration of medication accounted for higher kidney dysfunction. Regular screening and management are therefore recommended to avert progression to end-stage renal failure (ESRD).

1. Introduction

The global public health importance of renal dysfunction is increasing due to a host of reasons including an increasing number of patients progressing to end-stage renal disease (ESRD), high costs to public health systems, and its associated morbidity and mortality, particularly those associated with cardiovascular disease [1]. The prevalence of hypertension is on the rise in Sub-Saharan Africa where most people with the disease remain undiagnosed, untreated, or inadequately treated [2]. Available information on hypertension prevalence in Ghana indicates rates ranging from 7.5% to 25.4% [3, 4]. There exist a multidirectional relationship between increased blood pressure (BP) and kidney pathology. The kidneys participate in the development and perpetuation of essential hypertension [5]. On the other hand, hypertension of any aetiology can lead to renal impairment (benign or malignant nephrosclerosis) and increased BP accompanied by proteinuria is an important factor related to the progression of kidney dysfunction [6]. Elevated BP damages blood vessels within the kidney, impairing its ability to filter fluid and waste from the blood, leading to an increase of fluid volume in the blood thus causing an increase in BP [7]. Despite being a principal public health issue, there is no surveillance system capable of detecting renal dysfunction at any stage among the populace as pertained in other developing nations across the world [8]. Prior to this study, there was very little information in the literature about the burden of kidney dysfunction among Ghanaians living with hypertension in Hwidiem in the Asutifi-South District of the Brong-Ahafo Region. In view of this, there is an urgent need for identifying hypertensive individuals with less than optimum kidney function with the aim of enhancing management approaches to reversing the disorder. This study is therefore aimed at evaluating the burden of renal dysfunction among hypertensive patients seeking medical care at the St. Elizabeth Hospital in Hwidiem in the Asutifi-South District of the Brong-Ahafo Region, Ghana.

2. Materials and Methods

2.1. The Study Site.
Asutifi-South District is one of the administrative districts in the Brong Ahafo Region, Ghana. The District was carved out from the then Asutifi District in July 2012 with Hwidiem as the district capital. The dominant vocation of the district is agriculture with 71.8% of households engaged in activities such as crop farming, animal rearing, and fish farming. St. Elizabeth hospital is a Catholic Health delivery facility in the Goaso Diocese. It is located in the Asutifi-South District in the Brong Ahafo Region of Ghana, providing healthcare to all its neighboring communities. It started as a Leprosy camp in 1955 and evolved over the years into a District Hospital. The hospital provides the following services: curative, preventive and promotive, rehabilitative, diagnostic, and special programs [9].

2.2. Study Design.
A hospital-based, descriptive cross-sectional study was conducted between January and March 2018 at the Diabetes and Hypertension Clinic of St. Elizabeth Hospital in the Asutifi-South District of the Brong Ahafo Region.

2.3. Sample Population.
The study population consisted of male and female hypertensive participants who were of consent age (18 years and above) in the Asutifi-South District. The hypertensive registrants were conveniently and purposively sampled at the Diabetes and Hypertensive Clinic of the hospital.

2.4. Sample Size.
Using the average monthly attendance of hypertensive patients for three months (133), a total study population of 399 was generated for the three months study duration. Raosoft online sample size calculator (http://www.raosoft.com/samplesize.html) was used, and a recommended minimum sample of 197 participants was calculated at 95% confidence level, 5% margin of error, and a response distribution of 50%.

2.5. Study Data Collection

2.5.1. Socio-Demographic Data Capture (Questionnaire).
A self-reported semistructured questionnaire was administered to obtain primary data from consenting adult clients. Sociodemographic information captured included age, gender, marital status, educational level, and occupation. Diabetes status and therapeutic variables including type of antihypertensive medication used and the duration on medication were ascertained using patient folders.

2.6. Blood Pressure and Weight Measurement.
Blood pressure was measured in the nondominant arm using fully-automated blood pressure monitor (OMRON Healthcare, Intelli-Sense BP785, HEM-7222, USA) in sitting position after resting for 3–5 minutes. A single qualified nurse recorded the average of two consecutive blood pressure readings taken on different occasions. Weight of participants was measured in light clothing, without shoes, and standing upright using a digital weighing scale (Health O Meter, USA) to the nearest 0.1 kg.

2.7. Blood Sampling and Laboratory Analysis.
Venous blood sample was drawn from the antecubital veins of the arm of which three (3) milliliters was dispensed into a vacutainer® serum separator tube using the closed vacutainer system. The sample in the serum separator tube was allowed to clot, centrifuged at 2500 revolutions per minute (rpm) for 5 minutes at room temperature to obtain serum. The serum was stored at -20°C at the St. Elizabeth Hospital until analysis. Serum samples were then transported on ice to the St. John of God Hospital Laboratory, Duayaw-Nkwanta where it was thawed and creatinine was measured on a Random Access Fully Automated Dirui CS – T240 Chemistry Analyzer, China. The methods used to assay creatinine were predetermined by the reagent manufacturer (Dirui Industries Co., Ltd, China). The quality of the results was ensured by running daily quality control checks and regular calibration of the instruments used.

2.8. Estimated Glomerular Filtration Rate (eGFR) Calculation.
The eGFR was calculated from serum creatinine values using the following predictive equations:

(I) Cockroft-Gault (CG) [10]

$$\text{Males} = \frac{(140 - \text{Age}) \times \text{Weight}}{72 \times \text{Serum Creatinine (mg/dl)}}$$

$$\text{Females} = \frac{(140 - \text{Age}) \times \text{Weight}}{72 \times \text{Serum Creatinine}} \times 0.85$$

(1)

TABLE 1

Gender	Serum Creatinine μmol/L (mg/dL)	Estimated Glomerular Equation
Female	≤62 (≤0.7)	$eGFR = 166 \times \left(\dfrac{\text{Serum Creatinine}}{0.7^{-0.329}} \right) \times (0.993)^{Age}$
Female	>62 (>0.7)	$eGFR = 166 \times \left(\dfrac{\text{Serum Creatinine}}{0.7^{-1.209}} \right) \times (0.993)^{Age}$
Male	≤80 (≤0.9)	$eGFR = 163 \times \left(\dfrac{\text{Serum Creatinine}}{0.9^{-0.411}} \right) \times (0.993)^{Age}$
Male	>80 (>0.9)	$eGFR = 163 \times \left(\dfrac{\text{Serum Creatinine}}{0.9^{-1.209}} \right) \times (0.993)^{Age}$

TABLE 2

GFR Category	Description	Range (ml/min/1.73 m^2)
G1	Normal or high	≥90
G2	Mildly decreased	60 to 89
G3	Mildly to moderately decreased	30 to 59
G4	Severely decreased	15 to 29
G5	Kidney failure	<15

(II) Four-Variable Modification of Diet in Renal Disease (4v-MDRD) [11]

$$\text{Males} = 186 \times SCr^{-1.154} \times Age^{-0.203} \times (1.212)$$

$$\text{Females} = 186 \times SCr^{-1.154} \times Age^{-0.203} \times (1.212) \qquad (2)$$
$$\times \, 0.74$$

(III) Chronic Kidney Disease Epidemiology collaboration-CKD-EPI [12]; see Table 1.

2.9. Definition of Renal Impairment. The calculated GFR was used to classify study participants into various categories of renal function according to the Kidney Disease Improvement Global Outcome (KDIGO) Criteria [13]. Renal impairment was defined as eGFR < 60 mL/min/1.73 m^2 consistent with categories G3, G4, and G5 as indicated in Table 2.

2.10. Statistical Analysis. Normality of all continuous variables was tested. Continuous variables were expressed as their mean ± standard deviation. Gender variation in the prevalence of kidney function was performed using unpaired t-tests, chi-square ($\chi 2$) tests, or Fisher exact tests where appropriate. A level of p<0.05 was considered as statistically significant for all analyses. IBM Statistical Package for Social Sciences (SPSS Inc, Chicago, USA) (http://www.spss.com) version 22.00 and GraphPad Prism version 6.01 GraphPad software, San Diego, California USA (http://www.graphpad.com), for windows were used for statistical analysis

2.11. Ethical Consideration. Ethical approval was obtained from the Research Ethics Committee of the University of Health and Allied Sciences, Ho, Ghana **(UHAS-REC/A.5 [35] 17-18)**, as well as written approval from management of St. Elizabeth hospital, Hwidiem. Informed consent from all participants was obtained following explanations and

clarification of the purpose of the study. Data obtained from participants was kept confidential.

3. Results

Out of the two hundred (200) participants recruited into this study, 48 (24.00%) were males and 152 (76.00%) were females. The average age of the total population was 61 ± 10 years. Sixty-seven (33.50%) of the study participants were both diabetic and hypertensive while 133 (66.50%) were hypertensive only. Majority of the study population were married [127 (63.5%)], with only 22.00% attaining secondary level education or higher at the time of this study. Majority of the study participants were gainfully employed 161 (80.50%). The average weight of the study participants was 64.23 ± 13.2 kg with the difference in weight between participants presenting with both diabetes and hypertension and those suffering from only hypertension observed to be statistically comparable (see Table 3).

The prevalence of renal impairment ranged from 9.50% through 10.50 to 25.00% using the 4v-MDRD, CKD-EPI and CG equations respectively. About 50 (22.50%), 19 (8.00%), and 21 (8.50%) of study participants were found to present with mild to severely decreased GFR (G3) using CG, 4v-MDRD, and CKD-EPI, respectively, with less than 3% classified as having severely decreased GFR (G4) while none presented with kidney failure (G5). The prevalence of renal impairment was significantly tilted toward the diabetic and hypertensive group using the CG, 4v-MDRD, and CKD-EPI equations (see Table 4).

Significant gender variation in renal dysfunction was observed, with a higher prevalence tilted toward the female gender using the CG and 4v-MDRD equations except for CKD-EPI equation where the difference in the percentage scores was statistically comparable. The rate of renal impairment among the male participants ranged from 2.08% to

TABLE 3: Socio-demographic characteristic of the population under study stratified by disease status.

Parameter	Total	Diabetic and Hypertensive all together	Hypertensive only
Total Respondents	200 (100)	67 (33.5)	133 (66.5)
Age (years)	61 ± 10	62 ± 9	61 ± 10
Weight (kg)	64.23 ± 13.2	63.10 ± 13.8	64.80 ± 13.8
Gender			
Male	48 (24.0)	12 (17.9)	36 (27.1)
Female	152 (76.0)	55 (82.1)	97 (72.9)
Marital Status			
Single	3 (1.5)	1 (1.5)	2 (1.5)
Married	127 (63.5)	36 (53.7)	91 (68.4)
Divorced	9 (4.5)	5 (7.5)	4 (3.0)
Widowed	58 (29.0)	24 (35.8)	34 (25.6)
Separated	3 (1.5)	1 (1.5)	2 (1.5)
Educational background			
None	86 (43.0)	33 (49.3)	53 (39.8)
Basic	70 (35.0)	21 (31.3)	49 (36.8)
Secondary	21 (10.5)	9 (13.4)	12 (9.0)
Tertiary	23 (11.5)	4 (6.0)	19 (14.3)
Employment Status			
Unemployed	36 (18.0)	12 (17.9)	24 (18.0)
Employed	161 (80.5)	54 (80.6)	107 (80.5)
On Pension	3 (1.5)	1 (1.5)	2 (1.5)

Data is presented as mean ± standard deviation and frequency with percentage in parenthesis.

TABLE 4: Renal dysfunction categorization among study population using KDIGO eGFR Criteria stratified by disease status.

	eGFR Category		Total	Diabetic and Hypertensive all together	Hypertensive only	p-value
	G 1	(≥90)	73 (36.50)	22 (32.84)	51 (38.35)	
	G 2	(60 to 89)	77 (38.50)	25 (37.31)	52 (39.10)	
CG	G 3	(30 to 59)	45 (22.50)	17 (25.37)	28 (21.05)	
	G 4	(15 to 29)	5 (2.50)	3 (4.48)	2 (1.50)	
	G 5	(<15)	0 (0.00)	0 (0.00)	0 (0.00)	
	Renal impairment (3+4+5)		**50 (25.00)**	**20 (29.85)**	**30 (22.56)**	**0.3002**
	G 1	(≥90)	137 (68.50)	41 (61.19)	96 (72.18)	
	G 2	(60 to 89)	44 (22.00)	15 (22.39)	29 (21.80)	
4v-MDRD	G3	(30 to 59)	16 (8.00)	9 (13.43)	7 (5.26)	
	G4	(15 to 29)	3 (1.50)	2 (2.99)	1 (0.75)	
	G5	(<15)	0 (0.00)	0 (0.00)	0 (0.00)	
	Renal impairment (3+4+5)		**19 (9.50)**	**11 (16.42)**	**8 (6.02)**	**0.0227**
	G1	(≥90)	130 (65.00)	40 (59.70)	90 (67.67)	
	G2	(60 to 89)	49 (24.50)	16 (23.88)	33 (24.81)	
CKD-EPI	G3	(30 to 59)	17 (8.50)	8 (11.94)	9 (6.77)	
	G4	(15 to 29)	4 (2.00)	3 (4.48)	1 (0.75)	
	G5	(<15)	0 (0.00)	0 (0.00)	0 (0.00)	
	Renal impairment (3+4+5)		**21 (10.50)**	**11 (16.42)**	**10 (7.52)**	**0.00845**

Data is presented as frequency and percentage in parenthesis. 4v-MDRD – four variable Modification of Diet in Renal Disease, CG – Cockcroft-Gault, CKD-EPI – Chronic Kidney Disease Epidemiology collaboration, eGFR – estimated Glomerular Filtration Rate, CKD – Chronic Kidney Disease, G1-Category one, G2-Category two, G3-Category three, G4-Category four, G5-Category five.

TABLE 5: Renal dysfunction categorization among study population using KDIGO eGFR Criteria stratified by gender.

	eGFR Category		Male	Female	p-value
CG	G1	(≥90)	22 (45.83)	51 (33.55)	
	G2	(60 to 89)	20 (41.67)	57 (37.50)	
	G3	(30 to 59)	6 (12.50)	39 (25.66)	
	G4	(15 to 29)	0 (0.00)	5 (3.29)	
	G5	(<15)	0 (0.00)	0 (0.00)	
	Renal impairment (3+4+5)		**6 (12.50)**	**44 (28.95)**	**0.0222**
4v-MDRD	G1	(≥90)	38 (79.17)	99 (65.13)	
	G2	(60 to 89)	9 (18.75)	35 (23.03)	
	G3	(30 to 59)	1 (2.08)	15 (9.87)	
	G4	(15 to 29)	0 (0.00)	3 (1.97)	
	G5	(<15)	0 (0.00)	0 (0.00)	
	Renal impairment (3+4+5)		**1 (2.08)**	**18 (11.84)**	**0.0487**
CKD-EPI	G1	(≥90)	37 (77.08)	93 (61.8)	
	G2	(60 to 89)	9 (18.75)	40 (26.32)	
	G3	(30 to 59)	2 (4.17)	15 (9.87)	
	G4	(15 to 29)	0 (0.00)	4 (2.63)	
	G5	(<15)	0 (0.00)	0 (0.00)	
	Renal impairment (3+4+5)		**2 (4.17)**	**19 (12.50)**	**0.1136**

Data is presented as frequency with percentage in parenthesis. 4v-MDRD: four-variable modification of diet in renal disease, CG: Cockcroft-Gault, CKD-EPI: chronic kidney disease epidemiology collaboration, eGFR: estimated Glomerular Filtration Rate, CKD: chronic kidney disease, G1: category one, G2: category two, G3: category three, G4: category four, and G5: category five.

TABLE 6: Prevalence of renal dysfunction stratified by age and medication.

Parameter	CG	Rank	4v-MDRD	Rank	CKD-EPI	Rank
Age Category (years)						
<50	2 (7.40)	4th	1 (3.70)	4th	1 (3.70)	4th
50-59	11 (22.00)	2nd	10 (20.00)	1st	10 (20.00)	1st
60-69	19 (21.35)	3rd	5 (5.62)	3rd	6 (6.74)	3rd
≥70	18 (56.25)	1st	3 (9.38)	2nd	4 (11.76)	2nd
Antihypertensive Medication						
ACE Inhibitor	27 (24.32)	2nd	10 (9.01)	2rd	11 (9.91)	3rd
CC Blocker	36 (20.34)	4th	14 (7.91)	3rd	18 (10.17)	2nd
Diuretics	6 (23.08)	3rd	4 (15.38)	1st	4 (15.38)	1st
AR Blocker	17 (25.00)	1st	6 (8.82)	4th	6 (8.82)	4th
β-Blocker	1 (12.50)	5th	0 (0.00)	5th	0 (0.00)	5th
One	7 (29.17)	3rd	2 (8.33)	3rd	3 (12.50)	2nd
Two	24 (25.00)	4th	9 (9.38)	2nd	8 (6.56)	4th
Three	6 (31.58)	2nd	3 (15.79)	1st	8 (18.18)	1st
Four	1 (33.33)	1st	0 (0.0)	4rh	1 (10.00)	3rd

Data is presented as frequency with percentage in parenthesis. 4v-MDRD: four-variable modification of diet in renal disease, CG: Cockcroft-Gault, CKD-EPI: chronic kidney disease epidemiology collaboration. ACE inhibitor: angiotensin converting enzyme inhibitor, and CC blocker: calcium channel blocker.

12.50% as compared to 11.84% to 28.95% among their female counterparts. All the male participants presenting with renal impairment were in G3 category (see Table 5).

Using the predictive equations, renal dysfunction was found to be highest in participants aged 70 years or more except for the 4v-MDRD and CKD-EPI equations where the scores were highest among the 50-59 years age group. Among the hypertensive medications, patients on Diuretics and AR Blockers presented with the highest scores using the predictive CKD equations. Generally, study participants on combination therapy of three medications presented with the greatest percentage of kidney dysfunction (see Table 6). Among the respondents presenting with renal impairment, there was a significantly increasing number of respondents from the first quartile through to the fourth quartile of antihypertensive medication duration whereas the reverse was observed among participants without evidence of renal damage (p=0.0301).

4. Discussion

In the present study, the prevalence of renal impairment among the study population was estimated at 25.00%, 9.50%, and 10.50% using CG, 4v-MDRD, and CKD-EPI predictive equations, respectively. With the exception of CG equation (29.85% vs 22.56%; p=0.3002), the prevalence of renal impairment among participants presenting with both diabetes and hypertension was significantly higher compared to participants presenting with only hypertension (Table 4). Ephraim and colleagues recorded a 30% prevalence of kidney dysfunction using the CKD-EPI definitive criteria among a high-risk population in the Sekondi-Takoradi Metropolis in South-Western Ghana [14]. A similar investigation conducted among hypertensive patients in Donkorkrom in the Eastern Region yielded a prevalence of 50%, 43%, and 46% using CG, MDRD, and CKD-EPI equations, respectively [15]. In other jurisdictions, a high burden of renal dysfunction among hypertensive individuals was reported in Nigeria [16, 17], Cameroon [18, 19], Guinea [20], Brazil [21], and Qatar [22]. However, renal dysfunction prevalence rates lower than the findings of this study have been reported among some Ghanaian (4.1% and 0.5%) [23] and South African (7.8%) [24] populations.

Although information is dearth in the present study to explaining the difference in kidney disease burden between the current work and others in various jurisdictions, a host of factors have been suggested to contribute to this phenomenon including difference in population characteristics, geographical location, ethnicity, hereditary, type of definitive criteria used in estimating kidney dysfunction, laboratory method employed and the presence of other CKD risk profiles as well as disease severity [14, 23, 24].

Gender preponderance to impaired renal function has been shown to be skewed toward the female gender [19]. In the present study, a significant proportion of female respondents recorded higher percentage scores compared to their male counterparts using CG and 4v-MDRD equations except for CKD-EPI equation where the difference in the renal dysfunction scores was statistically comparable (Table 5). Our results could be partly attributed to the greater health seeking behaviour among Ghanaian hypertensive females than males recorded in this study, notwithstanding the results compared with our previous findings, where femininity significantly accounted for renal dysfunction among a hypertensive population in the Kumasi Metropolis [23]. Though the relationship which exists between the female gender and kidney dysfunction in hypertension is not fully understood, it is suggested that obesity associated with femininity may play an indirect role in mediating the pathophysiological process [25]. The proposed pathway linking obesity to kidney dysfunction in females includes glomerular hyperfiltration with resultant albuminuria and eventual segmental glomerulosclerosis [19].

In the present study, using the predictive CKD equations, renal dysfunction was found to be highest in participants aged 70 years or more except for 4v-MDRD and CKD-EPI equations where the CKD scores were highest among the 50-59 years age group (Table 6). This suggests that increasing age is associated with a decline in renal function of participants.

Age is widely documented as an independent risk factor for both hypertension and kidney dysfunction in the Ghanaian and other populations [14, 23, 26–28]. In advancing age, a fall in GFR is probably due to reductions in the glomerular capillary plasma flow rate, glomerular capillary ultrafiltration coefficient, afferent arteriolar resistance and increased glomerular capillary hydraulic pressure; the haemodynamic changes occur with structural alterations, including loss of renal mass; hyalinization of afferent arterioles and in some cases, development of efferent glomerular arterioles; increase in the percentage of sclerotic glomeruli and tubulointerstitial fibrosis [17, 29].

The advent of the Seventh Report of the Joint National Committee on Prevention, Detection, Evaluation, and Treatment of High Blood Pressure (JNC VII) 2003 guidelines has seen a surge in the treatment and control of hypertension with antihypertensive medications in people with kidney dysfunction [30]. However, there are recent reports indicating a probable role of antihypertensive medications in worsening kidney function [31, 32]. Among the antihypertensive medications used in this study, participants on Angiotensin II Receptor Blockers (ARB) (25.00%) and Thiazide Diuretics (15.38%) presented with the highest percentage scores using CG, 4v-MDRD, and CKD-EPI equations, respectively. Generally, study respondents on three combination therapy demonstrated greater percentage scores (Table 6). A significantly increasing number of respondents presenting with kidney dysfunction clustered at increasing quartile of duration of antihypertensive medication use (p=0.0301). [33]. Hawkins and Houston [34] observed a positive correlation between changes in the use of diuretics and increase in the occurrence of ESRD with a time lag of two years. Increased advanced stages of renal insufficiency, particularly among those with albuminuria after an increase in ARB polytherapy, have been reported [30].

The present study is limited in its cross-sectional design; hence causal relationship of renal impairment could not be established. Serum creatinine assay (picric acid method) adopted from the manufacturer was not traceable to the standardized isotope dilution mass spectrometry (IDMS). The study also relied on a single measurement of serum creatinine and estimation of GFR instead of two measurements three months apart in addition to urine protein estimation to determine urine albumin/creatinine ratio (ACR). This could lead to many missed cases of kidney damage.

5. Conclusion

The burden of renal dysfunction is high among Ghanaian hypertensive clients in the Asutifi-South District of the Brong-Ahafo Region. Females and participants presenting with comorbidity (both hypertension and diabetes) were most affected by renal dysfunction. Older age, thiazide diuretic and AR Blocker medications, increasing duration of antihypertensive therapy, and their combination were associated with greater kidney dysfunction. Regular screening and management are therefore recommended to avert progression to end-stage renal disease (ESRD).

Authors' Contributions

This work was carried out with the collaboration of all authors. Authors have reviewed and certified the final manuscript for submission.

References

[1] R. T. Gansevoort, R. Correa-Rotter, and B. R. Hemmelgarn, "Chronic kidney disease and cardiovascular risk: epidemiology, mechanisms, and prevention," *The Lancet*, vol. 382, no. 9889, pp. 339–352, 2013.

[2] F. Ataklte, S. Erqou, S. Kaptoge, B. Taye, J. B. Echouffo-Tcheugui, and A. P. Kengne, "Burden of Undiagnosed Hypertension in Sub-Saharan Africa," *A Systematic Review and Meta-Analysis*, 2014.

[3] S. H. Nyarko, "Prevalence and Sociodemographic Determinants of Hypertension History among Women in Reproductive Age in Ghana," *International Journal of Hypertension*, vol. 2016, Article ID 3292938, 6 pages, 2016.

[4] I. Solomon, M. Adjuik, and W. Takramah, "Prevalence and awareness of hypertension among urban and rural adults in Hohoe Municipality, Ghana," *Journal of Marketing Research*, vol. 3, no. 3, pp. 136–145, 2017.

[5] N. R. Pandey, Y.-Y. Bian, and S.-T. Shou, "Significance of blood pressure variability in patients with sepsis," *World Journal of Emergency Medicine*, vol. 5, no. 1, p. 42, 2014.

[6] D. S. Keith, G. A. Nichols, C. M. Gullion, J. B. Brown, and D. H. Smith, "Longitudinal follow-up and outcomes among a population with chronic kidney disease in a large managed care organization," *JAMA Internal Medicine*, vol. 164, no. 6, pp. 659–663, 2004.

[7] B. Leticia and R. Charlotte, "Chronic Kidney Disease and Hypertension: A Destructive Combination," 2012, http://www.medscape.com/viewarticle/766696_2.

[8] R. García-Trabanino, Z. Trujillo, A. V. Colorado, S. Magaña Mercado, and C. A. Henríquez, "Prevalence of patients receiving renal replacement therapy in El Salvador in 2014," *Nefrología (English Edition)*, vol. 36, no. 6, pp. 631–636, 2016.

[9] EHAR, St. Elizabeth Hospital Annual Report, Ed., 2017.

[10] D. W. Cockcroft and M. H. Gault, "Prediction of creatinine clearance from serum creatinine," *Nephron*, vol. 16, no. 1, pp. 31–41, 1976.

[11] A. S. Levey, J. P. Bosch, J. B. Lewis, T. Greene, N. Rogers, and D. Roth, "A more accurate method to estimate glomerular filtration rate from serum creatinine: a new prediction equation. Modification of Diet in Renal Disease Study Group," *Annals of Internal Medicine*, vol. 130, no. 6, pp. 461–470, 1999.

[12] NKF, The National Kidney Foundation recommended CKD-EPI Creatinine Equation (2009) GFR Calculator, Ed., 2017.

[13] KDIGO, KDIGO 2012 Clinical Practice Guideline for the Evaluation and Management of Chronic Kidney Disease, Ed., 2013.

[14] R. K. Ephraim, S. Biekpe, S. A. Sakyi, P. Adoba, H. Agbodjakey, and E. O. Antoh, "Prevalence of chronic kidney disease among the high risk population in South-Western Ghana; a cross sectional study," *Canadian Journal of Kidney Health and Disease*, vol. 2, no. 1, article 40, 2015.

[15] E. K. Mireku, Biochemical Correlates of Renal Dysfunction Among Non-Diabetic Hypertensives, Ed., 2012.

[16] E. Odum and E. Udi, "Evaluation of cardiovascular risk factors in patients with chronic kidney disease," *Port Harcourt Medical Journal*, vol. 11, no. 2, p. 60, 2017.

[17] M. R. Akpa and N. N. Unamba, "Asymptomatic chronic kidney disease and correlates in untreated hypertensive patients attending a referral hospital in Southern Nigeria," *Clinical Practice*, vol. 6, no. 1, pp. 9–13, 2017.

[18] F. F. Kaze, A.-P. Kengne, C. T. Magatsing, M.-P. Halle, E. Yiagnigni, and K. B. Ngu, "Prevalence and determinants of chronic kidney disease among hypertensive cameroonians according to three common estimators of the glomerular filtration rate," *The Journal of Clinical Hypertension*, vol. 18, no. 5, pp. 408–414, 2016.

[19] B. Hamadou, J. Boombhi, F. Kamdem et al., "Prevalence and correlates of chronic kidney disease in a group of patients with hypertension in the Savanah zone of Cameroon: A cross-sectional study in Sub-Saharan Africa," *Cardiovascular Diagnosis and Therapy*, vol. 7, no. 6, pp. 581–588, 2017.

[20] M. L. Kaba, M. Camara, M. Béavogui et al., "Risk factors for chronic kidney disease among patients admitted to the medical wards in Conakry," *Saudi Journal of Kidney Diseases and Transplantation*, vol. 27, no. 5, pp. 1073–1075, 2016.

[21] N. A. Pinho, R. d. Oliveira, and A. M. Pierin, "Hipertensos com e sem doença renal: avaliação de fatores de risco," *Revista da Escola de Enfermagem da USP*, vol. 49, no. spe, pp. 101–108, 2015.

[22] S. Suliman, M. Thomas, and E. Satti, "Predictors of chronic kidney disease in hypertensive patients: a oneyear prospective study at hamad general hospital, Qatar," *Journal of Nephrology and Therapeutics*, vol. 9, no. 6, pp. 1–7, 2016.

[23] C. Aryee, W. K. B. A. Owiredu, J. Osei-Yeboah, E. Owusu-Dabo, E. F. Laing, and I. K. Owusu, "An analysis of anthropometric indicators and modifiable lifestyle parameters associated with hypertensive nephropathy," *International Journal of Hypertension*, vol. 2016, Article ID 6598921, 14 pages, 2016.

[24] A. B. Adeniyi, C. E. Laurence, J. A. Volmink, and M. R. Davids, "Prevalence of chronic kidney disease and association with cardiovascular risk factors among teachers in Cape Town, South Africa," *Clinical Kidney Journal*, vol. 10, no. 3, pp. 363–369, 2017.

[25] Y. Wang, X. Chen, Y. Song, B. Caballero, and L. J. Cheskin, "Association between obesity and kidney disease: a systematic review and meta-analysis," *Kidney International*, vol. 73, no. 1, pp. 19–33, 2008.

[26] C. Okwuonu, I. Chukwuonye, O. Adejumo, E. Agaba, and L. Ojogwu, "Prevalence of chronic kidney disease and its risk factors among adults in a semi-urban community of South-East Nigeria," *Nigerian Postgraduate Medical Journal*, vol. 24, no. 2, p. 81, 2017.

[27] F. M. Tedla, A. Brar, R. Browne, and C. Brown, "Hypertension in chronic kidney disease: navigating the evidence," *International Journal of Hypertension*, vol. 2011, Article ID 132405, 9 pages, 2011.

[28] V. Van Der Meer, H. P. M. Wielders, D. C. Grootendorst et al., "Chronic kidney disease in patients with diabetes mellitus type 2 or hypertension in general practice," *British Journal of General Practice*, vol. 60, no. 581, pp. 884–890, 2010.

[29] J. R. Weinstein and S. Anderson, "The aging kidney: physiological changes," *Advances in Chronic Kidney Disease*, vol. 17, no. 4, pp. 302–307, 2010.

[30] M. Komaroff, F. Tedla, E. Helzner, and M. A. Joseph, "Antihypertensive medications and change in stages of chronic kidney disease," *International Journal of Chronic Diseases*, vol. 2018, Article ID 1382705, 10 pages, 2018.

[31] L. A. Tomlinson, G. A. Abel, A. N. Chaudhry et al., "ACE inhibitor and angiotensin receptor-II antagonist prescribing and hospital admissions with acute kidney injury: A longitudinal ecological study," *PLoS ONE*, vol. 8, no. 11, Article ID e78465, 2013.

[32] SPRINT Research Group, "A randomized trial of intensive versus standard blood-pressure control," *The New England Journal of Medicine*, vol. 373, no. 22, pp. 2103–2116, 2015.

[33] A. G. Ptinopoulou, M. I. Pikilidou, and A. N. Lasaridis, "The effect of antihypertensive drugs on chronic kidney disease: A comprehensive review," *Hypertension Research*, vol. 36, no. 2, pp. 91–101, 2013.

[34] R. G. Hawkins and M. C. Houston, "Is population-wide diuretic use directly associated with the incidence of end-stage renal disease in the United States? A hypothesis," *American Journal of Hypertension*, vol. 18, no. 6, pp. 744–749, 2005.

22

Hypertension and Associated Factors in Rural and Urban Areas Mali: Data from the STEP 2013 Survey

Hamidou Oumar Bâ ⓘ,[1] Youssouf Camara,[2] Ichaka Menta,[1]
Ibrahima Sangaré,[1] Noumou Sidibé,[1] I. B. Diall,[3] Souleymane Coulibaly,[3]
Maiga Asmaou Kéita,[4] and Georges Rosario Christian Millogo[5]

[1]CHU Gabriel Touré Bamako, Bamako, Mali
[2]CHU Kati, Kati, Mali
[3]CHU Point G, Bamako, Mali
[4]CHU Mère-Enfant, Bamako, Mali
[5]CHU YO, Ouagadougou, Burkina Faso

Correspondence should be addressed to Hamidou Oumar Bâ; bhamiba@yahoo.fr

Background. Our study aims to estimate hypertension (HTN) prevalence and its predictors in rural and urban area. *Methods.* We conducted a cross-sectional population-based study involving subjects aged 15 to 65 years. Collected data (sociodemographic, blood pressure, weight, height, and blood glucose) were analyzed using SPSS version 20. A logistic regression was conducted to look for factors associated with HTN. *Results.* Mean was 47 years. High blood pressure (HBP) prevalence was 21.1 and 24.7%, respectively, in rural and urban setting. In rural area age group significantly predicted hypertension with age of 60 years having more-than-4-times risk of hypertension, whereas, in urban area age group, sex and body mass index were predictors with OR: HTN raising from 2.06 [1.24–3.43] for 30–44 years old to 7.25 [4.00–13.13] for 60 years and more using <30 years as reference. Female sex was protective with OR of 0.45 [0.29–0.71] and using normal weight as reference OR for overweight was 1.54 [1.04–2.27] and 2.67 [1.64–4.36] for obesity. *Conclusion.* Hypertension prevalence is high and associated factors were age group in rural area and age group, female sex, and body mass index in urban area.

1. Introduction

Hypertension (HTN) as leading risk factor for cardiovascular diseases has been largely described by many authors in the world [1–4]. As in other parts of the world HTN is a public health problem of growing concern in Low- and Middle-Income Countries (LMIC) [5, 6] and particularly in Africa [7, 8]. Newer African data on prevalence from community-based studies are high and above 25% [9, 10] and up to 53% [11]. Many factors have been described as associated with HTN [2, 12, 13].

Published data and mostly those from population-based studies are either old or rare in Mali. Prevalence data based on a 2002 conducted survey found 26% in the urban

setting Bamako [14]. Recent data are therefore needed as well in urban as in rural areas. Our study aims to estimate hypertension prevalence and its risk factors in some rural and urban areas based on 2013 step survey data.

2. Materials and Methods

We conducted a cross-sectional population-based study, whose data stemmed from the 2013 STEPS-Survey in urban and rural areas. This approach has been described by the World Health Organization (WHO) [15].

2.1. Sampling and Data Collection. The study sample is based on the last STEPS-Survey which was conducted in 2013 with

TABLE 1

Commune	Number of clusters	Type of area	Quartiers/villages
II (Bamako)	3	Urban	Bakaribougou, Médina coura; Niarela
III (Bamako)	3	Urban	Bamakocourabolibana, Dravelila, N'Tomicorobougou
VI (Bamako)	6	Urban	Banankabougou, Magnanbougou, Missabougou, Niamakoro, Sogoniko; Yirimadjo
Koulikoro	5	Urban	Katibougou, Kasso, Kolebougou, Koulikoroba, Koulikoro garre I
Kati central	3	Rural	Kati coura, Malibougou, Sébénicoro
Ouélessébougou	2	Rural	Fanicodiana, Tinkele
Ségou	4	Urban	Bagadadji, Darsalam, Mission, Sidosonicoura
Sikasso	4	Urban	Boula hameau, Lafiabougou koko, Quartuier résidentiel, Wayerma I
Total	*30*		

2102 subjects aged from 15 to 65 years of whom 1543 (73.4%) in urban and 559 (26.6%) in rural areas.

It was conducted in administrative units known as communes and within each commune in towns/villages.

A two-stage cluster sampling method was used to select subjects from urban and rural areas. First clusters were obtained among communes in the three involved regions and second clusters from quartiers within these communes. Households were then randomly selected and all eligible adults in the household were interviewed and underwent physical exam and measurements.

The sample size was calculated using the formula

$$n = \frac{Z^2 pq}{i^2} \times d \qquad (1)$$

with n = sample size, Z = 1,96, p = 40% = 0.40, $q = 1 - p$ = 0.6, i = 3% = 0.03, d = 2.

A total of 30 clusters as given in Table 1 were obtained.

2.2. Data Collection. The following data were recorded for each study participant:

(i) Sociodemographic

(ii) 3 blood pressures and heart rate measures in 5 min interval, using their mean as systolic, diastolic blood pressure, respectively, SBP, DBP, and HR

(iii) Fasting/postprandial glycemia

(iv) Weight in kilogram (Kg) and height in centimeter (cm) allowing calculation of body mass index (BMI) in Kg/m^2 as weight (Kg)/height (cm)^2

(v) Waist circumference (WC) and hip circumference (HC) all in cm

(vi) Waist-to-hip ratio (rWH) as WC in cm divided by HC in cm

(vii) Mean blood pressure from 3 measures

For the filling of the survey formulary and performing measurements, medical teams were built and trained for the household visit (and second visit in case household members were not present). Each subject was interviewed and different measures were obtained according to guidelines of the WHO STEPS approach for chronic disease surveillance [15].

Interviews were performed by medical staff and focused on sociodemographic characteristics, lifestyle, cardiovascular risk factors, personal and family history of cardio-vascular diseases, or other chronic illnesses.

Height was measured without shoes to the nearest centimeter with subject stand on the footplate with back against stadiometer rule.

Weight was measured to the nearest 0.1 kg on an electronic scale with the subject wearing light clothing and no shoes.

Waist circumference (WC) and hip circumference (HC) were measured with a stretch-resistant tape that is wrapped snugly around the subject, but not constricting.

WC was measured at the midpoint between the lower border of the rib cage and the iliac crest with the subject being light clothed.

HC was measured around the widest portion of the buttocks.

We used for blood pressure measurements a Frangly® aneroid sphygmomanometer with a medium and large cuff size and performed measures at rest, the subject being in sitting position on the right arm. The mean of the two blood pressure readings was used for each subject in this study. A third measure was performed in some cases if blood pressure values were borderline.

2.3. Definitions. Education level was graded as follows:

(i) Level 0: no school attending

(ii) Level 1: school attending for 1–6

(iii) Level 2: school attending for 7–9

(iv) Level 3: school attending for 10–12

(v) Level 4: school attending for 12 and more years

Hypertension was defined as systolic blood pressure (SBP) ≥ 140 mmHg and/or diastolic blood pressure (DBP) ≥ 90 mmHg or self-reported use of antihypertensive drug irrespective of measured blood pressure [16].

Mean arterial blood pressure (mBP) was calculated with the following formula: DBP + ((SBP – DBP)/3).

General obesity was defined by body mass index (BMI) and further central obesity through the waist circumference (WC) [17].

BMI served to define weight disorders as follows:

(i) Underweight (UW): <18.5

(ii) Normal weight (NW): 18.5–24.99

(iii) Overweight (OW): ≥25.00–29.99

(iv) Obesity (OB): ≥30.00

Based on waist circumference, OW was defined as WC ≥90 cm and ≥80 respectively for men and women and OB as waist ≥102 cm for men and ≥88 cm for women [18].

For waist-to-hip ratio (rWH) Men with a rWH 0.90–0.99 and women with a rWH 0.80–0.84 were classified as overweight, whilst men with a rWH ≥ 1.00 and women with a rWH ≥ 0.85 were classified as obese [18].

Diabetes was assessed with a glucometer (one-touch ultra Bayer®), fastened or postprandial with cutting values of 1.26 and 2 g, respectively, and the use of antidiabetic medicine.

2.4. Data Analysis. Statistical analysis was done using analytical software SPSS version 20. Results were expressed as either mean values (standard deviation) or proportions. *t*-test for continuous variables and chi-square or Fisher test analysis for categorical variables were used. Level of significance was set at 0.05.

After a prevalence estimation in rural and urban setting, hypertensive subjects were selected to compare them regarding sociodemographics and descriptives variables.

Finally a logistic regression was conducted to look for predictors of hypertension in rural and in urban setting using age group, marital status, sex, educational level, tobacco smoking, alcohol consumption, body mass index, waist circumference, and waist-to-hip ratio and diabetes as independent variables.

For logistic regressions the following references were used: <30 years, single, Female, unschooled, nonsmoker, no alcohol consumption, normal weight for BMI, WC, and rWH, no diabetes, and resting HR > 90/min

3. Results

From the 2102 study participants, 495 were hypertensive subjects of whom 118 (23.8%) resided in rural area.

Mean age of the sample was 47.78±13.230 (47.00±13.214 in rural and 48.03 ± 13.243 in urban area with$p$ = 0.451). Height and Glycemia were slightly higher in urban areas with 167.60 versus 165.76 cm and 120.18 versus 116.23 mg/l with p value of 0.074 and 0.536. rWH was not significantly different with 0.91 in urban and 0.92 in rural area and p value of 0.634 (Table 2).

Weight, BMI, WC, and HC were higher in urban areas compared to those in rural areas, 75.47 versus 68.50 kg, 26.29 versus 24.83 kg/m^2, 92.79 versus 85.45 cm, and 102.2 versus 93.45 cm, respectively. All p values were highly significant with 0.0001 (Table 2).

Age group showed the same profile, increasing proportion up to 59 years in urban as in rural areas. Age group

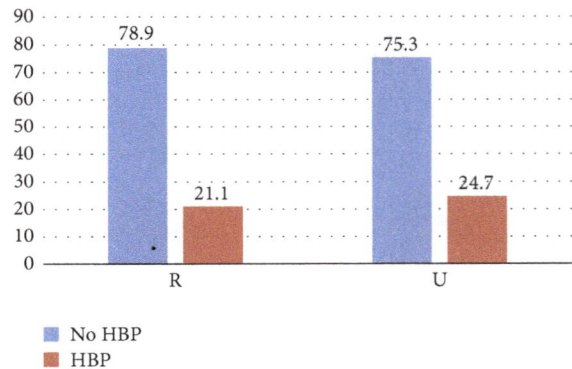

FIGURE 1: Blood pressure profile in rural and urban area.

45–59 y made 37% (9.5 in rural and 27.5% in urban areas). But differences did not reach significant level (Table 3).

Female sex and the status married represented 60.2 and 81.4% of the sample, respectively, but with p value of 0.086 and 0.676 whereas almost half of the sample was unschooled (p < 0.0001) (Table 3).

HBP prevalence was 21.1 and 24.7%, respectively, in rural and urban setting (Figure 1).

Among blood pressure parameters, heart rate was lower in urban areas (78.8%) versus 81.25% in rural areas with a p value of 0.040. Systolic, diastolic, and mean arterial pressure were slightly higher in urban areas with, respectively, 151.23 mmHg, 94.62 mmHg, and 113.49 mmHg versus 150.94 mmHg, 94.10 mmHg, and 113.04 mmHg in rural areas. Corresponding p values were, respectively, 0.900, 0.675, and 0.753 (Table 4). Pulsed pressure was in the same level with 56.84 mmHg in rural areas and 56.61 mmHg in urban areas (p = 0.904).

Using logistic regression, age group was found to be a significant predictor for hypertension (χ^2 = 139.13, df = 22, and p < 0.001) in rural areas. The OR were 2.60, 4.97, and 9.70 for 30–44 y, 45–59 y, and above 60 years old, respectively, with under 30 years as reference (Table 5).

Whereas in urban area age group, sex, and BMI were found as predictors for hypertension, hypertension increased in age group from 2.06 CI [95% 1.24-3.43] for 30–44 y to 7.25 CI [95% 4.00-13.13] for 60 y and above (p < 0.0001). Female sex was protective with OR of 0.45 IC [95% 0.29-0.71] and BMI showed an increase of hypertensive subjects with increasing BMI. OR for overweight was 1.54 IC [95% 1.04-2.27] and 2.67 IC [95% 1.64-4.36] for obesity.

4. Discussion

In the study with a large data sample, we first estimated HTN prevalence in rural and urban area and then conducted a logistic regression to look for predictors of HTN. To our knowledge it is the first time that community-based data are analyzed in such a way. Previous studies are either community-based in urban area [14] or from hospital based data.

TABLE 2: Description of sociodemographic characteristics of 495 hypertensive subjects in the 2013 STEP survey in Mali.

| Variables | Setting | | | | Total | | p |
| | Rural | | Urban | | | | |
	N	%	N	%	N	%	
Age groups (years)							
16–29	14	2.8	41	8.3	55	11.1	
30–44	28	5.7	97	19.6	125	25.3	0.845
45–59	47	9.5	136	27.5	183	37.0	
60 and more	29	5.9	103	20.8	132	26.7	
Sex							
Male	39	7.9	158	31.9	197	39.8	0.086
Female	79	16.0	219	44.2	298	60.2	
Marital status							
Unmarried	8	1.6	32	6.5	40	8.1	
Divorced	0	0.0	1	0.2	1	0.2	0.676
Married	95	19.2	308	62.2	403	81.4	
Widowers	15	3.0	36	7.3	51	10.3	
Education level							
Level 0	79	16.0	165	33.3	244	49.3	
Level 1	11	2.2	84	17.0	95	19.2	
Level 2	14	2.8	51	10.3	65	13.1	<0.0001
Level 3	13	2.6	63	12.7	76	15.4	
Level 4	1	0.2	14	2.8	15	3.0	

TABLE 3: Description of continuous variables of 495 hypertensive subjects in rural and urban setting in Mali.

| | Rural | | | Urban | | | Total | | | p |
	Mean	N	SD	Mean	N	SD	Mean	N	SD	
Age	47.00	118	13.214	48.03	377	13.243	47.78	495	13.230	0.451
Weight (Kg)	68.50	116	13.305	75.47	376	16.510	73.83	492	16.076	<0.0001
Height (cm)	165.76	118	09.708	167.60	375	09.711	167.16	493	9.732	0.074
BMI	24.83	116	04.346	26.29	374	05.516	26.41	490	5.330	<0.0001
WC	85.48	114	11.819	92.79	368	14.123	91.06	482	13.952	<0.0001
HC	93.50	115	12.914	102.31	334	15.315	100.05	449	15.218	<0.0001
rWH	0.92	111	0.087	0.91	328	0.108	0.92	439	0.103	0.634
Glycemia	116.23	117	29.638	120.18	363	66.882	119.22	480	59.968	0.536

BMI: body mass index; WC: waist circumference; HC: hip circumference; rWH: waist-to-hip ratio.

TABLE 4: Blood pressure related parameters in the sample of 495 hypertensive subjects.

| | Rural | | | Urban | | | Total | | | p |
	Mean	N	SD	Mean	N	SD	Mean	N	SD	
SBP	150.94	118	22.734	151.23	377	21.630	151.16	495	21.875	0.900
DBP	94.10	118	13.193	94.62	377	11.310	94.49	495	11.774	0.675
HR	81.25	118	16.177	78.03	377	14.368	78.80	495	14.866	0.040
PP	56.84	118	17.421	56.61	377	18.224	56.67	495	18.019	0.904
mBP	113.04	118	14.862	113.49	377	12.939	113.38	495	13.408	0.753

SBP: systolic blood pressure; DBP: diastolic blood pressure; HR: heart rate; PP: pulsed pressure; mBP: mean blood pressure.

TABLE 5: Logistic regression predicting hypertension in rural setting.

Variables	B	S.E.	df	Sig.	OR	95% CI for OR	
						Lower	Upper
Age group: <30 years as reference			3	.000			
30–44	.955	.462	1	.039	2.60	1.05	6.42
45–59	1.603	.468	1	.001	4.97	1.99	12.42
60 and more	2.272	.535	1	.000	9.70	3.40	27.66
Marital status: single as reference			2	.904			
Married	.018	.544	1	.974	1.02	0.35	2.96
Widower	.220	.706	1	.755	1.25	0.31	4.97
Sex	−.811	.414	1	.050	0.44	0.20	1.00
Educational level: unschooled as reference			4	.595			
Level 1	−.336	.441	1	.446	0.71	0.30	1.70
Level 2	−.123	.403	1	.761	0.88	0.40	1.95
Level 3	.008	.426	1	.986	1.01	0.44	2.32
Level 4	−1.654	1.092	1	.130	0.19	0.02	1.63
Tobacco smoking	.042	.389	1	.914	1.04	0.49	2.24
Alcohol consumption	−.242	.713	1	.735	0.79	0.19	3.18
BMI: Underweight as reference			3	.887			
Normal weight	.395	.661	1	.550	1.49	0.41	5.43
Overweight	.537	.702	1	.445	1.71	0.43	6.78
Obesity	.411	.803	1	.608	1.51	0.31	7.28
WC: normal as reference			2	.211			
Overweight	.390	.350	1	.265	1.48	0.74	2.94
Obesity	.711	.408	1	.082	2.04	0.91	4.53
rWH: normal as reference			2	.054			
Overweight	.296	.431	1	.491	1.35	0.58	3.13
Obesity	1.066	.465	1	.022	2.90	1.17	7.23
Diabetes	.133	.383	1	.728	1.14	0.54	2.42
Resting HR > 90/min	1.551	.652	1	.017	4.72	1.32	16.94

4.1. Prevalence of Hypertension. HTN prevalence remains high in rural and urban setting with values above 20% as shown in Figure 1. There is more HTN in urban area than in rural area as found by many other authors [13, 19, 20]. Previous data [14] was conducted only in the urban city of Bamako. Compared to others parts of the world [5] our prevalence is relatively low. Trends over the time due to unavailability of data cannot be assessed as done for west African countries [21].

4.2. Hypertension in Rural Area. Our data suggest high prevalence of HTN as found in other rural areas in Africa [19, 22] but remains low compared to data from Ghana [23] with near twice our prevalence. This is opposed to data from rural areas in Sudan with near 16% [24].

Our high prevalence could be due to either a real increase in HTN prevalence due to changing in behaviors (less physical activity, diet modifications) or modification in the population.

Looking for predictive factors, we found that only age group and resting heart rate significantly predicted HTN, with OR for age group increases with increasing age from 1.05 to 3.4 as shown in Table 5. This also conforms to what is known about HTN and it increases with aging. Many factors are found to be associated with HTN such that in our study (Table 6) age and BMI were predictors for HTN as found by Abebe et al. [13] and Neupane et al. [25]. Fasting glucose [13] and income and educational level [23] were factors found by these authors.

4.3. Hypertension in Urban Area. The same finding of a high HTN prevalence was confirmed with our data. Our prevalence of 24.7% is practically equal to that found on data from the 2002 study which was conducted using the same WHO STEPwise approach and had involved only population of the urban city of Bamako.

In their systematic analysis Adeloye and Basquill [8] gave prevalence for countries of different regions Africa. Our prevalence was similar to that of sub-Saharan Africa as found by Adeloye and Basquill. Elsewhere, we see large differences in prevalence, but increase is constant [25, 26]. Some authors reported stable prevalence like in Switzerland [27], Turkey [28].

Opposed to finding in rural area, age, female sex, and body mass index were found to be predictive for HTN.

TABLE 6: Logistic regression predicting hypertension in urban setting.

Variables	B	S.E.	df	Sig.	OR	95% CI for OR Lower	Upper
Age group: <30 years as reference			3	.000			
30–44	.724	.259	1	.005	2.06	1.24	3.43
45–59	1.459	.261	1	.000	4.30	2.58	7.18
60 and more	1.981	.303	1	.000	7.25	4.00	13.13
Marital status: single as reference			3	.369			
Married	.224	.269	1	.404	1.25	0.74	2.12
Widower	.420	.408	1	.303	1.52	0.68	3.38
Divorced	−1.346	1.121	1	.230	0.26	0.03	2.34
Female sex	−.789	.228	1	.001	0.45	0.29	0.71
Educational level: unschooled as reference			4	.284			
Level 1	−.079	.209	1	.705	0.92	0.61	1.39
Level 2	−.030	.257	1	.907	0.97	0.59	1.61
Level 3	−.372	.223	1	.096	0.69	0.44	1.07
Level 4	−.622	.370	1	.093	0.54	0.26	1.11
Tobacco smoking	.087	.261	1	.738	1.09	0.65	1.82
Alcohol consumption	.083	.334	1	.803	1.09	0.57	2.09
BMI: Normal as reference			2	.000			
Overweight	.429	.200	1	.032	1.54	1.04	2.27
Obesity	.983	.249	1	.000	2.67	1.64	4.36
WC: normal as reference			2	.054			
Overweight	.451	.258	1	.080	1.57	0.95	2.60
Obesity	.665	.281	1	.018	1.95	1.12	3.37
rWH: normal as reference			2	.407			
Overweight	.199	.232	1	.391	1.22	0.77	1.92
Obesity	.334	.250	1	.182	1.40	0.86	2.28
Diabetes	.069	.225	1	.760	1.07	0.69	1.67
Resting HR > 90/min	.274	.476	1	.564	1.32	0.52	3.35

For age group the OR increases with age from 2.06 (30–44 years) to 7.25 (60 and more) which is similar finding in most studies [10, 13, 23] in Africa.

Female sex appeared to be protective in our study with an OR of 0.45.

Lastly BMI was the third predictive factor that we found with OR 1.54 for overweight and 2.67 of obese subjects. This increasing of HTN with increasing BMI has been described by many authors [13, 23].

4.4. Strength and Limits. Our data provide recent and community-based data on hypertension prevalence in rural and urban areas in Mali, using the WHO STEPwise survey strategy, and contribute to covering the need of such data.

We faced some difficulties which can be considered as limits. First, due to financial reason, lipid profile was not included in the 2013 STEPS-Survey. Second we also have been unable to take into account income and lastly comparison was difficult due to the lack of previous data.

5. Conclusion

Hypertension prevalence is high in rural and urban area and associated factors were age group in rural area and age group, female sex, and body mass index in urban area. Our data could be used as reference and serve to initiate more extensive studies permitting to get robust data for deciders. It is also important to find financial support to include lipid profile in the next STEPS-Survey.

Conflicts of Interest

The authors declare that there are no conflicts of interest regarding the publication of this paper.

Acknowledgments

Thanks are due to Dr. Nazoum Diarra, who led for years the Non-Communicable Disease section at the Ministry of Health, for giving us opportunity to publish these data.

References

[1] P. M. Kearney, M. Whelton, K. Reynolds, P. Muntner, P. K. Whelton, and J. He, "Global burden of hypertension: analysis of worldwide data," *The Lancet*, vol. 365, no. 9455, pp. 217–223, 2005.

[2] M. M. Ibrahim and A. Damasceno, "Hypertension in developing countries," *The Lancet*, vol. 380, no. 9841, pp. 611–619, 2012.

[3] 2013, World Health Organization, A global brief on Hypertension: silent killer global public health crises (World Health Day 2013). Geneva: WHO.

[4] R. G. Victor, Systemic hypertension-mechanisms and Diagnosis in Braunwald heart Disease p 934-952.

[5] A. M. Sarki, C. U. Nduka, S. Stranges, N.-B. Kandala, and O. A. Uthman, "Prevalence of hypertension in low- and middle-income countries: A systematic review and meta-analysis," *Medicine (United States)*, vol. 94, no. 50, article no. 1959, 2015.

[6] L. Fourcade, P. Paule, and B. Mafart, "Hypertension Artérielle en Afrique subsaharienne. Actualité et Perspectives," *Medecine Tropicale*, vol. 67, pp. 559–567, 2007.

[7] M. Thorogood, M. D. Connor, G. L. Hundt, and S. M. Tollman, "Understanding and managing hypertension in an African sub-district: A multidisciplinary approach," *Scandinavian Journal of Public Health*, vol. 35, no. 69, pp. 52–59, 2007.

[8] D. Adeloye and C. Basquill, "Estimating the prevalence and awareness rates of hypertension in Africa: a systematic analysis," *PLoS ONE*, vol. 9, no. 8, Article ID e104300, 2014.

[9] D. Guwatudde, J. Nankya-Mutyoba, R. Kalyesubula et al., "The burden of hypertension in sub-Saharan Africa: A four-country cross sectional study," *BMC Public Health*, vol. 15, no. 1, article no. 2546, 2015.

[10] A. Awoke, T. Awoke, S. Alemu, and B. Megabiaw, "Prevalence and associated factors of hypertension among adults in Gondar, Northwest Ethiopia: a community based cross-sectional study," *BMC Cardiovascular Disorders*, vol. 12, article 113, 2012.

[11] A. A. Alsheikh-Ali, M. I. Omar, F. J. Raal et al., "Cardiovascular risk factor burden in Africa and the Middle East: the Africa Middle East Cardiovascular Epidemiological (ACE) study," *PLoS ONE*, vol. 9, no. 8, article e102830, 2014.

[12] J. L. Fleg, "Age-associated changes in cardiovascular structure and function: a fertile milieu for future disease," *Heart Failure Reviews*, vol. 17, no. 4-5, pp. 545–554, 2012.

[13] S. M. Abebe, Y. Berhane, A. Worku, and A. Getachew, "Prevalence and associated factors of hypertension: a crosssectional community based study in Northwest Ethiopia," *PLoS ONE*, vol. 10, no. 4, Article ID e0125210, 2015.

[14] H. O. Bâ, Y. Camara, I. Menta et al., "Hypertension in urban population over 20 years in Bamako, Mali," *Heart and Cardiol*, vol. 2, no. 7, 2016.

[15] World Health Organisation. L'approche STEPwise de l'OMS pour la surveillance des facteurs de risque des maladies chroniques (STEPS) https://www.who.int/chp/steps. Consulté le 29.01.17.

[16] A. V. Chobanian, G. L. Bakris, H. R. Black et al., "The seventh report of the joint national committee on prevention, detection, evaluation, and treatment of high blood pressure: the JNC 7 report," *The Journal of the American Medical Association*, vol. 289, no. 19, pp. 2560–2572, 2003.

[17] WHO. Overweight and obesity http://www.who.int/entity/mediacentre/factsheets/fs311/en/ accessed 21.11.2017 10H39 AM.

[18] WHO. Waist Circumference and Waist–Hip Ratio: Report of a WHO Expert Consultation Geneva, 8–11 December 2008 http://www.who.int/entity/nutrition/publications/obesity/WHO_report_waistcircumference_and_waisthip_ratio/en/, 21.11.2017 10H41 AM.

[19] M. E. Hendriks, F. W. N. M. Wit, M. T. L. Roos et al., "Hypertension in Sub-Saharan Africa: cross-sectional surveys in four rural and urban communities," *PLoS ONE*, vol. 7, no. 3, Article ID e32638, 2012.

[20] N. Kodaman, M. C. Aldrich, R. Sobota et al., "Cardiovascular disease risk factors in Ghana during the rural-to-urban transition: A cross-sectional study," *PLoS ONE*, vol. 11, no. 10, Article ID e0162753, 2016.

[21] Iwelunmor et al. Globalization and Health 2014, 10:42 http://www.globalizationandhealth.com/content/10/1/42.

[22] L. D. Yan, B. H. Chi, N. Sindano, S. Bosomprah, J. S. Stringer, and R. Chilengi, "Prevalence of hypertension and its treatment among adults presenting to primary health clinics in rural Zambia: Analysis of an observational database," *BMC Public Health*, vol. 15, no. 1, article no. 2258, 2015.

[23] K. Z. Gebreselassie and M. Padyab, "Epidemiology of hypertension stages in two countries in sub-sahara africa: factors associated with hypertension stages," *International Journal of Hypertension*, vol. 2015, 12 pages, 2015.

[24] S. A. Balla, A. A. Abdalla, T. A. Elmukashfi, and H. A. Ahmed, "Hypertension among Rural Population in Four States: Sudan 2012," *Global Journal of Health Science*, vol. 6, no. 3, pp. 206–212, 2014.

[25] D. Neupane, C. S. McLachlan, R. Sharma et al., "Prevalence of hypertension in member countries of South Asian Association for Regional Cooperation (SAARC): systematic review and meta-analysis," *Medicine*, vol. 93, no. 13, p. e74, 2014.

[26] L. Yang, J. Yan, X. Tang, X. Xu, W. Yu, and H. Wu, "Prevalence, Awareness, Treatment, Control and Risk Factors Associated with Hypertension among Adults in Southern China, 2013," *PLoS ONE*, vol. 11, no. 1, Article ID e0146181, 2016.

[27] I. Guessous, M. Bochud, J.-M. Theler, J.-M. Gaspoz, and A. Pechère-Bertschi, "1999–2009 trends in prevalence, unawareness, treatment and control of hypertension in Geneva, Switzerland," *PLoS ONE*, vol. 7, no. 6, Article ID e39877, 2012.

[28] S. Sengul, T. Akpolat, Y. Erdem et al., "Changes in hypertension prevalence, awareness, treatment, and control rates in Turkey from 2003 to 2012," *Journal of Hypertension*, vol. 34, no. 6, pp. 1208–1217, 2016.

23

S-Amlodipine: An Isomer with Difference—Time to Shift from Racemic Amlodipine

Jamshed Dalal ⓘ,[1] J. C. Mohan,[2] S. S. Iyengar,[3] Jagdish Hiremath,[4] Immaneni Sathyamurthy,[5] Sandeep Bansal,[6] Dhiman Kahali,[7] and Arup Dasbiswas[8]

[1]Centre for Cardiac Sciences, Kokilaben Dhirubhai Ambani Hospital, Mumbai, India
[2]Fortis Hospital, Shalimar Bagh, New Delhi, India
[3]Manipal Hospital, Bangalore, India
[4]Ruby Hall Clinic, Pune, India
[5]Apollo Hospitals, Chennai, India
[6]Department of Cardiology, VMMC & Safdarjung Hospital, New Delhi, India
[7]B M Birla Heart Research Centre, Kolkata, India
[8]NRS Medical College and Hospital, Kolkata, India

Correspondence should be addressed to Jamshed Dalal; jjdalal@hotmail.com

Academic Editor: Tomohiro Katsuya

Calcium channel blockers are among the first-line drugs for treatment of hypertension (HTN). S-amlodipine (S-AM), an S-enantiomer of amlodipine, is available in India and in other countries like China, Korea, Russia, Ukraine, and Nepal. Being clinically researched for nearly two decades, we performed in-depth review of S-AM. This review discusses clinical evidence from total 42 studies (26 randomized controlled trials, 14 observational studies, and 2 meta-analyses) corroborating over 7400 patients treated with S-AM. Efficacy and safety of S-AM in HTN in comparison to racemic amlodipine, used as monotherapy and in combination with other antihypertensives, efficacy in angina, and pleiotropic benefits with S-AM, are discussed in this review.

1. Introduction

Management of hypertension (HTN) involves different therapeutic approaches. Among the medications for treating HTN, calcium channel blockers (CCBs) are one of the first-line agents as recommended by recent Joint National Committee 8 (JNC-8) guidelines [1]. Besides efficacy, occurrence of adverse effects (AEs) plays an important role in maintaining adherence with medications [2]. Occurrence of peripheral edema is the major reason for poor adherence with amlodipine. The Anglo-Scandinavian Cardiac Outcomes Trial-Blood Pressure Lowering Arm (ASCOT-BPLA) [3] reported peripheral edema in 23% patients receiving amlodipine. This suggests that nearly 1 out of 4 patients treated with amlodipine may develop peripheral edema. Conventionally used amlodipine is a mix of S- and R-enantiomers. Development of separate enantiomers improves pharmacokinetics (PK) and avoids undesirable AEs [4]. From R- and S-isomers of amlodipine, S-enantiomer has nearly 1000 times greater affinity for the receptor site. Further, S-amlodipine (S-AM) has less variable PK, lower intrasubject variation, and longer half-life [5]. S-AM is equally efficacious at half-dose with better tolerability and lesser incidence of peripheral edema than racemic amlodipine (Amlo) [6].

S-AM is marketed world-wide. The central drugs standards control organization (CDSCO), India, approved S-AM on 16 August 2002 for its use in HTN [7]. Globally, S-AM has been approved and is being used in countries like China [8], Korea [9], Ukraine [10], Philippines [11], and Nepal [12]. Besides these, S-AM is marketed in nearly 47 countries [13]. Since S-AM approval in China (1999) [14] and in India (2002) [7], it has been studied extensively. As being researched for nearly two decades, we performed an in-depth review of clinical evidence of S-amlodipine and provided key summary with identification of areas for further research.

2. Search Methodology and Literature Details

We performed search using terms "S-Amlodipine" or "levamlodipine" across electronic databases like PUBMED, Google Scholar, and clinical trials registry, http://www .clinicaltrials.gov. Additionally, a general search at Google search engine was performed. Clinical studies including randomized trials and observational and postmarketing studies before June 2017 were included in the review. Journals articles available only as print copies were also included in the review. For non-English literature articles, information available from the abstracts was captured.

After an extensive search, we included total 42 studies. In these, 26 were RCTs (20 monotherapy and 6 combination studies), 14 were observational studies (13 monotherapy studies and 1 combination study) and two were meta-analyses. From these, a maximum number of studies ($n = 18$) were from China followed by 11 from India, 6 from Korea, 3 each from Russia and Ukraine, and one from Sri Lanka. Combined from all the studies, over 7400 patients had received S-AM either alone or in combination with other antihypertensives. In these studies, racemic amlodipine was the major comparator in 26 studies and in two meta-analyses as well. As monotherapy and/or combination therapy, other comparator molecules from 10 studies were lercanidipine (Lercan), nifedipine sustained release (Nifed-SR), cilnidipine (CLD), ramipril (Rami), enalapril (Enala), losartan (Los), telmisartan (Telmi), and indapamide. In five observational studies, there was no comparator to S-AM. In two combination studies, the combination treatment was compared to S-AM monotherapy.

3. S-Amlodipine in Hypertension

For its use in HTN, S-AM has been evaluated in various RCTs (total 22) and observational studies (total 9) either as monotherapy (total 25) or in combination (total 6 RCTs only). Two meta-analyses were performed in 2010 and 2015 with 15 and 8 studies of S-AM (levamlodipine), respectively. Major findings from the RCTs, observational studies, and meta-analyses are summarized in Tables 1, 2, and 3, respectively. Most of these studies were comparing S-AM (2.5 to 5 mg) to racemic amlodipine (5 to 10 mg) and found near equal antihypertensive efficacy with lower incidence of side effects. Two RCTs especially evaluated ankle (peripheral) edema with S-AM in comparison to Amlo and reported significantly lower incidence of edema with better tolerability of S-AM [15, 16]. Besides racemic amlodipine, S-AM was compared to lercanidipine [17, 18] and ramipril [19] in three trials. S-AM had nearly similar efficacy and tolerability to lercanidipine. However, its efficacy and safety were better than that of ramipril (Table 1). A study from Chen et al. [20] needs a special mention as they compared higher-dose (5 mg) to the lower-dose (2.5 mg) of S-AM (Table 1). After 8-week treatment, 24-hour ambulatory systolic BP (SBP) reduction was significantly greater in 5 mg group than in 2.5 mg of S-AM (between group difference: 2.1 mmHg, $p = 0.02$). However, 24-hour diastolic BP (DBP) reduction was similar (between group difference: 0.9 mmHg, $p = 0.17$). Interestingly, the incidence of overall AEs was similar (20.0% versus 17.0%, resp., $p = 0.05$) in both

groups and proportion of individual AEs was nearly equal in both doses. This perpetuates that S-AM can be safely used of high-dose of 5 mg per day with incremental efficacy.

All nine observational studies were monotherapy trials (Table 2). In these, racemic amlodipine was comparator in four studies, lercanidipine in one, and cilnidipine in one trial. Four studies were single arm trials with no comparator. Four studies without any comparator, the safety and efficacy of S-amlodipine (SESA) studies, were the postmarketing trials that reported significant BP reduction with significantly less or no occurrence of pedal edema in Indian hypertensive patients (Table 2) [21–24]. Occurrence of edema with S-AM in comparison to Amlo and cilnidipine was evaluated in another observational study from India. Incidence of peripheral edema with S-AM and cilnidipine was significantly lower than racemic amlodipine in males (6.7% and 0.0% versus 36.7%, resp.) and in females (10.0% and 3.3% versus 43.3%, resp.) ($p < 0.001$ for both drug comparisons in either gender) (Table 2) [25].

S-AM was also assessed in combination with other antihypertensives like atenolol [26, 27] and telmisartan [28, 29] and in patients receiving both angiotensin converting enzyme inhibitor or angiotensin receptor blocker (ACEI/ARB) and beta blocker (BB) [16]. In studies of combination with atenolol and ACEI/ARB + BB, S-AM had similar antihypertensive efficacy compared to racemic amlodipine (Table 1). However, in two separate studies, combination of S-AM and telmisartan (40–80 mg) was associated with greater BP reduction compared to monotherapy of telmisartan 80 mg or S-AM 2.5 mg (Table 1). Tolerability of telmisartan-based combinations was reported to be similar or better than the comparative monotherapy treatments (Table 1).

In a meta-analysis (Table 3) of 15 trials, Liu et al. [30] reported similar effect of S-AM (2.5 mg) on BP compared to racemic amlodipine (5 mg). From three high-quality RCTs included in the meta-analysis, weighted mean difference (WMD) of SBP and DBP was −2.84 (95% confidence interval (CI), −6.42 to 0.74) and −1.71 (95% CI, −3.48 to 0.06), respectively, after 4-week treatment (one RCT) whereas it was −1.13 (95% CI, −5.29 to 3.03) and −1.34 (95% CI, −2.67 to −0.01), respectively, after 8-week treatment (two RCTs). Further, S-Amlo was associated with significantly less edema than racemic amlodipine (risk difference, −0.02; 95% CI, −0.03 to 0.00). Another meta-analysis performed recently by Zhao and Chen [31] involving 1456 patients from eight studies reported that levamlodipine (S-AM) was efficacious (odds ratio (OR) 2.19, 95% CI 1.61–2.97; $p < 0.01$) and safer (OR 0.51, 95% CI 0.34–0.77; $p < 0.01$) than racemic amlodipine. Thus, available evidence from RCTs, observational studies, and meta-analyses finds equivalent BP lowering efficacy of S-AM against racemic amlodipine with better tolerability. Incidence of pedal edema is found to be significantly lesser with S-AM than racemic amlodipine.

4. S-Amlodipine in Angina

The antianginal effects of racemic amlodipine are known. Systemic vasodilation with reduction afterload reducing cardiac workload and dilatation of coronary vasculature and

TABLE 1: Randomized controlled trials of S-amlodipine in hypertension.

Author (year)	Country	S-AM (mg)	Comparator (mg)	n	Duration (weeks)	Antihypertensive efficacy	AEs
Monotherapy Studies (n = 16)							
Liu et al. (2001) [44]	China	2.5	Amlo (5)	30/30	4	Equivalent	NA
Fang (2002) [45]	China	2.5	Amlo (5)	140/140	40	Equivalent	NR
Cheng et al. (2002) [46]	China	2.5–5	Amlo (5–10)	60/60	5	Equivalent	No difference, milder with S-AM
Hiremath and Dighe (2002) [47]	India	2.5	Amlo (5)	25/25	6	Mean change of SBP/DBP (S-AM Vs Amlo) Standing: −24.21/−13.08 vs −21.6/−13.44 Supine: −27.13/−14.17 vs −22.04/−13.68 Sitting: −26.86/−14.17 vs −23.06/−14.28	None
Kerkar (2003) [48]	India	2.5	Amlo (5)	25/25	6	Mean change of SBP/DBP (S-AM Vs Amlo) Standing: −22.6/−12.72 vs −21.96/−13.24 Supine: −22.84/−13.18 vs −22.32/−13.4 Sitting: −20.16/−13.76 vs −22.24/−15.0	None
Pathak et al. (2004) [49]	India	2.5	Amlo (5)	97/91	6	Mean change of SBP/DBP (S-AM Vs Amlo) Standing: −19.22/−13.63 vs −19.14/−12.76 Supine: −19.69/−13.95 vs −19.24/−13.33 Sitting: −19.87/−14.31 vs −19.24/−13.05	None
Zhang (2006) [50]	China	2.5–5	Amlo (5–10)	36/36	8	S-AM: 165.30/98.22 to 132.70/81.87 Amlo: 164.30/99.30 to 134.10/85.61	Number: 1 vs 6
Bae et al. (2008) [51]	Korea	2.5	Amlo (5)	58/60	8	SBP: −24.27 ± 11.55 vs −25.24 ± 12.47 DBP: −14.73 ± 8.9 vs −14.56 ± 9.28 S-AM non-inferior to Amlo	No significant differences
Zhu et al. (2008) [52]	China	2.5–5	Amlo (5–10)	44	8	Mean change in SBP: 156.26 to 131.50 vs 158.23 to 131.74 DBP: 98.48 to 83.28 vs 99.18 to 83.19	None

TABLE 1: Continued.

Author (year)	Country	S-AM (mg)	Comparator (mg)	n	Duration (weeks)	Antihypertensive efficacy	AEs
Youn et al. (2010) [17]	Korea	2.5	Lercani	32/29	8	Mean change sSBP: -20.5 ± 13.6 vs -19.93 ± 14.5 sDBP: -14.03 ± 8.07 vs -12.93 ± 8.68	None
Kim et al. (2011) [19]#	Korea	2.5	Rami (2.5–5)	68/70	8	Mean change SBP: -18.1 ± 7.91 vs -14.3 ± 11.96 ($p = 0.047$) DBP: -12.7 ± 7.02 vs -9.6 ± 7.38 ($p = 0.023$) BP normalization rate: 81.3% vs 61.4% ($p = 0.017$)	5.8% vs 14.2% ($p = 0.012$)
Shengye (2012) [53]	China	2.5–5	Amlo (5–10)	90/90	8	Equivalent	Milder with S-AM
Oh et al. (2012) [15]	Korea	2.5–5	Amlo (5–10)	17/17*	12	Mean change sSBP: -21.82 ± 8.76 vs -26.82 ± 11.89 ($p = 0.172$) sDBP: -14.71 ± 6.94 vs -10.88 ± 5.81 ($p = 0.091$)	Significant improvement in ankle edema with S-AM (AFV difference: -70.26 mL, $p = 0.028$)
Zhao (2013) [54]	China	NA	Nifed-SR	61/61	NA	Significant reduction in BP in both groups Overall response rate: 91.8% vs 80.33% ($p < 0.05$)	Lower with S-AM: 6.56% vs 18.03% ($p < 0.05$)
Parvathi et al. (2014) [55]	India	2.5	Amlo (5)	54/54	12	SBP change: -32.4 vs -26.9 DBP change: -13.4 vs -12.0	Edema significantly lower with S-AM: mean change AC: 0.26 vs 0.02 ($p < 0.009$)
Chen et al. (2017) [20]	China	2.5	S-AM (5)	263/260	8	SBP: 6.0 vs 8.1 ($p = 0.02$) DBP: 3.8 vs 4.7 ($p = 0.17$) Target BP achievement: SBP: 81.8% vs 90.8% DBP: 84.0% vs 94.2% SBP&DBP: 75.7% vs 87.3% ($p \leq 0.003$)	17.0% vs 20.0 ($p = 0.05$)

TABLE 1: Continued.

Author (year)	Country	S-AM (mg)	Comparator (mg)	n	Duration (weeks)	Antihypertensive efficacy	AEs
Combination Studies (n = 6)							
Rajanandh et al. (2013) [26] [+Atenolol 50 mg]	India	2.5	Amlo (5)	32/32	24	Mean change SBP: 40 vs 40 DBP: 28 vs 34 Non-significant difference	No difference: 21.9% vs 31.3%
Maksimova et al. (2013) [27] [+Atenolol]	Russia	2.5	Amlo (5)	Total: 31		LSM reduction SBP: −15.9 vs −12.7 DBP: −7.3 vs −5.3 HR: −3 vs −4	Number: 8 vs 16
Hu and Xiao (2013) [56] [S-AM + Irbesartan vs Indapamide + Irbesartan]	China	NA	Indapamide	83	12–24	At 12 and 24 weeks Lower 24-h DBPV, day-time SBPV with S-AM than Indapamide At 24 weeks Significantly lower morning SBP, 24-h DBPV and SBPV	NA
Ihm et al. (2016) [28] [Telmisartan + S-AM FDC (CKD-828): 2.5/40 and 2.5/80]	Korea	2.5	S-AM 2.5	63/63/61	8	Mean NP change in groups: 2.5/40 & 5/40 vs S-AM 2.5 SBP: −12.89, −13.79 vs −4.55 ($p < 0.0001$) DBP: −9.67, −10.72 vs −4.93 Differences in mean change: SBP: −4.34 ($p = 0.0028$) and −5.61 ($p < 0.0001$) DBP: −4.73 ($p = 0.0002$) and −5.79 ($p < 0.0001$) Achieving BP <140 or <90 mmHg: 60.32% ($p = 0.0004$), 60.66% ($p = 0.0003$) vs 28.33%	9.52% ($p = 0.0086$), 14.29% ($p = 0.0632$) vs 27.87%
Park et al. (2016) [29] [Telmisartan + S-AM FDC: 2.5/40 and 2.5/80 mg]	Korea	2.5 & 5	T (80)	61/60/62	8	2.5/40 & 5/40 Vs T80 SBP: −10.56, −12.32 vs −2.44 DBP: −8.12, −9.58 vs −1.76 ($p < 0.0001$ for both) Achieving target BP <140 or <90: 35.59%, 40.68% vs 11.86%	No differences: 18.6%, 20.0% vs 22.6%
Galappatthy et al. (2016) [16] [ACEI/ARB + BB]	Sri Lanka	2.5–5	Amlo (5–10)	76/70	16	Responders Rate: Similar- 98.57% vs 98.68%	New pitting edema: 31.40 vs 46.51% ($p = 0.0301$); ARR: 15.1% Increase in pitting edema score ($p = 0.038$) & patient rated edema score ($p = 0.036$) with Amlo

AC: ankle circumference, ACEI/ARB: angiotensin converting enzyme inhibitor/angiotensin receptor blocker, AEs: adverse effects, AFV: ankle-foot volume, Amlo: racemic amlodipine, ARR: absolute risk reduction, AT: atenolol, BB: beta blocker, BP: blood pressure, DBP: diastolic BP, DBPV: DBP variability, FDC: fixed-dose combination, HR: heart rate, LSM: least square mean, Nifed-SR: nifedipine sustained release, NA: not available, NR: not reported, RRR: relative risk reduction, RR: risk reduction, S-AM: S-amlodipine, SBP: systolic BP, SBPV: SBP variability, and T: telmisartan; * only females; # chlorthalidone 12.5 mg was added to treatments if BP remained uncontrolled with study medications.

TABLE 2: Observational studies of S-amlodipine in hypertension.

Author (year)	Country	S-AM (mg)	Comparator (mg)	n	Duration (weeks)	Antihypertensive efficacy	AEs
SESA (2003) [21]	India	2.5–5	-	1859 2.5: 1514 5: 345	4	2.5 mg: 161/100 to 129/84 5 mg: 179/107 to 137/86 $p < 0.0001$ for both	Rate: 1.61% Edema: 0.75%
SESA-II (2005) [22]	India	2.5–5	-	2230	4	SBP: −26.65 DBP: −13.30 HR: −3.51	Reduction in pedal edema: 93% cases, RRR: 95.4%
SESA-IV (2007) [23]	India	2.5–5	-	1076	4	SBP: −24.27 ($p < 0.0001$) DBP: −13.28 ($p < 0.0001$) HR: −4.87 ($p < 0.0001$)	Edema: 1.77%
SESA-IVA (2007) [24]	India	2.5–5	-	30	4	2.5 mg: 150.48/92.28 to 128.57/80.86 5 mg: 165.78/95.55 to 132/82.22 $p < 0.0001$ for both	None
Bobroff et al. (2007) [57]	Ukraine	2.5–10	Amlo (5–10)	60/38	12	SBP: −30.7 versus −29.2 DBP: −13.7 versus −14.0 Target of <140/90: 83.3% versus 84.2% In both groups, significant reduction in Average daily BP Daytime BP Nighttime BP	Peripheral edema; 1.6% versus 7.8%
Basu (2007) [58]	India	5	Amlo (10)	10/10	4	SBP: 154.4 to 130.4 versus 157.6 to 132.4 DBP: 99.1 to 77.5 versus 87.2 to 78.4 Equal efficacy in Daytime MAP Nighttime MAP	None
Sierkova et al. (2009) [59]	Ukraine	NA	Amlo	31/32	NA	Equal BP reduction with 2 times lower dose of S-AM	Lesser with S-AM
Koval et al. (2013) [18]	Russia	NA	Lercani	NA	NA	Similar efficacy in reducing BP in HTN with obesity	Lower with lercani
Mohanty et al. (2016) [25]	India	2.5–5	Amlo (5–10) and CLD (10–20)	60/60/60	12	NR	Incidence of Edema M: 6.7% vs 36.7% and 0.0% F: 10.0% vs 43.3% and 3.3%

AEs: adverse effects, Amlo: racemic amlodipine, BP: blood pressure, CLD: cilnidipine, DBP: diastolic BP, F: females, HR: heart rate, HTN: hypertension, Lercani: lercanidipine, M: males, MAP: mean arterial pressure, NA: not available, RRR: relative risk reduction, S-AM: S-amlodipine, SESA: safety and efficacy of S-Amlodipine, and SBP: systolic BP.

TABLE 3: Meta-analyses of S-amlodipine in hypertension.

Author (year)	Country	S-AM (mg)	Comparator (mg)	n	Duration (weeks)	Antihypertensive efficacy	AEs
Liu et al. (2010) [30]	China	2.5	Amlo (5)	15 trials	4–40	All trials: Similar efficacy Only high-quality trials: WMD for decrease in SBP/DBP at 4 weeks: −2.84/−1.71 8 weeks: −1.38/−1.33	Similar; RD: all trials: −0.04; High quality: −0.04
Zhao and Chen (2015) [31]	China	NA	Amlo	8 trials: 732/724	NA	Significantly better efficacy of S-AM than Amlo: OR 2.19 ($p < 0.01$)	Significantly lower rate of AEs: OR 0.51 ($p < 0.01$)

AEs: adverse effects, Amlo: racemic amlodipine, BP: blood pressure, DBP: diastolic BP, NA: not available, OR: odds ratio, RD: risk difference, S-AM: S-amlodipine, and SBP: systolic BP.

reduction in cardiac oxygen consumption underlie the relief in anginal cases. Being an isomer of amlodipine, S-AM has also shown efficacy in angina. In SESA-Angina study (2005) [32] conducted in India, patients of ischemic heart disease (IHD) with history of angina and positive stress test (n = 25) were included. No other concomitant treatments were allowed during the treatment period of 8 weeks. S-AM (2.5–5 mg/d) treatment was associated with significant reduction in average number angina attacks in every 15 days (p < 0.0001) and significant improvement in anginal symptoms (94.1%). After treatment, there was significant increase in exercise capacity (p < 0.0001) and nonsignificant increase in time required for 1.5 mm ST-segment depression (p = 0.1764) and maximum workload achieved (p = 0.1170). No AEs were reported in any patient. This emphasizes efficacy and safety of S-AM in management of angina.

5. S-Amlodipine and Pleiotropic Benefits

5.1. Effect on Arterial Stiffness and Endothelial Function. Efficacy of S-AM for change in arterial stiffness and endothelial function was assessed in four RCTs [33–36] and in one observational study [37]. In a 12-week randomized study, Liangjin et al. (2013) [33] compared levamlodipine (S-AM, 2.5–5 mg, n = 40) to nifedipine sustained release (Nifed-SR, 10 mg, n = 40) for its effect on BP variety ratio (BPVR) and CIMT. Compared to baseline, systolic and diastolic BPVR was significantly better with S-AM than Nifed-SR at 12 weeks. CIMT was reduced significantly with S-AM (p < 0.05) but not with Nifed-SR (Table 4). There was significant correlation of BPVR with CIMT in S-AM group. Changes in lipid parameters and C-reactive protein were nonsignificant in both groups.

One RCT [34] reported significant improvements in flow mediated dilatation [FMD] after 6-week treatment with S-AM and racemic amlodipine. Continued treatment for 12 weeks was found to lower serum cholesterol equally in both groups. Guo et al. [35] reported significant improvements in the central BP components, brachial-ankle pulse-wave velocity (PWV), ambulatory arterial stiffness index (AASI), and the variability of ambulatory BP in both S-AM and racemic amlodipine treatment. However, both treatments were not associated with significant changes in CIMT. Thus, the benefits with S-AM on vascular function are similar to those exerted by racemic amlodipine. In another 6-week, randomized, crossover trial, Si et al. [36] reported that FMD%, nitric oxide (NO) and endothelial nitric oxide synthase (eNOS) levels were significantly improved in both groups with no between treatment differences. Increase in NO levels in cultured human umbilical vein endothelial cells was significant with both treatments but more marked in Amlo. Authors concluded that, with S-AM, probably antihypertensive effect is the cause of improved vascular function and S-AM may exert its protective effect on endothelial function by unknown mechanism. However, a 6-month study which assessed effects of S-AM (5–10 mg/d) and enalapril (10–20 mg/d) combination compared to enalapril alone on endothelial dysfunction in patients with chronic pulmonary heart disease (CPHD) and HTN (n = 65) observed that S-AM

added to enalapril is associated with further improvements in endothelial function than enalapril alone in HTN. This was probably because of more pronounced reduction in endothelin-1 (ET-1) level after treatment with two drugs (3.86 ± 0.24 to 1.95 ± 0.19 pg/mL, p < 0.05) compared to enalapril alone (3.32 ± 0.27 to 1.83 ± 0.21 pg/mL, p < 0.05). Therefore, though there remains uncertainty about possible mechanisms, S-AM may exert some protection effect on endothelium by improving eNOS levels and reducing ET-1 levels [37].

5.2. Effect on Structure and Function of Left Ventricle and Brachial Artery. Iskenderov and Saushkina (2013) [38] assessed S-AM (n = 61) and Amlo (n = 66) in stages 1-2 HTN patients using left ventricular (LV) and brachial artery structural and functional parameters. After 24-week treatment, S-AM was associated with comparable BP reduction to Amlo, but the mean dose was significantly lower (7.5 ± 0.8 versus 11.6 ± 1.4 mg/day; p < 0.01). Significant improvement in LV structure and function and brachial artery function were reported. Reductions in atherogenic lipoproteins and total cholesterol were also significant with S-AM.

5.3. Efficacy in Renal Transplant Patients. Tang et al. (2003) [39] observed that, in kidney transplant patients with HTN (n = 20), S-AM (2.5 to 5 mg) treatment for 2 months was associated with significant reduction in SBP (p < 0.01), DBP (p < 0.01), and blood nitrogen (p < 0.05) with no increase of serum creatinine (p > 0.05). Normalization of BP was reported in 85% of patients.

5.4. Efficacy in Insulin Resistance. In a randomized, double-blind, prospective cohort study in type 2 diabetes (T2D) patients, Xiao et al. [40] compared effects of S-AM (2.5–5 mg/d, n = 112) and losartan (50–100 mg/d, n = 115) after treatment for 36 months (156 weeks). They had followed patients at first, second, and third year of the study. Difference in the reduction in SBP and DBP at the end of 12 months was statistically significant between two groups. However, there were no significant differences between the groups when assessed at the end of 24 or 36 months. Change in fasting insulin levels (mIU/L) and insulin sensitivity index (ISI) was significant with both S-AM and losartan by the end of 3 years (p < 0.05). This establishes equivalent efficacy of S-AM to an ARB, losartan in improvement of insulin sensitivity in patients with HTN and impaired fasting glucose.

5.5. Effect on Platelet Aggregation. In patients of HTN and T2D, Li et al. (2013) [41] studied effect of levamlodipine on platelet aggregation and expression of matrix metalloproteinase (MMP) 9 and MMP 2. In 32 patients treated, platelet aggregation maximal assessed by coagulation instrument TYXN-91A reduced significantly (p < 0.05) from 47.77 ± 11.92 (pretreatment) to 40.78±13.97 (posttreatment). Platelet inhibition rate was 13.50 ± 25.23%. There was no effect on levels of MMP 9 and MMP 2. This study highlights that S-AM has potential to prevent platelet aggregation in high-risk patients like HTN with T2D.

TABLE 4: Pleiotropic effects of S-amlodipine.

Author (year)	Country	S-AM (mg)	Comparator (mg)	n	Duration (weeks)	Antihypertensive efficacy	Pleiotropic effect
Effect on Arterial stiffness and Endothelial function							
RCTs							
Liangjin et al. (2013) [33]	China	2.5–5	Nifed-SR (10)	40/40	12	SBPVR (mmHg) S-AM: 14.7 ± 3.1 to 12.1 ± 2.7 ($p < 0.05$) Nifed-SR: 14.8 ± 2.9 to 13.7 ± 3.2 ($p > 0.05$) DBPVR (mmHg) S-AM: 10.2 ± 1.8 to 8.5 ± 1.9 ($p < 0.05$) Nifed-SR: 10.2 ± 1.9 to 9.8 ± 2.5 ($p > 0.05$)	CIMT (per mm) S-AM: 1.24 ± 0.41 to 1.08 ± 0.28 ($p < 0.05$) Nifed-SR: 1.23 ± 0.31 to 1.22 ± 0.33
Zhang et al. (2003) [34]	China	2.5	Amlo (5)	60	6	NA	FMD% S-AM: 4 ± 4 to 3 ± 4 ($p = 0.01$) Amlo: 6.7% to 6.8% ($p = 0.01$)
Guo et al. (2012) [35]	China	NA	Amlo	126/106	24	S-AM: 153.88/94.03 to 132.59/81.96 ($p < 0.001$ for both) Amlo: 152.21/93.3 to 133.22/82.47 ($p < 0.001$ for both)	Significant improvements in central BP components baPWV ambulatory arterial stiffness index variability of ambulatory BP (all $P < 0.0001$) CIMT: No significant changes
Si et al. (2014) [36] [crossover trial, 2-week washout]	China	2.5	Amlo (5)	24	6 × 6	SBP: 162 to 132 (Amlo) and 131 (S-AM) ($p < 0.01$ for both) DBP: 95 to 81 (Amlo) and 82 (S-AM) ($p < 0.01$ for both) HR: 76 to 72 (Amlo) and 73 (S-AM) ($p < 0.05$ for both)	FMD%: 5.7 to 8.0 (Amlo) and 7.3 (S-AM) ($p < 0.01$ for both) NMD%: 13.6 to 12.9 (Amlo) and 14.1 (S-AM) NO μmol/L: 42 to 62 (Amlo) and 59 (S-AM) ($p < 0.01$ for both) eNOS μL: 20 to 26 (Amlo) and 24 (S-AM) ($p < 0.01$ for both)

TABLE 4: Continued.

Author (year)	Country	S-AM (mg)	Comparator (mg)	n	Duration (weeks)	Antihypertensive efficacy	Pleiotropic effect
Observational study							
Nestorovich (2013) [37] [S-AM + Enalapril versus enalapril]	Ukraine	5–10	E (10–20)	33/32	24	NR	Combination therapy had greater changes in Maximal speed (Vmax) of bloodstream in BA (i) initial (22.8 and 17.6 cm/sec) (ii) after reactive hyperaemia (41.7 and 31.6 cm/sec), Speed of retrograde wave: (i) initial (19.6 and 14.3 cm/sec) (ii) after reactive hyperaemia (25.9 and 20.2 cm/sec) (iii) post-occlusive dilatation (5.2% and 3.4%) Changes in endothelin-1 levels (i) Combination: 3.86 ± 0.24 to 1.95 ± 0.19 pg/mL, $p < 0.05$ (ii) Enalapril alone: 3.32 ± 0.27 to 1.83 ± 0.21 pg/mL, $p < 0.05$
Effect on LV and BA function							
Iskenderov and Saushkina (2013) [38]	Russia	-	Amlo	61/66	24	Comparable BP reduction at lower dose of S-AM	S-AM was associated with - Complete regression of LVH: 51% cases Normalization of LV diastolic function: 62.4% cases Significant improvement in BA vasomotor function Significant reduction in atherogenic lipoproteins and TC
Efficacy in renal transplant cases							
Tang et al. (2003) [39]	China	2.5–5	Amlo	20	8	Significant reduction in SBP ($p < 0.01$) DBP ($p < 0.01$) BUN ($p < 0.05$)	Normalization of BP in 85% cases Improved renal function
Effect on insulin resistance [RCT]							
Xiao et al. (2016) [40]	China	2.5–5	Losartan (50–100)	112/115	156	BP reduction was significant and similar in both groups	In both groups, significant reduction in fasting insulin Increase in insulin sensitivity index
Effect on platelet aggregation and expression of MMP 2 and MMP 9							
Li et al. (2013) [41]	China	NA	-	32	NA	NA	Reduced platelet aggregation maximal (%): 47.77 ± 11.92 to 40.78 ± 13.97 ($p < 0.05$) Platelet inhibition rate (%): 13.5 ± 25.23 No effect on MMP levels

AEs: adverse effects, Amlo: racemic amlodipine, BA: brachial artery, baPWV: brachial artery pressure wave velocity, BP: blood pressure, BUN: blood urea nitrogen, CIMT: carotid intima media thickness, DBP: Diastolic BP, DBPVR: DBP variety ratio, eNOS: endothelial nitric oxide synthase, FMD: flow-mediated dilation, HR: heart rate, LV: left ventricle, LVH: left ventricular hypertrophy, MMP: matrix metalloproteinase, NA: not available, Nifed-SR: nifedipine sustained release, NMD: nitroglycerine-mediated dilatation, NO: nitric oxide, NR: not reported, OR: odds ratio, RD: risk difference, S-AM: S-amlodipine, SBP: systolic BP, SBPVR: SBP variety ratio, and TC: total cholesterol.

6. S-Amlodipine and Pedal Edema

CCBs are associated with a considerable risk of peripheral oedema that may reduce patient compliance or necessitate switching to a different drug. It has been now well-established that S-AM is associated with lower incidence of pedal edema and improved compliance to therapy as evident from studies discussed above. Of note is a recent RCT from Galappatthy et al. (2016) [16] where the incidence of leg edema was the primary outcome assessed. Patients uncontrolled with BB and ACEI/ARB ($n = 172$) were randomized to S-AM 2.5–5 mg ($n = 86$) and racemic amlodipine 5–10 mg ($n = 86$). With S-AM, absolute risk reduction of new edema was 15.1%, relative risk reduction was 32.47%, and number needed to treat was seven (NNT = 7). In SESA trial, edema was resolved in 98.72% patients after switching from racemate amlodipine to S-AM [21]. In SESA-II study done in 2230 patients with HTN, incidence of pedal edema was reported in 41.90% patients who were taking racemic amlodipine before switching over to S-AM [22]. When patients were switched over to S-AM, resolution of pedal edema was noted in 93.07%. Overall incidence of pedal edema was 1.92% with S-AM and the relative risk reduction of pedal edema after S-AM switch was 95.4%. Thus, the evidence convincingly suggests minimal incidence of edema with S-AM compared to racemate amlodipine. The confirmatory evidence is observed in a meta-analysis of 15 RCT of S-AM where Liu et al. [30] reported that S-AM ($n = 907$) was associated with significantly less edema than racemic amlodipine ($n = 897$) (risk difference [RD], −0.02; 95% CI, −0.03 to 0.00; test for overall effect: $Z = 2.20$; $p = 0.03$).

Higher incidence of pedal edema is likely to result in higher degree of discomfort. Therefore, use of chirally pure S-AM would be advantageous due to lower incidence of edema which could result in improved adherence to therapy and hence optimum BP control. Amlodipine causes mainly precapillary vasodilatation without proportional increase of postcapillary blood flow, which leads to peripheral edema. Although R-amlodipine does not have calcium channel blocking properties, it reduces activity of postural vasopressor reflex, which increases the pressure in capillary vessels that activates egress of fluid into surrounding tissues. Studies have shown that nitric oxide (NO) released by the inducible nitric oxide synthase is responsible for development of edema. R (+) amlodipine is involved in local NO formation through the kinin pathway and this may lead to loss of the precapillary reflex vasoconstriction and development of edema when racemate mixture is used. S-AM at any concentration was not found to release NO and does not affect postural vasopressor reflex [42].

7. S-Amlodipine and Cost-Effectiveness

From China, Hu et al. (2014) [43] conducted a retrospective cost-effectiveness analysis from two multicentre RCTs of S-AM (2.5 mg/d, $n = 110$) and Amlo (5 mg/d, $n = 104$). With 4–8 weeks of treatment, efficacy rate of both drugs was similar (84.91% and 77.45%, resp.). Cost figures observed for 1 mmHg reduction with S-AM and Amlo were 8.1 Yuan (~1.2 $) and 10 Yuan (~1.5 $) for SBP and 16.9 Yuan (~2.5 $) and 21.7 Yuan (~3.2 $) for DBP, respectively. Reported AEs were 4.6% and 10.3% in two groups, respectively. Thus, study suggests S-Amlo is more cost-effective than racemic amlodipine.

8. Summary

Compared to racemic amlodipine, S-AM had equivalent antihypertensive efficacy *at half-dose*. Evidence suggests efficacy of S-AM in 24-hour ambulatory BP reduction, including day-time and nigh-time BP reduction. It was also found to be effective in nocturnal HTN showing its effectiveness in nondippers. Meta-analyses showed equivalent efficacy of S-AM compared to racemic amlodipine with similar or lower rates of AEs. Significantly lower incidence of peripheral edema suggests a better tolerability of S-AM and absolute risk reduction of 15.1% in peripheral edema is seen. Otherwise, overall incidence of AEs was nearly similar with two treatments. Compared to cilnidipine, incidence of edema was found to be nearly similar with S-AM, whereas it was significantly lesser in both drugs when compared to racemic amlodipine. Higher-dose S-AM (5 mg) was more effective and equally safe as that of lower-dose (2.5 mg). In *combination* with telmisartan, atenolol, and enalapril, S-AM showed greater antihypertensive effect with better safety and tolerability. Besides HTN, S-AM was found effective and safe in angina. It lowers numbers of attacks and improves symptoms. S-AM had shown BP lowering efficacy in renal transplant cases with no significant adverse effect on functional renal parameters.

Besides being potent antihypertensive, S-AM showed various pleiotropic benefits. These include improvement in endothelial function, slowing of CIMT progression or reversal of increased CIMT, improvement in arterial stiffness, regression of LVH and improvement in LV diastolic function, improvement in lipid profile, improvement in insulin sensitivity, and reduction in platelet aggregation.

Analysis from China identified S-AM as the cost-effective therapy with economic savings compared to racemic amlodipine.

9. Limitations

Although we did extensive search of literature, there is likely chance of missing on non-English literature not covered under the databases searched. Most of the non-English articles were available as abstracts only.

10. Conclusion

An equivalent antihypertensive efficacy to racemic amlodipine with lesser or negligible peripheral edema proves S-amlodipine as a cost-effective treatment option in HTN. It is effective, safe, and well-tolerated in combination with other antihypertensives as well. Besides HTN, its efficacy in angina makes it suitable agent in patient with both comorbidities. Pleiotropic benefits like improvement in endothelial function and insulin sensitivity show its promise in patients with comorbidities like diabetes. Given its positive effects on BP, endothelial function, platelet aggregation, insulin sensitivity, and atherogenic lipids, S-AM is likely to lower the adverse cardiovascular outcomes. The evidence from this review clearly suggests that S-amlodipine may be considered as one of the first-choice antihypertensive in patients with HTN including those with heightened cardiovascular risk. Future research should focus on cardiovascular outcomes with S-AM in patients with HTN and other comorbidities.

Acknowledgments

The authors are thankful to medical team of Emcure Pharmaceuticals Ltd., Pune, India, for their assistance in procuring the literature evidence and assistance in conceptualization of this article. They also thank Dr. Vijay M. Katekhaye, Quest MedPharma Consultants, Nagpur, India, for his assistance in drafting and editing this manuscript.

References

[1] P. A. James, S. Oparil, B. L. Carter et al., "2014 Evidence-based guideline for the management of high blood pressure in adults: report from the panel members appointed to the Eighth Joint National Committee (JNC 8)," *Journal of the American Medical Association*, vol. 311, no. 5, pp. 507–520, 2014.

[2] K. Rahimi, C. A. Emdin, and S. MacMahon, "The Epidemiology of Blood Pressure and Its Worldwide Management," *Circulation Research*, vol. 116, no. 6, pp. 925–935, 2015.

[3] B. Dahlöf, P. S. Sever, N. R. Poulter et al., "Prevention of cardiovascular events with an antihypertensive regimen of amlodipine adding perindopril as required versus atenolol adding bendroflumethiazide as required, in the Anglo-Scandinavian Cardiac Outcomes Trial-Blood Pressure Lowering Arm (ASCOT-BPLA): a multicentre randomised controlled trial," *The Lancet*, vol. 366, no. 9489, pp. 895–906, 2005.

[4] Y. K. Agrawal, H. G. Bhatt, H. G. Raval, P. M. Oza, and P. J. Gogoi, "Chirality - A new era of therapeutics," *Mini-Reviews in Medicinal Chemistry*, vol. 7, no. 5, pp. 451–460, 2007.

[5] L. Pathak, "Chiral switches in the management of hypertenison," *BMJ (South Asia edition)*, vol. 21, pp. 668-669, 2005.

[6] H. P. Thacker, "S-Amlodipine - The 2007 Clinical Review," *J Indian Med Assoc*, vol. 105, pp. 180–190, 2007.

[7] http://www.cdsco.nic.in/writereaddata/list_of_drugs_approved_during_200.

[8] "Levamlodipine besylate," http://app1.sfda.gov.cn/datasearcheng/face3/base.jsp?tableId=85&tableName=TABLE85&title=Database%20of%20approved%20Active%20Pharmaceutical%20Ingredients%20(APIs)%20and%20API%20manufacturers%20in%20China&bcId=136489131226659132460942000667.

[9] "Korea Innovative Pharmaceutical Company Directory," Korea Health Industry Development Institute, Ministry of Health & Welfare. Ahngook Pharm, http://www.khidiuae.org/images/Korea%20Pharmaceutical%20Company.pdf.

[10] "SAMLOPIN., Instructions for medical use. Approved. The Order of Ministry of Health of Ukraine," http://www.gladpharm.com/images/mod_catalog_prod_files/24311/Samlopin_tabl_insert_eng_03.06.2016.pdf.

[11] "Amlobes – S(-)amlodipine besylate 5 mg tablet," *VerHeiLen GmbH - Farma Iberica, http://farmaiberica.com/products/amlobes/.*

[12] R. Paudel, P. Kishore, P. Mishra, S. Palaian, and B. C. Dwari, "Urticarial Skin Reaction Induced by Oral Clonidine," *Journal of Pharmacy Practice and Research*, vol. 36, no. 3, pp. 218-219, 2006.

[13] "Chiral Drugs – S-Amlodipine, Calcium channel Blocker," Asomex, http://www.chiralemcure.com/pop/S-amlodipine_globalpresence.html.

[14] "Levamlodipine Beslate Accounts for Half of Chinese Antihypertension Drug Market," 2017, http://www.en-cphi.cn/news/show-20651.htm.

[15] G.-C. Oh, H.-Y. Lee, H.-J. Kang, J.-H. Zo, D.-J. Choi, and B.-H. Oh, "Quantification of Pedal Edema During Treatment With S(-)-Amlodipine Nicotinate Versus Amlodipine Besylate in Female Korean Patients With Mild to Moderate Hypertension: A 12-Week, Multicenter, Randomized, Double-Blind, Active-Controlled, Phase IV Clinical Trial," *Clinical Therapeutics*, vol. 34, no. 9, pp. 1940–1947, 2012.

[16] P. Galappatthy, Y. C. Waniganayake, M. I. M. Sabeer, T. J. Wijethunga, G. K. S. Galappatthy, and R. A. Ekanayaka, "Leg edema with (S)-amlodipine vs conventional amlodipine given in triple therapy for hypertension: A randomized double blind controlled clinical trial," *BMC Cardiovascular Disorders*, vol. 16, no. 1, article no. 168, 2016.

[17] J. S. Youn, Y. S. Ahn, Y. J. Hwang, H. M. Jung, W. J. Kim, and M. G. Lee, "Phase IV Clinical Trial for the Comparison of Efficacy and Safety between S- (-) -Amlodipine Nicotinate and Lercanidipine HCl in patients with hypertension," *Korean Hypertension*, vol. 16, pp. 18–30, 2010.

[18] SN. Koval, IA. Bozhko Snegurskaya, and SV. Salnikova, *Comparative Efficacy and Tolerability of Lercanidipine and S-isomer of Amlodipine in Patients with Essential Hypertension Associated with Abdominal Obesity. Arterial Hypertension*, [ABSTRACT], Arterial Hypertension, 2013.

[19] M. S. Kim, M. H. Jeong, M. G. Lee et al., "The Phase 4 Randomized, Public, Parallel, Comparative, Clincial Trial to Compare Efficacy and Safety of S-(-)-Amlodipine Nicotinate with Ramipril in Hypertensive Patients," *Journal of the Korean Society of Hypertension*, vol. 17, no. 3, pp. 103–113, 2011.

[20] Q. Chen, Q. Huang, Y. Kang et al., "Efficacy and tolerability of initial high vs low doses of S-(-)-amlodipine in hypertension," *The Journal of Clinical Hypertension*, vol. 19, no. 10, pp. 973–982, 2017.

[21] "Safety and Efficacy of S-Amlodipine: SESA study," in *JAMA-India*, vol. 2, pp. 87–92, 2003.

[22] "The SESA-II Study: Safety and Efficacy of S (-) Amlodipine in the Treatment of Hypertenison," in *Indian Medical Gazette*, pp. 529–533, SESA-II Study group, 2005.

[23] "SESA IV: Results of a Multicentric Post-marketing Surveillance Study on Safety and Efficacy of S-amlodipine in the Treatment of Hypertension," in *Cardiology Today*, vol. XI, pp. 1–4, SESA-IV Study group, 2007.

[24] K. Singh, "Safety and Efficacy of S(-)Amlodipine in the Management Stage-I and Stage-II Hypertension: The SESA-IVA Experience at Imphal," *Indian Medical Gazette*, pp. 230–234, 2007.

[25] M. Mohanty, K. P. Tripathy, S. Sarkar, and V. Srivastava, "Comparative Analysis On Incidence Of Pedal Oedema Between Amlodipine, Cilnidipine And S-Amlodipine In Mild To Moderate Hypertensive Individuals Of Either Sex," *IOSR Journal of Dental and Medical Sciences*, vol. 15, pp. 24–34, 2016.

[26] M. G. Rajanandh, A. S. Parihar, and K. Subramaniyan, "Comparative Effect of Racemic Amlodipine and its Enantiomer with Atenolol on Hypertensive Patients-A Randomized, Open, Parallel Group Study," *Journal of Experimental and Clinical Medicine(Taiwan)*, vol. 5, no. 6, pp. 217–221, 2013.

[27] M. A. Maksimova, Y. V. Lukina, and S. Y. Martsevich, "The role of S-amlodipine in arterial hypertension therapy with combination of calcium channel blockers and beta-blockers," in *Ration Pharmacother Cardiol*, vol. 9, pp. 236–240, 2013.

[28] S.-H. Ihm, H.-K. Jeon, T.-J. Cha et al., "Efficacy and safety of two fixed-dose combinations of S-amlodipine and telmisartan (CKD-828) versus S-amlodipine monotherapy in patients with hypertension inadequately controlled using S-amlodipine monotherapy: An 8-week, multicenter, randomized, double-blind, Phase III clinical study," *Drug Design, Development and Therapy*, vol. 10, pp. 3817–3826, 2016.

[29] C. G. Park, T. H. Ahn, E. J. Cho et al., "Comparison of the Efficacy and Safety of Fixed-dose S-Amlodipine/Telmisartan and Telmisartan in Hypertensive Patients Inadequately Controlled with Telmisartan: A Randomized, Double-blind, Multicenter Study," *Clinical Therapeutics*, vol. 38, no. 10, pp. 2185–2194, 2016.

[30] F. Liu, M. Qiu, and S. Zhai, "Tolerability and effectiveness of (S)-amlodipine compared with racemic amlodipine in hypertension: A systematic review and meta-analysis," *Current Therapeutic Research*, vol. 71, no. 1, pp. 1–29, 2010.

[31] Z. G. Zhao and Y. Chen, "Efficacy and Saftey of Amlodipine vs. Levamlodipine for Mild to Moderate Hypertension: A Syetmatic Review," in *Evaluation and Analysis of Drug-use in Hospitals of China*, vol. 15, pp. 318–321, 2015, https://www.cabdirect.org/cabdirect/abstract/2063216081.

[32] J. S. Hiremath, "The SESA-Angina Study — Safety and Efficacy of S (-) Amlodipine in Angina," *Indian Medical Gazette*, pp. 403–408, 2005.

[33] G. Liangjin, Z. Hanlin, L. Yaqian, S. Menga, and H. Yan, "Effect of Levamlodipine besylate and nifedipine sustained-release tablets on blood pressure variety ratio and carotid intima media thickness in patients with primary hypertension," *Modern Journal of Integrated Traditional Chinese*, p. 22, 2013.

[34] H. Zhang, KS. Liu, RG. Gao, C. Liu, and HY. Xue, "Effects of l-amlodipine and amlodipine on vascular endothelial function and serum cholesterol in patients with essential hypertension," *Chinese Journal of New Drugs and Clinical*, 2003.

[35] J. Guo, Y. Gong, and Y. Li, "858 The effectiveness of s(-)-amlodipine on vascular function," *Journal of Hypertension*, vol. 30, p. e251, 2012.

[36] D. Si, Y. He, C. Yang et al., "The effects of amlodipine and S(-)-amlodipine on vascular endothelial function in patients with hypertension," *American Journal of Hypertension*, vol. 27, no. 1, pp. 27–31, 2014.

[37] S. V. Nestorovich, "Correction of endothelial dysfunction under the influence of treatment complex of S (-) Amlodipine and ACE-inhibitor Enalapril in patients with chronic pulmonary heart disease with arterial hypertension," *Journal of Scientific & Innovative Research*, p. 716, 2013.

[38] B. G. Iskenderov and S. V. Saushkina, "Organoprotective and metabolic effects of S-amlodipine in patients with arterial hypertension," *Kardiologiya*, vol. 53, no. 10, pp. 24–29, 2013.

[39] S. D. Tang, J. Qi, W. Han, and Z. L. Ming, "P-257 Levamlodipine Therapy for Hypertension After Kidney Transplantation," *American Journal of Hypertension*, p. 16, 2003.

[40] W.-Y. Xiao, N. Ning, M.-H. Tan et al., "Effects of antihypertensive drugs losartan and levamlodipine besylate on insulin resistance in patients with essential hypertension combined with isolated impaired fasting glucose," *Hypertension Research*, vol. 39, no. 5, pp. 321–326, 2016.

[41] J. Li, L. Fu, G-J. Lao, C. Yang, M. Ren, and L. Yan, "Effects of Levamlodipine on Platelet Aggregation and Expression of MMP-9 / MMP-2 in Patients with Type 2 Diabetes and Hypertension," *Journal of Sun Yat-Sen University (Medical Sciences)*, vol. 35, pp. 35–270, 2014.

[42] X.-P. Zhang, E. L. Kit, S. Mital, S. Chahwala, and T. H. Hintze, "Paradoxical release of nitric oxide by an L-type calcium channel antagonist, the R+ enantiomer of amlodipine," *Journal of Cardiovascular Pharmacology*, vol. 39, no. 2, pp. 208–214, 2002.

[43] S. Hu, Y. Zhang, J. He, and L. Du, "A Retrospective Cost-Effectiveness Analysis of S-Amlodipine in China," *Value in Health*, vol. 17, no. 7, p. A758, 2014.

[44] G. S. Liu, K. Wang, and M. H. Zhnag, "Comparative effect of amlodipine and levamlodipine on nocturnal hypertension in hypertensive patients," *Bulletin of Medical Postgraduate*, p. 6, 2001.

[45] Z. G. Fang, "Clinical evaluation of levamlodipine in treatment of 140 patients with essential hypertenison," *Chinese New Drugs Journal*, p. 12, 2002.

[46] Y-Z. Cheng, Wu. X-G, X-Y. Chen, and W. Fu, "Clinic study of the efficacy and adverse reactions levamlodipine besylate in treatment of hypertension," *Chinese Journal Medicianl Guide*, p. 03, 2002.

[47] M. S. Hiremath and G. D. Dighe, "A Randomized, Double-blind, Double-dummy, Multicentric, Parallel Group, Comparative Clinical Trial of S-amlodipine 2.5 mg versus Amlodipine 5 mg in the Treatment of Mild to Moderate Hypertension," *JAMA-India*, vol. 8, pp. 86–92, 2002.

[48] PG. Kerkar, "Clinical Trial of S-Amlodipine 2.5 mg versus Amlodipine 5 mg the Treatment of Hypertension," *Indian Journal of Clinical Practice*, p. 13, 2003.

[49] L. Pathak, M. S. Hiremath, P. G. Kerkar, and V. G. Manade, "Clinical Trial of S-Amlodipine 2.5 mg Versus Amlodipine 5 mg in the treatment of Mild to Moderate Hypertenison - A Randomized, Double-blind Clinical Trial," *Journal of the Association of Physicians of India*, vol. 52, pp. 197–202, 2004.

[50] L. Zhang, "Study of Action and Adverse Drug Reaction of Levamlodipine Besylate and Amlodipine Besylate," *Chinese Journal of Pharmacoepidemiology*, p. 06, 2006.

[51] J.-H. Bae, J.-E. Jun, M.-M. Lee, C.-H. Kim, M-S. Hyon, K. H. Choe et al., "Double-blind, Randomized, Multi-center Trial for the Comparison of Efficacy and Safety between S-Amlodipine Besylate and Amlodipine Besylate in Patients with Hypertension," *Korean Hypertension J*, vol. 14, pp. 28–36, 2008.

[52] Y. Zhu, Z. Hua, K. Shi, Z. Tan, L. Gong, and Y. Zhuo, "Effect and safety of levoamlodipine maleate tablets on patients with mild-to-moderate hypertension," *Chinese Journal of Clinical Pharmacy*, p. 02, 2008.

[53] Y. Shengye, "Efficacy Observation of Amlodipine and Levamlodipine for Mild to Moderate Hypertension," *Chinese Journal of Medicinal Guide*, p. 09, 2012.

[54] G-H. Zhao, "Clinical efficacy of levamlodipine besylate in treatment of primary hypertension," in *Cardiovascular Disease Prevention and Control*, vol. 9, 2013.

[55] T. Parvathi, J. E. Ramya, and B. Meenakshi, "Prospective Study to Compare the Efficacy and Tolerability of S-Amlodipine 2.5 mg versus Racemic Amlodipine 5 mg in Mild to Moderate Hypertension. Research And Reviews?: Journal Of Pharmacology And Toxicological Studies," *Journal Of Pharmacology And Toxicological Studies*, vol. 2, pp. 26–33, 2014.

[56] X. Hu and C. Xiao, "Effects of irbesartan combined with levamlodipine or indapamide regimen on blood pressure variation in patients with primary hypertensive," *Clinical Cardiology*, p. 03, 2013.

[57] V. A. Bobroff, O. I. Davydova Medvedenko, and L. V. Klimenko, "Application of S-amlodipine in treatment of patients with mild to moderate arterial hypertension," *Health of Ukraine*, vol. 12, pp. 1–5, 2007.

[58] D. Basu, "Comparative Study to Evaluate the Effect of S-Amlodipine versus Amlodipine on Office and Ambulatory Blood Pressure in Mild to Moderate Hypertensives," *Indian Medical Gazette*, pp. 493–497, 2007.

[59] V. K. Sierkova, N. V. Kuz'minova, and I. S. K. Alshantti, "Comparative estimation of efficiency and safety of racemic amlodipine and its S-enantiomer in hypertensive patients," *Lik Sprava*, no. 3-4, pp. 39–44, 2009.

Permissions

All chapters in this book were first published in IJH, by Hindawi Publishing Corporation; hereby published with permission under the Creative Commons Attribution License or equivalent. Every chapter published in this book has been scrutinized by our experts. Their significance has been extensively debated. The topics covered herein carry significant findings which will fuel the growth of the discipline. They may even be implemented as practical applications or may be referred to as a beginning point for another development.

The contributors of this book come from diverse backgrounds, making this book a truly international effort. This book will bring forth new frontiers with its revolutionizing research information and detailed analysis of the nascent developments around the world.

We would like to thank all the contributing authors for lending their expertise to make the book truly unique. They have played a crucial role in the development of this book. Without their invaluable contributions this book wouldn't have been possible. They have made vital efforts to compile up to date information on the varied aspects of this subject to make this book a valuable addition to the collection of many professionals and students.

This book was conceptualized with the vision of imparting up-to-date information and advanced data in this field. To ensure the same, a matchless editorial board was set up. Every individual on the board went through rigorous rounds of assessment to prove their worth. After which they invested a large part of their time researching and compiling the most relevant data for our readers.

The editorial board has been involved in producing this book since its inception. They have spent rigorous hours researching and exploring the diverse topics which have resulted in the successful publishing of this book. They have passed on their knowledge of decades through this book. To expedite this challenging task, the publisher supported the team at every step. A small team of assistant editors was also appointed to further simplify the editing procedure and attain best results for the readers.

Apart from the editorial board, the designing team has also invested a significant amount of their time in understanding the subject and creating the most relevant covers. They scrutinized every image to scout for the most suitable representation of the subject and create an appropriate cover for the book.

The publishing team has been an ardent support to the editorial, designing and production team. Their endless efforts to recruit the best for this project, has resulted in the accomplishment of this book. They are a veteran in the field of academics and their pool of knowledge is as vast as their experience in printing. Their expertise and guidance has proved useful at every step. Their uncompromising quality standards have made this book an exceptional effort. Their encouragement from time to time has been an inspiration for everyone.

The publisher and the editorial board hope that this book will prove to be a valuable piece of knowledge for researchers, students, practitioners and scholars across the globe.

List of Contributors

Ettore Malacco
L. Sacco Hospital, 20157 Milano, Italy

Stefano Omboni
Italian Institute of Telemedicine, Solbiate Arno, 21048 Varese, Italy

Gianfranco Parati
Istituto Auxologico Italiano and University of Milano-Bicocca, 20149 Milano, Italy

Náyade del Prado-González
Instituto de Investigación Sanitaria, Hospital Clínico San Carlos (IdISSC), Madrid, Spain

Arturo Corbatón-Anchuelo, María Teresa Martínez-Larrad, Cristina Fernández-Pérez and Manuel Serrano-Ríos
Instituto de Investigación Sanitaria, Hospital Clínico San Carlos (IdISSC), Madrid, Spain
Spanish Biomedical Research Centre in Diabetes and Associated Metabolic Disorders (CIBERDEM), Madrid, Spain

Rafael Gabriel
Escuela Nacional de Salud, ISCIII, Spain

Tegwindé R. Compaoré
Centre de Recherche Biomoléculaire Pietro Annigoni (CERBA), BP 364, Ouagadougou 01, Burkina Faso
Laboratoire de Biologie et Génétique Moléculaires (LABIOGENE), Université de Ouagadougou, BP 7021, Ouagadougou 03, Burkina Faso

Daméhan Tchelougou, Simplice D. Karou, Maléki Assih and Virginio Pietra
Centre de Recherche Biomoléculaire Pietro Annigoni (CERBA), BP 364, Ouagadougou 01, Burkina Faso
Laboratoire de Biologie et Génétique Moléculaires (LABIOGENE), Université de Ouagadougou, BP 7021, Ouagadougou 03, Burkina Faso
Ecole Supérieure des Techniques Biologiques et Alimentaires (ESTBA-UL), Université de Lomé, BP 1515, Togo

Florencia W. Djigma, Djeneba Ouermi and Jacques Simpore
Centre de Recherche Biomoléculaire Pietro Annigoni (CERBA), BP 364, Ouagadougou 01, Burkina Faso
Laboratoire de Biologie et Génétique Moléculaires (LABIOGENE), Université de Ouagadougou, BP 7021, Ouagadougou 03, Burkina Faso

Centre Médical Saint Camille (CMSC), BP 444, Ouagadougou 09, Burkina Faso

Cyrille Bisseye
Centre de Recherche Biomoléculaire Pietro Annigoni (CERBA), BP 364, Ouagadougou 01, Burkina Faso
Laboratoire de Biologie et Génétique Moléculaires (LABIOGENE), Université de Ouagadougou, BP 7021, Ouagadougou 03, Burkina Faso
Laboratoire de Biologie Moléculaire et Cellulaire (LABMC), Université des Sciences et Techniques de Masuku (USTM), BP 943, Franceville, Gabon

Patrice Zabsonré
Service de Cardiologie, CHU-Yalgado Ouédraogo, BP 7022, Ouagadougou 03, Burkina Faso

Jonas K. Kologo and Valentin N. Yaméogo
Service de Cardiologie, CHU-Yalgado Ouédraogo, BP 7022, Ouagadougou 03, Burkina Faso
Centre Médical Saint Camille (CMSC), BP 444, Ouagadougou 09, Burkina Faso

Mohsen Janghorbani, Ashraf Aminorroaya and Masoud Amini
Isfahan Endocrine and Metabolism Research Center, Isfahan University of Medical Sciences, Isfahan, Iran

Homamodin Javadzade, Azam Larki and Mahnoush Reisi
Department of Health Education and Health Promotion, Bushehr University of Medical Sciences, Bushehr, Iran

Rahim Tahmasebi
Department of Biostatistics, Bushehr University of Medical Sciences, Bushehr, Iran

Pan Yang
School of Public Health, Sun Yat-sen University, Guangzhou, China
Guangdong Provincial Institute of Public Health, Guangdong Provincial Center for Disease Control and Prevention, Guangzhou, China

Wenjun Ma and Hualiang Lin
Guangdong Provincial Institute of Public Health, Guangdong Provincial Center for Disease Control and Prevention, Guangzhou, China

Yiqing Zheng and Haidi Yang
Department of Otolaryngology, Sun Yat-sen Memorial Hospital, Sun Yat-sen University, Guangzhou, China

Shoko Takahashi
Medical Affairs, Global Established Pharma Business, Pfizer Japan Inc., Shinjuku Bunka Quint Building, 3-22-7 Yoyogi,Shibuya-ku, Tokyo 151-8589, Japan

Megumi Hiramatsu
PMS Planning&Operation, Pfizer Japan Inc., Shinjuku Bunka Quint Building, 3-22-7 Yoyogi, Shibuya-ku, Tokyo 151-8589, Japan

Shinichi Hotta and Yukie Watanabe
Clinical Informatics and Innovation, Pfizer Japan Inc., Shinjuku Bunka Quint Building, 3-22-7 Yoyogi, Shibuya-ku,Tokyo 151-8589, Japan

Osamu Suga
Medical Writing and Document Management, Pfizer Japan Inc., Shinjuku Bunka Quint Building, 3-22-7 Yoyogi, Shibuya-ku, Tokyo 151-8589, Japan

Yutaka Endo
Clinical Statistics, Pfizer Japan Inc., Shinjuku Bunka Quint Building, 3-22-7 Yoyogi, Shibuya-ku, Tokyo 151-8589, Japan

Isamu Miyamori
University of Fukui, 23-3 Matsuokashimoaizuki, Eiheiji-cho, Yoshida-gun, Fukui Prefecture 910-1193, Japan

Yijun Yu, Yanling Xu, Mingjing Zhang, Yuting Wang, Wusong Zou and Ye Gu
Department of Cardiology, Wuhan Fourth Hospital, Puai Hospital Affiliated to Tongji Medical College, Huazhong University of Science and Technology, Wuhan 430030, China

Marina Njelekela
Department of Physiology, Muhimbili University of Health and Allied Sciences, Dar es Salaam, Tanzania

Akum Aveika and Guerino Chalamila
Management and Development for Health, HIV/AIDS Care and Treatment Program, Dar es Salaam, Tanzania

Alfa Muhihi
Management and Development for Health, HIV/AIDS Care and Treatment Program, Dar es Salaam, Tanzania
Africa Academy for Public Health, Dar es Salaam, Tanzania

Donna Spiegelman
Department of Epidemiology, Harvard TH Chan School of Public Health, Boston, MA, USA
Department of Biostatistics, Harvard TH Chan School of Public Health, Boston, MA, USA

Wafaie Fawzi
Department of Epidemiology, Harvard TH Chan School of Public Health, Boston, MA, USA
Department of Nutrition, Harvard TH Chan School of Public Health, Boston, MA, USA
Department of Global Health and Population, Harvard TH Chan School of Public Health, Boston, MA, USA

Claudia Hawkins
Feinberg School of Medicine, Northwestern University, Chicago, IL, USA

Catharina Armstrong
Tufts University School of Medicine, Boston, MA, USA

James Okuma
Department of Nutrition, Harvard TH Chan School of Public Health, Boston, MA, USA

Enju Liu
Department of Nutrition, Harvard TH Chan School of Public Health, Boston, MA, USA
Department of Global Health and Population, Harvard TH Chan School of Public Health, Boston, MA, USA

Sylvia Kaaya
Department of Psychiatry and Mental Health, Muhimbili University of Health and Allied Sciences, Dar es Salaam, Tanzania

Ferdinand Mugusi
Department of Internal Medicine, Muhimbili University of Health and Allied Sciences, Dar es Salaam, Tanzania

Raja Ram Dhungana
Nepal Family Development Foundation, Kathmandu, Nepal

Achyut Raj Pandey and Bihungum Bista
Nepal Health Research Council, Kathmandu, Nepal

Suira Joshi
Ministry of Health and Population, Kathmandu, Nepal

Surya Devkota
Manmohan Cardiothoracic, Vascular and Transplant Centre, Institute of Medicine, Tribhuvan University, Kathmandu, Nepal

Jeanette Sessoms, Kathryn Reid, Ishan Williams and Ivora Hinton
University of Virginia School of Nursing, McLeod Hall, Charlottesville, VA 22908-0782, USA

Pietro A. Modesti, Ilaria Marzotti, Danilo Malandrino, Maria Boddi and Sergio Castellani
Department of Experimental and Clinical Medicine, University of Florence, Florence, Italy

Maria Calabrese
Diabetology Unit, Ospedale Misericordia e Dolce, Prato, Italy

Hushao Bing
Associazione Culturale Cinese di Fujian in Italia, Prato, Italy

Dong Zhao
Department of Epidemiology, Capital Medical University Beijing Anzhen Hospital and National Institute of Heart, Lung & Blood Disease, Beijing, China

João M. Pedro
Centro de Investigação em Sáude de Angola (CISA), Caxito, Angola
EPIUnit, Instituto de Sáude Pública, Universidade do Porto, Rua das Taipas, No. 135, 4050-600 Porto, Portugal

Miguel Brito
Centro de Investigação em Sáude de Angola (CISA), Caxito, Angola
Health and Technology Research Center, Escola Superior de Tecnologia da Sáude de Lisboa, Instituto Polit´ecnico de Lisboa, Av. D. João II, Lote 4.69.01, 1990-096 Lisboa, Portugal

Henrique Barros
EPIUnit, Instituto de Sáude Pública, Universidade do Porto, Rua das Taipas, No. 135, 4050-600 Porto, Portugal
Faculdade de Medicina, Universidade do Porto, Al. Prof. Hern^ani Monteiro, 4200-319 Porto, Portugal

Wichai Aekplakorn
Department of Community Medicine, Faculty of Medicine, Ramathibodi Hospital, Mahidol University, Bangkok 10400,Thailand

La-or Chailurkit and Boonsong Ongphiphadhanakul
Department of Medicine, Faculty of Medicine, Ramathibodi Hospital, Mahidol University, Bangkok 10400,Thailand

Yaa Obirikorang
Department of Nursing, Faculty of Health and Allied Sciences, Garden City University College (GCUC), Kenyasi, Kumasi, Ghana

Michael Opoku Boateng and Dari Pascal Dapilla
Department of Nursing, Faculty of Health and Allied Sciences, Garden City University College (GCUC), Kenyasi, Kumasi, Ghana
Department of Nursing, Kintampo Municipal Hospital, Kintampo, Ghana

Christian Obirikorang, Selorm Philip Segbefia, Peter Kojo Brenya, Bright Amankwaa, Emmanuel Nsenbah Batu and Beatrice Amoah
Department of Molecular Medicine, School of Medical Science, Kwame Nkrumah University of Science and Technology (KNUST), Kumasi, Ghana

Emmanuel Acheampong and Enoch Odame Anto
Department of Molecular Medicine, School of Medical Science, Kwame Nkrumah University of Science and Technology (KNUST), Kumasi, Ghana
School of Medical and Health Science, Edith Cowan University, Joondalup, Australia

Daniel Gyamfi and Evans Asamoah Adu
Department of Medical Laboratory Technology, Faculty of Allied Health Sciences, KNUST, Ghana

Adjei Gyimah Akwasi
Department of Community Health, School of Medical Sciences, KNUST, Ghana

Oluwaseun A. Akinseye
Department of Medicine, Icahn School of Medicine at Mount Sinai, Queens Hospital Center, 82-68 164th Street, Jamaica, NY 11432, USA

Stephen K. Williams, Azizi Seixas, Seithikurippu R. Pandi-Perumal, Julian Vallon, Ferdinand Zizi and Girardin Jean-Louis
Center for Healthful Behavior Change, Department of Population Health, NYU School of Medicine, 227 East 30th Street, New York, NY 10016, USA

Jenifer d'El-Rei, Ana Rosa Cunha, Michelle Trindade and Mario Fritsch Neves
Department of Clinical Medicine, State University of Rio de Janeiro, 20551-030 Rio de Janeiro, RJ, Brazil

Nafees Ahmad
Faculty of Pharmacy and Health Sciences, University of Balochistan, Balochistan, Pakistan

Amer Hayat Khan and Irfanullah Khan
Discipline of Clinical Pharmacy, School of Pharmaceutical Sciences, Universiti Sains Malaysia, Pulau Pinang, Malaysia

Amjad Khan
Department of Pharmacy, Quaid-e-Azam University, Islamabad, Pakistan

Muhammad Atif
Department of Pharmacy,The Islamia University, Bahawalpur, Pakistan

Christos Papageorgiou, Efstathios Manios, Efstathios Manios, Eleni Koroboki, Maria Alevizaki, Meletios-Athanasios Dimopoulos and Nikolaos Zakopoulos
Department of Clinical Therapeutics, National and Kapodistrian University of Athens, Medical School, Athens, Greece

Eleftheria Tsaltas
1st Department of Psychiatry, National and Kapodistrian University of Athens, Medical School, "Eginition" Hospital, 115 28 Athens, Greece

Elias Angelopoulos and Charalabos Papageorgiou
1st Department of Psychiatry, National and Kapodistrian University of Athens, Medical School, "Eginition" Hospital, 115 28 Athens, Greece University Mental Health Research Institute (UMHRI), Athens, Greece

Aiah Lebbie, Richard Wadsworth and Camilla Bangura
Department of Biological Sciences, Njala University, PMB, Freetown, Sierra Leone

Janette Saidu
Institute of Food Technology, Nutrition & Consumer Studies, Njala University, PMB, Freetown, Sierra Leone

Sylvester Yao Lokpo, James Osei-Yeboah and Romeo Asumbasiya Aduko
Department of Medical Laboratory Sciences, School of Allied Health Sciences, University of Health and Allied Sciences, Ho, Ghana

William K. B. A. Owiredu
Department of MolecularMedicine, School of Medical Sciences, Kwame Nkrumah University of Science and Technology, Kumasi, Ghana
Department of Clinical Biochemistry, Diagnostic Directorate, Komfo Anokye Teaching Hospital, Kumasi, Ghana

Francis Abeku Ussher
Faculty of Health and Allied Sciences, Koforidua Technical University, Koforidua, Eastern Region, Ghana

Verner Ndudiri Orish
Department of Microbiology and Immunology, School of Medicine, University of Health and Allied Sciences, Ho, Ghana

Felix Gadzeto and Paul Ntiamoah
Laboratory Department, St. Elizabeth Hospital, Catholic Health Services, Hwidiem, Brong Ahafo Region, Ghana

Felix Botchway
Department of Chemical Pathology, University of Ghana, Accra, Ghana

Ivan Muanah
St. Elizabeth Hospital, Catholic Health Services, Hwidiem, Brong Ahafo Region, Ghana

Hamidou Oumar Bâ, Ichaka Menta, Ibrahima Sangaré and Noumou Sidibé
CHU Gabriel Touré Bamako, Bamako, Mali

Youssouf Camara
CHU Kati, Kati, Mali

I. B. Diall and Souleymane Coulibaly
CHU Point G, Bamako, Mali

Maiga Asmaou Kéita
CHU Mére-Enfant, Bamako, Mali

Georges Rosario Christian Millogo
CHU YO, Ouagadougou, Burkina Faso

Jamshed Dalal
Centre for Cardiac Sciences, Kokilaben Dhirubhai Ambani Hospital, Mumbai, India

J. C. Mohan
Fortis Hospital, Shalimar Bagh, New Delhi, India

S. S. Iyengar
Manipal Hospital, Bangalore, India

Jagdish Hiremath
Ruby Hall Clinic, Pune, India

Immaneni Sathyamurthy
Apollo Hospitals, Chennai, India

Sandeep Bansal
Department of Cardiology, VMMC & Safdarjung Hospital, New Delhi, India

Dhiman Kahali
B M Birla Heart Research Centre, Kolkata, India

Arup Dasbiswas
NRS Medical College and Hospital, Kolkata, India

Index

Organ Damage, 1, 4-5, 9, 57-58, 67, 89, 93, 170
Organ Dysfunction, 51
Oxidative Stress, 57, 112

P
Pharmacological Therapy, 19
Pharmacological Treatment, 1, 14, 91, 103-106
Polymorphisms, 24-29, 142, 145

R
Racemic Amlodipine, 199-200, 204-206, 209, 211-212
Renal Dysfunction, 184-190
Renin, 8, 12, 24, 27, 29-30, 54

S
S-amlodipine, 199-201, 204-207, 209-212
Self-care Intervention, 38-39, 42

Serum Bisphenol, 109, 115
Serum Creatinine, 10, 32, 185-186, 189-190, 206

T
Threonine, 25
Tinnitus, 44-50
Triglyceride, 31-34, 36, 61, 63, 65-66, 132
Type 2 Diabetes, 27, 31-32, 43, 48, 76, 101-102, 116, 142, 145, 156, 206, 211

U
Urinary Albumin, 10

V
Vascular Homeostasis, 24, 141

Z
Zofenopril, 1-12